D1083370

THE GREAT WAR
AND
THE BIRTH OF MODERN MEDICINE

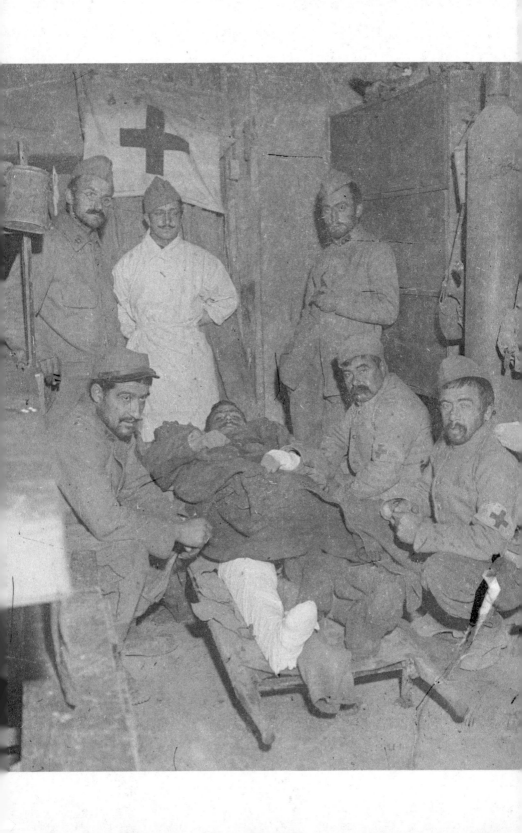

THE GREAT WAR
AND THE BIRTH OF
MODERN MEDICINE

A HISTORY

THOMAS HELLING, MD

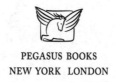

PEGASUS BOOKS
NEW YORK LONDON

THE GREAT WAR AND THE BIRTH OF MODERN MEDICINE

Pegasus Books, Ltd.
148 West 37th Street, 13th Floor
New York, NY 10018

Copyright © 2022 by Thomas Helling, MD

First Pegasus Books cloth edition March 2022

Interior design by Maria Fernandez

frontispiece: First aid post (*poste de secours*) in Fort Vaux, Verdun sector, November 1916. (ECPAD, Agence d'Images de la Defense, Paris)

ISBN: 978-1-64313-899-2

10 9 8 7 6 5 4 3 2 1

Printed in the United States of America
Distributed by Simon & Schuster
www.pegasusbooks.com

For all those men and women
who must confront the horrors of war.

From the Evils of Mankind Comes Improbable Redemption.

Contents

ONE

The Fury of War

"A War . . . of Mankind"

"It is a war not of nations, but of mankind. It is a war to exorcise a world-madness and end an age." So spoke H. G. Wells in 1914 of the unfolding conflagration that came to be known as the Great War.[1] It was a war of Prussian aggression, a war of imperialism, a war of ambition and treaties and madness, a war filled with horror and slaughter and anguish. Indeed, Wells felt that the German state had slipped into "physical and moral brutality,"[2] becoming a boil on the earth that must be lanced. And all so that peace might be restored. It would be a crusade for peace.

But before 1914, before the slaughters began, war was seen as a glorious adventure, the mark of masculinity, of patriotism, of passion, even. So, European citizenry applauded. Just before the first waves of German troops crossed the Belgian border the morning of August 4, 1914, the Belgian King Albert had delivered a stirring speech to parliament, and the throngs of people outside became delirious with fervor, incensed at the German insolence and chanting for Belgian independence. Lieutenant General de Coune, commanding the Garde Civique, "rose in his stirrups, waving his sword . . . What a sacred and unforgettable emotion stirred the hearts of those Belgians."[3] What aplomb, what chivalry!

In Paris, the fury of war was also in the air. The two houses of France's parliament met in joint session. First, President Raymond Poincaré, then Prime Minister René Viviani, spoke, lashing out in moral terms, insisting war now was a matter of "right and liberty." The applause was deafening. The Senate and Chamber of Deputies unanimously voted for war.[4] According to historian Barbara Tuchman, "French soldiers in red trousers and big-skirted, dark blue coats . . . chanted as they marched through the streets" demanding the return of Alsace and Lorraine, lost in the war of 1870–71. Companies of volunteers cheered prancing cavalry regiments in anachronistic gleaming breastplates and medieval-style helmets with shouts of death to Germans.[5] American novelist Edith Wharton, witnessing the French reaction in Paris, wrote that "the sudden flaming up of national life . . . seemed to penetrate the throngs who streamed up and down the Boulevards till late into the night," apparently oblivious to the realities of war.[6]

To the east, enthusiasm was just as shameless. At the Reichstag in Berlin, amid frantic applause, Chancellor Theobald von Bethmann-Hollweg bellowed: "We are at war with Russia and France—a war that has been forced upon us."[7] It was all so grand and bellicose.

◆

Within a month, as tens of thousands of Europe's finest youth lay mangled and rotting in the fields of Belgium and France, maimed and mutilated by new, powerful munitions of destruction, the military and the public would be seized by the terrors of modern warfare. And those wounded who were lucky enough to be snatched alive from the battlefield would sadly find the medical men and women assigned to help them ill prepared to cope with the sheer magnitude of the carnage and even less equipped to reassemble the deranged anatomy, physiology, and psychology that this war had spawned. "These frightful sights would work havoc with one's brain," nurse Julia Stimson exclaimed.[8] It was a "carnival of death," wrote Canadian historian Modris Eksteins years later, "a war now in the realm of the unreal, the make-believe." Yet, he maintained, "the 1914 war, when it broke out, was seen as an opportunity for both change and confirmation."[9] No truer than for the fate of its victims.

Even worse, the wretched injured languished in filthy encampments or side-railed boxcars, as if discarded refugees from Dante's *Inferno*, waiting their turn to enter overcrowded field hospitals, where overworked surgeons were often at a loss to sort through the innumerable wounded—who needed treatment first, who could be saved, who were hopelessly damaged? The horribly mangled—both in body and spirit—were left to wonder if their fate was not truly one worse than death. James Judd, an American volunteer physician serving in France, recalled one French soldier who had been wounded in Belgium and was taken by the Germans to a field hospital and dumped on the floor. The young poilu told him: "Here I lay for three days on the stone floor with some water and a few pieces of bread to sustain me. I saw limbs cut off without anesthesia. The shrieks of the sufferers were terrible."[10] At a base hospital in 1914 Boulogne, a British nurse observed a poorly ventilated, unsanitary infirmary:

It is distinctly unhealthy, and the odours [sic] in the place are indescribable and never to be forgotten [at her clearing station]. There is no lavatory accommodation—although latrines are situated along the quay, whither the blind are led by the armless, the lame carried on orderlies' backs.[11]

The French writer and poet César Méléra, in 1916 around Verdun, described the blatantly unromantic realities of this conflict:

A fetid mud sometimes reaches your ankles, disgorging an awful smell and a heavy, opaque air. He who has not seen the wounded emitting their death rattle on the field of battle . . . drinking their urine to appease their thirst . . . has seen nothing of war.[12]

Such realities would sorely challenge the medical profession to face the truths of a modern form of warfare that was more arbitrary and brutal than in past conflicts. Yet, this Great War would bring forth an accelerated revolution in medicine that began in the laboratories of the celebrated European physiologists of the 19th century, the likes of Xavier Bichat, Claude Bernard, Johannes Müller, and Carl Ludwig, who were intent on unraveling and understanding the elaborate machinery of living animals. Yet now their heirs, the 20th-century scientists, would study not animals but human beings embroiled in life-or-death struggles. Both government and industry would call on these men and women in the nascent fields of experimental science to uncover and put to work techniques and therapeutics on a scale heretofore unknown, and that would form the foundations of medicine for generations to come, even to the present day. In the words of the French physicist Charles Nordmann, "French science [will have] the honor of seeing its battalions crowded around the masters in the laboratories invited to the defense of the homeland."[13]

In those first horrid days of August, as casualties poured in, physicians could do little but sift through the rows of infirmed, inspect, bandage, and move on. Doctors were at a loss for how to treat them all. Yet public outcry demanded better. The sight of the ragged, bleeding forms crowding train depots and makeshift hospitals, many with neglected, infected wounds, was intolerable to a citizenry whose youth were thrown like ripened grapes into the vats of a promiscuous war. Doctors improvised. A system of sorting developed; surgeons rummaged through packed first aid stations and frontline hospitals to find those in most need of treatment—those who, without some help from surgeons, were doomed to die. The French would have a name for the whole process, a name that would carry through to the present day—*triage* (literally, sorting).

As the war ground on, the immediacy of terrible wounds demanded surgeons be closer to the battle, literally on the fringes of combat. Here, huddled under thunderous artillery exchanges, in dingy dugouts, surgeons explored, trimmed, cleaned, and repaired wounds that otherwise might have proved fatal. Perhaps all sides recognized the importance, but it was the French who popularized it and gave it license. Visionary pioneers like French surgeons Maurice Marcille and Antonin Gosset rushed entire surgical teams in rickety trucks almost to the trenches themselves so that surgeons could begin work. Then, once stabilized, those same wounded were hustled to the rear, to better-equipped, expansive hospital compounds, where specialists continued the repair work. The British quickly followed suit, sending surgical crews scrambling from their battlefield hospitals ever closer to frontline fortifications. Even Germans moved their *Feldlazaretten*—their field hospitals—nearer and nearer, until they, too, were within earshot of the cannons. Later, doctors of the arriving American Expeditionary Force would model the French and British hospital systems. American military called this echeloned care, a phased approach to match urgency and complexity with available specialists as patients processed from battlefield to intermediate staging areas to civilian hospitals along routes of evacuation. It would all begin far forward, though, in sandbagged dugouts, squalid cellars, or deserted family dwellings, with the smell of cordite in the air, the crack of automatic weapons, and the flickering lights of oil lamps.

The wounds inflicted were horribly complex, of a kind not seen before in the history of warfare. High-energy shells showered victims with flesh-tearing shrapnel. Rapid-fire machine guns tore at muscle and bone and riddled guts, literally chopping troops to pieces. Weaponry had outstripped medical science. Surgeons scrambled to keep up with the results of munitions that the new industrial age lavishly rolled off assembly lines. From mountainous stockpiles to artillery tubes and gun magazines, weaponry showered battlefields and anyone in it with instant destruction. The magnitude of trauma inflicted by these exploding and penetrating projectiles unroofed any number of derangements that doctors scrambled to address. The human frame recoiled from such insults with frightening severity; blood poured in rivulets, causing profound sinking of vital functions, with lethal consequences. Hearts beat with desperation, and organs starved for oxygen-rich hemoglobin quickly withered. It was this urgency that provoked intense focus by surgeons. Indeed, it was such human wreckage—such disordered anatomy and physiology—that compelled doctors to scramble for solutions, to bring to bear the full weight of scientific genius. Faced with such unraveling of the machinery of life, surgeons accomplished the unbelievable: literal resurrection from the throes of death. Newfound techniques allowed doctors to instill bottles of blood from the veins of others—red blood cells capable of revitalization. That gray, moribund appearance of the shock patient then gave rise to a suffusion of color and the restoration of a failing heart: vitality, once again. It was there in those impromptu hospitals that fatigued surgeons labored over their fading patients, pouring in sustaining transfusions, paving the way to forestall that most primitive danger of the battlefield: the scourge of hemorrhage. Pioneering American surgeon George Crile, the most vocal advocate for transfusions, was passionate about their worth:

It [blood transfusion] became so obvious a method for the prevention and treatment of shock and for compensating hemorrhage, that before the end of the war blood was gathered from
the wounded and stored at the casualty clearing stations. [14]

As for those sullied gashes of the battlefield, bathed in the mud of
France's manured farmland, a grim, rancid process took hold, sending
scientists scurrying to their microscopes to unravel the invisible mysteries
of stubborn, flagellating bacteria that were the cause of such odious happenings and the demise of so many victims. Gas gangrene, one of the
sentinel features of the Great War, seemed everywhere. Yes, surgery was
the first reaction, cutting away bruised and battered skin and muscle,
but clinicians married their knife-born skills to laboratory science in
devising agents that would eradicate and kill the offending microbes. It
was a pivotal demonstration of therapy emerging from the intense workings of laboratory researchers and their pragmatic applications by clinical
practitioners. Nobel Laureate Alexis Carrel brought it all to fruition at
his swank hotel-hospital outside Compiègne, in northern France.

Then, over Flanders in 1915, billows of poisonous gas drifted across
Allied lines—the first time in the history of warfare that toxic clouds
were released on a massive scale. Soldiers choked and coughed and
panicked at the sight and smell. Some died an awful death, turning blue,
tearing at their throats, and frothing. Agents like chlorine and phosgene
ripped at lungs, suffocating victims. Germans loved the stuff; their scientists worked feverishly to design better chemicals and better delivery
systems. The whole business sparked an outpouring of research from
Allies, too, that, on one hand, assembled protective masks and adjusted
trench precautions, and on the other hand, engineered new kinds of gas
even more effective in penetrating those same masks. It was truly an evil
collaboration of science and industry: chemists intent on fabricating
toxins and industry intent on delivering them. Yet gas masks could be
lifesavers and would characterize the war; the denizens of the trenches
took on a troglodyte look, as if goggle-eyed aliens had finally populated
Earth. At last, the ultimate appeared: dichlorodiethyl sulfide: mustard
gas. Shot from artillery shells, it lathered troops in an oily, blistering

substance, blinding and scorching exposed flesh and lungs. Long daisy chains of stumbling troops, eyes swollen shut and wrapped tight, made their way to aid stations to await the consequences of their chemical burns. Gas wrecked soldiers physically and psychologically, driving them from their dugouts at the mere suggestion of a vaporous attack. Never would nations forget. The use of gas would always be a feared and deadly accompaniment of aggression.

There were the awakenings of new surgical specialties. The skill and cunning of the great Harvard neurosurgeon Harvey Cushing brought treatment of brain injuries to the forefront, cutting in half the death rate for those wounds. He was held in awe by fellow surgeons and laid the fundamentals for all surgery on the brain, traumatic and otherwise. His careful, meticulous handling of that delicate tissue formed the framework of what we now know as the specialty of neurosurgery. German, French, and British surgeons took on reconstruction of devastating and disfiguring facial injuries—so common in trench warfare—establishing the specialty of plastic surgery as not just a cosmetic luxury but an indispensable element in convalescence for these abhorrent wounds. They were particularly disturbing, those injuries to the face—borne as a hideous mask of the sins of war. For the victims, barely able to chew or drink or talk, reconstruction was paramount—but their wounds also struck inward, distorting image and worth and acceptance. James Judd saw these poor souls, too. Such a pitiful sight, he felt:

> There were some horrible wounds, especially the jaw cases. It does not seem possible a man could be alive with such wounds. One boy was shot through the shoulder at close range, then the ball tore open his neck and carried away a good part of the lower jaw, floor of the mouth and tongue. He was a nervous little chap and suffered greatly. [15]

The New Zealand surgeon Harold Gillies performed wonders for these people. A man of exquisite compassion, he not only tended to destroyed anatomy but also the damage of disfigurement and disgust. Under his guidance, his patients' care was holistic and persevering. For him, healing occurred on the surface and much deeper, returning for his patients not only their appearance, but also their dignity. Gillies's surgical inquisitiveness, mastery, and efforts to rehabilitate earned him the title "Father of Plastic Surgery."[16]

Necessity catalyzed other achievements. The pragmatic orthopedic surgeon Hugh Owen Thomas of Liverpool, England (Owen Thomas, as he was familiarly known), befuddled colleagues with his amazingly simple and universal splint, crucial in management of fractures of the leg. Yes, injuries to limbs were often survivable, but dangerous. In particular, fractures of the thick thighbone—the femur—could carry grave consequences. Unless immobilized, these injuries caused exquisite pain to their victims and, with their jiggling, jagged bony fragments, tore at tissue, escalating damage and stress—even to a deadly level. With Thomas's splint, broken ends were aligned and secured. Damage ceased, and some degree of comfort was restored. Lethality even lessened. Of course, there was also Wilhelm Röntgen and the introduction of his mysterious rays. Suddenly, doctors could peer into the depths of the human body. It became, literally, a fad of the war; Röntgen's machines were loaded onto trucks and carted off to the battlefield, aiding surgeons in diagnosis and treatment of previously hidden wounds. That provocative celebrity of Paris, Marie Curie, setting aside her research into radioactivity, would hear nothing less than the expansion of this fabulous technology to reach hospitals almost on the lips of trenches. From her enthusiasm and that of her colleagues, the Great War launched radiology as a decisive component of modern medicine.

And who has not heard of "shell shock"? The psychological trauma of Great War combat wore heavily and quickly on combatants. Day in and day out bombardments by high explosives and near suicidal infantry charges broke men, some reduced to babbling, contorted creatures shamelessly cowering in dugouts, trenches, and tents. Hysteria, doctors claimed, that catchall term referring to the fictitious angst blamed on the peculiar female gender. Thankfully, more compassionate figures arose, among them the kind gentleman William Rivers, a physician who better understood the complexities of the human psyche and the horrors of this Great War. From his efforts an understanding of what is now called post-traumatic stress developed—albeit imperfectly—which would be the foundation of future dealings with disturbed victims of terrible tragedies.

There would be one parting gasp for a world bludgeoned by this grand conflagration. It was the first global pandemic of modern history, as much a part of the Great War as bombs and bullets. The influenza epidemic of 1918 and 1919 struck troops of all nations with such voracity as to contribute to the eventual demise of the designs of Imperial Germany and lead to the Armistice of November 1918. Indeed, it was not the giant arsenals of mighty armies that ushered in victory and defeat, but invisible viruses so tiny as to escape the scrutiny of even the most powerful microscopes. These living particles ravaged healthy lungs of young men and soon spread to civilian populations whose only protection was the now-familiar axioms of mask wearing and social distancing. Lessons from the pandemic of the Great War would be dusted off for the next viral pandemic a century later.

The Greek philosopher Heraclitus called war "the father of all things."[17] In truth, this may very well apply to the First World War more than any other. The Great War could be looked upon as the Father of Modern Medicine. As author Alex Roland argued in his treatise "Science and War," science and technology did not impact the war as much as the war itself impacted science and technology.[18] Governments and private enterprises came to assist white-coated researchers to explore the nuances of physiology disrupted to the utmost. Doctors in uniform, literally under the enemy's guns, would figure it all out and make monumental changes in the management of mass casualties, blood loss, tissue damage, and wound infections. These men, indeed, would forevermore accompany warmongers, lending their reparative solutions as an imperative of modern medicine. Of course, it had always been that way, it seems. At the dawn of the American Revolution, patriot surgeon John Jones said of the carnage soon to begin:

> The practical good man will endeavor to employ himself
> in alleviating those evils which he finds incident to human
> nature, without too vain and curious an inquiry into causes,

the nature and operation of which, lie far beyond the narrow
limits of human understanding.[19]

Yes, as John Jones knew, in war there is damnation and redemption. Can we ever balance the scales? Can we ever justify the costs?
Was there any redeeming value to this Great War—the War to End
All Wars? British surgeon and historian Vincent Zachary Cope
devised a bizarre calculus of human calamities driving medical
therapeutics—a perverted balance sheet of bereavements and benefits.
For World War I Cope's so-called medical balance sheet, with all the
carnage and millions of lives lost, was yet decidedly on the positive
side.[20] Medicine—and untold future millions—would still profit
for generations to come. Yes, it was true. British historian Perrin
Selcer succinctly summarized: "[a]t war's end George Stewart, the War
Department Hospital's director, declared that surgeons had surpassed
armament-makers. 'The War has taught us how to save more lives
than the war cost.'"[21]

And so thought that venerable American surgeon William Williams
Keen, whose career spanned the Civil War and the Great War. He thus
provided a unique perspective. "Never in the history of the world," he
pronounced in 1918, "have such splendid efforts been made to reconstruct
and re-educate the inevitable wreckage of war . . . It is one of the real
benefits to the credit side of the great war."[22]

George Crile would echo the sentiments of many scientists and
physicians about this Great War's generation. "[T]he World War
has been my outstanding experience. It has given me a new impetus
in research. It has given new viewpoints on medicine as a whole and
more particularly in surgery and its organization for efficiency," George
Crile went on to say after his departure from France in January 1919.[23]
Other physicians might agree. Those who toiled in tents and canvas
hospitals and makeshift operating rooms in mud and rain struggling
to find exotic ways to keep men alive knew the power of their efforts.
Now and then, new skills and new technology did, in fact, save the
hopelessly injured.

British Surgeon General George Makins said aptly, after the war, that:

> The man of science has been living under the same roof and under the same conditions as the surgeon . . . Never before have the physiologist and the pathologist come into such close contact either with the practitioner or the patient.[24]

Together, chemists and physicists and doctors and technology and compassion united in one grand effort to propel medicine into a modern age—an age of collaboration and evidence and truth—and from the ashes of catastrophe wrought by the evils of mankind would, in fact, come redemption.

TWO

Marcille, Mignon, and Verdun: The Peculiar Metamorphosis of Battlefield Surgery

"A picture of human pity . . . "
—Alfred Mignon, 1916

The abomination of the Great War pulled many an obscure figure to the forefront. These would be the men of redemption. The story of this particular individual begins with an ending.

On a chilly January day in 1936—befitting such a somber occasion—in the small Loire Valley town of Tours, an elderly gentleman eased back in his chair and, without the great fanfare to which he had once been accustomed, passed away as privately as he had lived in his later years, alone in a modest apartment and largely forgotten. Long gone were the days of Verdun, when he had masterminded a medical system that up till then was in utter disarray, when he had sent young surgeons near the ravaged ravines, hillocks, and trenches of that scorched land to resurrect and reassemble the victims of modern warfare. And when he had so skillfully coordinated the movement of those same fallen soldiers swiftly away to hospitals along the chain of evacuation, as if pieces on a chessboard, so that they needn't lay in the muck and grime certain to fatally fester their wounds. That military bearing he so deeply cherished had bent and grayed over those twenty years since. Yes, twenty—even thirty—years before, he had been worshipped by his students and admired by fellow physicians. He was a master of his trade and an honored officer of France's military. Alfred Mignon, now eighty-one years old, relinquished this earth for the remembrances of the ages.[1]

In an excursion to the western front at the end of August 1914 the outspoken and flamboyant French surgeon Eugène-Louis Doyen found a horrific collection of gravely wounded men, suffering from flagrant infections of joints and limbs, some with those ballooning bullae so characteristic of gas gangrene, and surely waiting to die. "One operates very little at the front," he had been told when inquiring why his skills were not required near the battle lines. These poor soldiers had been deprived of surgical care, Doyen learned, because of the preachings of that renowned French military surgeon Edmond Delorme. Delorme, of course, had directed that wounds be bandaged only. Let there be a minimum of fiddling, that curiosity of overly ambitious doctors who turned healthy wounds into festering caverns of pestilence and death. Fingers searching through gaps in skin only brought to bear invisible microbes of destruction. It was he who had assured his minions that simple gunshot wounds undoubtedly healed by nature's own intent rather than the unnecessary meddling of doctors. It was, according to Delorme, *l'attitude abstentionniste*, the abstentionist attitude. In fact, he had emphasized this in a communiqué as recent as August 10, 1914, calling it the "catechism of abstention."[2] It was all part of a rather farcical series of regulations issued first in 1910 outlining proper behavior of the French Service de santé (Health Service). These dictates, of course, were based largely on experiences of the Franco-Prussian War of 1870–71. All well and good, perhaps, if those same critically injured men could be evacuated quickly to surgical hospitals. Doyen soon learned that was impossible. Transportation was hard to find, physicians nonexistent, delays intolerable, and care provided largely by "public charity"—spotty at best. "The number of wounded exceed all availabilities," he observed. His poor patients and their savage wounds were dutifully treated only by application of bandages and not the radical surgery they sorely needed. Doyen chafed at it all. Not one to mince words, he had sharp comments about the Service de santé and even more to say about the likes of Edmond Delorme. "Delorme, an incompetent surgeon . . . propagated, by his presumption, the most harmful errors to our wounded," Doyen declared before the senate on July 7, 1915.[3] More than 50 percent of deaths were the faulty organization of the Service de santé, he claimed.

His was not a lone voice. Former prime minister Georges Clemenceau, a physician himself, was highly critical of the Service de santé at the outbreak of war. Using his newspaper, *L'Homme libre*, as a vehicle for his vitriol, Clemenceau protested the inefficiencies of handling the enormous numbers of casualties, observing that "the wounded have had to travel simply lying on the black straw of the wagons that had just been used for the transport of the horses." Despite government retorts appearing in *Le Temps* a few weeks later that the problem lay not with the Service de santé but with the barbarous Germans who insisted on shelling even hospitals housing hundreds of wounded, Clemenceau gave no quarter. In a later article published in *L'Homme enchaîné*, he pointed out that vicious activities by the enemy were isolated incidents. No excuse, he exclaimed. The inordinate number of wounded mounting at the front simply overwhelmed an ill-prepared system of evacuation and nothing else.[4]

Why were such passions aroused? Frontline conditions were abominable. Nobody had anticipated the destructive force of 20th century weaponry. Nobody had seen so many casualties, falling literally in heaps. It was all a fault of totally inept battlefield tactics. Grand infantry assaults, in colorful orderly rows—called by the French *attaque à outrance* ("attack to excess")—allowed defensive forces equipped with deadly *mitraillettes* (machine guns) and *éclat d'obus* (splintering shrapnel) to mow down lines of charging, bayonet-laden troops. Far too few medics were sent to fetch them and far too few doctors waited in field stations for them. Hours, sometimes days, elapsed before they could be retrieved. By then, even simple lacerations and puncture wounds, injected with all the bacteria of France's manured soil, had festered and harbored madly multiplying anaerobic Welch and Fraenkel bacilli. Gas gangrene would soon become a battlefield epidemic.

THE STERILE WOUND

Before 1914, the last large-scale conflict fought by the French, the Franco-Prussian War, was a military medical disaster. France's armies had no means to swiftly evacuate sick and wounded. Such efforts often fell to private initiatives. Unsanctioned *ambulances*—field hospitals—sprang up all over Paris. However, while the lightly wounded were eagerly sought after by these providers, the more seriously maimed and those with contagions such as smallpox and typhoid were "mercilessly shunned."[5] A system of medical care for injured and sick soldiers was totally lacking. Fortunately, in the years leading up to the Great War, there had been deep adjustments in the state-supervised military health service, the Service de santé. New plans instigated in 1910 assigned doctors of the Service de santé to various military zones set up by the French military. Forward, in areas of combat, would be the *zone des armées*, strictly under military control. Commanders further subdivided the *zone des armées* into the *zone de l'avant*, the frontlines; the *zone des étapes*, or marshalling areas; and the *zone de l'arrière*, or rear areas—communications, supply depots, and rest areas. Far to the back was the vast civilian area, called the *zone de l'intérieur* (interior) under control by the minister of war. Medical issues such as hygiene, sorting of casualties (triage), evacuation, distribution of supplies, and organization of health installations were included in the plan. Near the front lines, in the *zone de l'avant*, casualties would be carried by stretcher bearers to aid stations, called *postes de secours*, where wounds were inspected and bandaged, and patients packaged for transport. Little surgery was done other than the most emergency of measures. Field hospitals—*ambulances*—along the way might also inspect the wounded, but, again, few trained surgeons were available to give any kind of meaningful care—rarely needed, went the common wisdom. Wounded would, sooner or later, arrive at so-called evacuation hospitals known as Hôpitaux d'Origine d'Étapes, or HOEs, which were little more than large holding pens adjacent to railway lines. Here wounded were put aboard trains to take them farther to the rear to large military hospitals in the *zone de l'intérieur*. It might not be until then that patients received any type of reparative surgical care at all.[6]

This all made sense at the time. From experiences in previous wars, including the Russo-Japanese War of 1904–05 and those in the Balkans (1912–13), most wounds, over 85 percent, it was thought, were from bullets and considered relatively clean. Opening and probing such wounds was considered dangerous and likely to infect instead of cleanse. There was no need, then, for surgeons to be much nearer the front lines, as there would be little for them to do. They were best positioned in larger hospitals much farther away. In fact, numbers of divisional and corps field hospitals were drastically reduced to conform to a war of movement, the so-called *attaque à outrance*, or a massed attack by infantry meant to startle and overpower any opponent. They were wars of mobility and maneuver, not given to stationary facilities, including hospitals.[7] "As they are mobile and must follow the movements of the division, [*ambulance*] doctors will only operate in cases of absolute urgency," the instructions read.[8]

And anyway, it had been long held that rampant epidemics laid far more troops low than enemy gunfire. Sanitary measures and preventative hygiene were the primary concerns of field commanders: absolve the dregs of dysentery and distempers taking troops from the firing lines to their bunks.

The aging surgeon Edmond Delorme, former director of the Service de santé, set the standard. After all, he had written the two-volume seminal text on military surgery, *Traité de Chirurgie de Guerre*, in 1888. Bullet wounds were innocuous, he insisted, and as recently as August 1914 had convinced the prestigious Société nationale de chirurgie de Paris of such. There was no doubt about his stance on early surgery for war wounds:

> At present, war surgery must be conservative in the vast majority of cases, in almost all bullet wounds . . . The characteristic of the practice in the lines of the front is the simplicity.

> The mass of the wounded who suddenly invade the health facilities and demand almost simultaneous care requires it. [9]

In fact, he was right on that point. Surgeons were simply overwhelmed by the flood of wounded. Inspecting, cleaning, and bandaging the injuries meshed well with their workload. There was no time for anything else. Even ominous wounds of the abdomen were ignored. Delorme went on to say that for those injuries, "immediate laparotomy is to be rejected . . . the most recent wars . . . affirmed its harmfulness." Belly wounds were uncommon issues anyway, Delorme claimed. Few, maybe one in ten, suffered from them. Instead, ship the casualty off. Even in Paris, all were in agreement. A surgeon at the Val-de-Grâce—the major military hospital in Paris—emphasized "preventive debridement [surgery] of wounds to the 'soft parts' are to be rejected." "Do not explore the wound," he admonished. [10]

In their starched collars, with fat cigars and in smoke-filled chambers, European colleagues agreed. The Prussian empire to the east was the self-proclaimed center of medical research and innovation in the new 20th century. [11] Considering their reputation, the opinion of German surgeons held sway. Foremost among them, the iconic Ernst von Bergmann, urged similar restraint in the care of war wounds. Almost fanatically concerned with cleanliness, Bergmann had maintained, of course, that simple bullet wounds were likely sterile. Proper management with meticulous cleansing and coverage with sterile bandages would be enough. He insisted surgeons not meddle—it would only invite infection. A cult following quickly developed. His pupil, Curt Schimmelbusch, joined in. In 1893 he, too, urged surgeons to apply conservatism to injuries, that needless snooping would only foster, not inhibit, infection. [12] The famous Carl Langenbuch, veteran army surgeon of the Franco-Prussian War of 1870–71 and the Russo-Turkish War of 1877–78, warned of similar perils: explore wounds only if there are life-threatening problems such as bleeding, otherwise stay away. [13] Even after war began in 1914, German surgeons had not changed their tune. In those first bloody encounters in Belgium and France, they still argued that bullet wounds healed without interference: "they are quickly cured by means of aseptic application of bandages." One veteran army surgeon of the western front gave this counsel as late as 1916:

> [In shot wounds] Be careful not to touch them or to clean the neighboring area; let dirt, hair, blood intentionally sit on the surrounding skin, pinch the edge of the wound with iodine tincture or mastisol, a piece of bandage stuffed on it—and have the sensation to have done everything necessary.[14]

Little was different from 1870.
The automobile would change all that.

LE VOITURE CHIRURGICALE[15]

The exceedingly wealthy Anne de Rochechouart de Mortemart was bewitched by the new automobile. Heiress to the Veuve Clicquot Champagne house, she was the great-granddaughter of Madame Clicquot Ponsardin, whose husband died in 1805 leaving her as the sole proprietress of champagne production, soon to be recognized as the *Veuve* (widow) Clicquot house. As for Anne, the great-granddaughter, with her marriage to Emmanuel de Crussol, the twelfth Duc d'Uzès, in 1867, she became the Duchesse d'Uzès only to lose her husband eleven years later in 1878. Never to remarry, she remained the dowager duchess. Anne was a woman of diverse curiosities, not given to idleness or inane dalliances. Instead, she was driven by authentic passions. And indeed, they were fiery emanations from the spirit, ranging far and wide, from elaborate fox hunts to political intrigue, backing the charismatic royalist Georges Boulanger who left her "speechless" at their first meeting. (Was there a romance? Who would know, but he flirtatiously answered her request for another visit with "Whenever you want.") A staunch advocate of women's rights, she was one of the founding contributors to l'Union française pour le suffrage des femmes (The French Union for the Suffrage of Women),[16] and dabbled in artistic expression with sculpting—a talent not often witnessed in the aristocracy. Through it all, she remained a righteous feminist, insisting on feminine individuality regardless of social position:

> It is difficult to admit that a woman of the world can have talent. How many have said, in front of my sculptures: "Bah, it's not she who did this! We know how they work, the women of the world! It would damage their fingers . . ."[17]

The Duchesse was to exhibit her sculpturing at the World's Columbian Exhibition in Chicago in 1893, the statue of Saint Hubert, a replica she had made for the Basilica of the Sacred Heart at Montmartre in Paris. But it was the automobile that drew her attention. "I, who have always loved horses had promised myself I would never have such horrible machines," she wrote. But then, there she was in 1898, the first French woman to earn an automobile license at the wheel of her sleek Delahaye, accompanied by three examiners. The Parisian press commented, "wearing a little black felt hat that she wore slanted over her ear, [the Duchesse] held the steering wheel and maneuvered very skillfully." "How much fun did I have with my little 'break' [Delahaye, type 1]." She went on to report to the journal *Les Annales politiques et littéraires* on May 8, 1898: "[t]he impressions I have felt, ask me; they were delicious; first to go at the pace that I liked, to overtake quickly, quickly, the other cars, adroitly enough not to hit them." So delicious, it seems, that she was awarded one of the first speeding tickets in the Bois de Boulogne driving her Delahaye at the incredible speed of ten miles per hour.[18] Her transgression was eagerly reported in *Le Figaro* on July 5, 1898, which divulged that she and her son, the Duke d'Uzès, were "victims of that unfortunate infringement which lurks for drivers of automobiles." Her punishment? A fine of 28 francs.[19]

And, at the outset of hostilities that August of 1914, la Société de bienfaisance russe à Paris (the Russian colony in Paris) graciously organized a Russian *ambulance* for the wounded of the French Army. The hospital was placed under the patronage of Russia's Empress Dowager Maria Feodorovna. It was at this time that the Duchesse d'Uzès was persuaded to assemble and preside over a Franco-Russian surgical unit, perhaps because of her acquaintance with Feodorovna or perhaps it was the dashing, pro-French Russian ambassador, Alexander Izvolsky, who had recently exclaimed about the looming enmities, *"C'est ma guerre!"* (This is my war!) It was all great festivity, the titled aristocracy begetting sums of wealth to a more humane effort than afternoon tea. Yet the Duchesse was moved by deeper motives, opening her château at Bonnelles, southwest of Paris, for scores of wounded, she herself would qualify as a nurse at age sixty-seven. And in this political and social maelstrom was one obscure French surgeon, heretofore unknown, who had peculiarly caught the attention of Paris's well-heeled. He was in love with the automobile as well. Would it not be seductive, with her passion for motorized conveyances, that the use of this new automobile for France's maimed be put before the Duchesse?

Enter that other dramatis persona in this play of events. Born in the small French village of Jouy-le-Châtel in the Seine-et-Marne region just outside of Paris, Maurice Marcille was himself the son of a physician. He had been an apprentice in the laboratories of the great French surgeon Louis-Hubert Farabeuf and the renowned anatomist Paul Poirier in 1902, where he delved into the intricacies of the inguinal and pelvic lymphatics that earned him his doctorate in medicine.[20] Maurice Marcille was a gifted, if not a bit impetuous, surgeon, having trained as an intern at three great Parisian hospitals: Charité, under Paul Tillaux; the Saint-Antoine under Charles Monod; and the Necker under the illustrious urologic surgeon Jean-François-Auguste Le Dentu. He had been described as an excellent intern, very intelligent. But there was a bit of a maverick in him, a flare for the dramatic. In those opening days of the new century all of Paris was abuzz at the dashing élan of this young doctor who won his bride, the young Cordélia Le Play, by whisking her away in his grand automobile sans consent of her father (today, eloping might be a better term), at least according to fellow surgeon Georges Duhamel, who proclaimed the affair with appropriate aplomb.[21] Marcille had, as they said, earned a reputation as a purveyor of "mauvaises plaisanteries, des lubies et des inventions cocasses" ("bad jokes, fads, and comical inventions"). Yet, despite a witty behavior, his demeanor was one of focused attention; he had an angular face, at once handsome and penetrating, the eyes riveted on his immediate occupation. His social adventures notwithstanding, this intensity earned him a coveted position as *Chirurgien des Hôpitaux de Paris* (Surgeon of the Hospitals of Paris)[22] in 1912, all without the usual connections of patrician Paris. That is, of course, until mobilization with the onset of war. His more plebian legacy would earn him only, at age forty-three even, a lowly military rank of *médecin aide-major de 2e class* (second lieutenant). Marcille chafed at this, a position distinctly unbecoming to someone of his self-acclaimed importance that, no doubt, rankled his equanimity.

On a more eclectic note, it was not just an infatuation with motor cars. Marcille had, in fact secured a patent for the revolutionary pneumatic tire in 1906, "the combination of a wheel rim, a tire cover, a gripping band, sleeves . . . adapted to engage with the studs."[23] Perhaps in this capacity as aficionados they came together, Marcille and the lady Anne de Rochechouart. She might have been drawn to a character so out of the ordinary, much like herself, a visionary with implacable energy. An intense man, he would approach her with his idea, formulated in the mundane dwellings of his military inactivity as a junior-grade officer—a continued affront to his self-assessed genius. With his subordinate rank, he had no hope of sharing his ideas with the surgical aristocracy or ministerial spheres. So it was here he laid at the Duchesse's feet the plans for his mobile operating theater, a team carried by automobiles right to the front, to spare the lives of fallen soldiers not long to live without surgical skills. Possibly a combination of jaunty self-confidence, an excitement, and a worry over the torments of injured men won her over. It ignited her interest and soon he had access to notables such as Aristide Briand, then minister of justice; Paul Deschanel, speaker of the House of Deputies; Louis Barthou, former prime minister; and Joseph Reinach, former vice president of the armed forces committee in the Chamber of Deputies. Tall and robust-appearing, Marcille could command his audience. As his acquaintance Georges Duhamel put it "he did not intend his expedition to be short of publicity and therefore he was acting accordingly."[24] Armed with this portentous support he then approached *médecin inspecteur général* François Troussaint, appointed by the Seventh Directorate (Health Ministry) as health service supervisor in the *zone de l'intérieur*, and *médecin inspecteur général* Paul Chavasse, recently appointed director of the Service de santé in the *zone des armées*.

From whence did Marcille's concept of a mobile surgical unit arise? He may have very well been familiar with the work of engineer Paul Boulant, employed by that pioneering automobile manufacturer Théophile Schneider and his prospering company, who had already developed a "mobile operating theater" in 1912. In fact, Boulant had obtained a patent for his *voiture chirurgicale* that very year. Motorized movement of wounded by trucks able to store up to eight litter patients was already commonplace. But there were those gravely wounded men, particularly with belly wounds, who need urgent surgery. For these sorry souls, motor transport would only "inflict further atrocious torture" and likely be fatal. The "legendary devotion and high standards of military doctors" would then make little difference. Some visionaries, though, knew the solution, even before war began. A particular distinguished and respected *médecin inspecteur* (senior military medical officer), Alfred Mignon, speaking at a conference at the Val-de-Grâce in May 1913, had said: "A seriously wounded . . . will have to stay in place, in an ambulance in the zone of the armies, right on the battlefield . . . [they] might have to stay 15 days, two months if necessary."[25] In other words, such cases must be treated early on and, therefore, near where they had fallen—near the field of battle. Paul Boulant indeed envisioned such a mobile unit that could bring surgery to those critical patients. He somehow persuaded his employers at Schneider's firm to start construction of a surgical truck that could accommodate roving surgeons and assistants. They chose the same chassis found on Parisian omnibuses and partitioned the cabin into three parts, the rear area being the operating "room" equipped with generator, electricity, sterilizer, and surgical accoutrements. Up to forty-five horsepower and a four-cylinder engine drove the five-ton truck at a cruising speed of almost twenty miles per hour.[26] Expanding side walls on this motorized camion would provide tentage to temporarily shelter the wounded. The unit would afford the Service de santé the most modern and advanced surgical technology available. Boulant's Schneider prototype was rolled out in the gardens of the Val-de-Grâce in the summer of 1912. It would be positioned just behind infantry divisions in the field and sent even farther forward, closer to the battle lines, as the need arose.[27]

Or, perhaps in that late summer of 1914 Marcille might have already heard of the terrible reports from Belgium and northern France. Accounts began surfacing describing the slaughter. Official censored reports sterilized the whole affair, but the truth leaked to journalists anyway. The novelist Jean Cocteau summarized those first ugly days in his book *Thomas l'imposteur*. He said that for France, "La guerre commença dans le plus grand désordre" ("the war began in the greatest disorder").[28] Even individual letters from soldiers were found and published:

> Our losses are appalling . . . You cannot know, my beloved mother, what man can do against man . . . my shoes are soiled with human brains, I squash chests and slip on entrails.[29]

What leveled lines of advancing troops, filled with naïve élan, rifles at the ready, bayonets gleaming, was the sheer efficiency of well-positioned machine-gun fire and the hailstorm of falling artillery shells spewing deadly shrapnel. It all was so intense that one infantryman testified from Charleroi in August 1914, "Il plut des marmites" (it rained shells).[30] During four days of combat on the borders of France and Belgium, from August 21 to 25, French forces recorded 140,000 casualties.[31] As appalling was the fate of the wounded. Surgeons reported that it was a "deplorable and lamentable situation" to witness "those unfortunates, exhausted by fatigue and pain, lying on a stretcher or, more often, straw for two, three, four days of an infernal trip."[32] The numbers of stricken men simply stunned health workers, unable to care for the multitude or even evacuate them in a timely fashion. Léon Werth, then a private in a brutal sector of the front, related that "there were not enough doctors. They [the wounded] were there, filthy, covered in lice, worms crawled in their wounds and into their bellies."[33] American nurse Mary Borden, working as a volunteer behind the lines, described it well:

> There had been a harvest. Crops of men were cut down in the fields of France where they were growing. They were mown

down with a scythe, were gathered into bundles, tossed about with pitchforks, pitchforked into wagons and transported great distances and flung into ditches . . .[34]

Alfred Mignon, then in charge of the Service de santé for Joseph Joffre's Third Army near the Argonne, wrote that "ambulances [at the front] were chambers of horrors . . . The smell of the rooms was disgusting and the grave signs of visceral or limb injuries gave a picture of human pity."[35]

It was all a mess. Transition of care, that smooth movement of casualties from one hospital to another, stalled. Key to this was speed and sorting, an all-important step of finding and solving urgent problems along the chain of evacuation. It didn't happen. Doctors thought little beyond the confines of their dingy field hospitals and too often were inclined to pass off moribund patients in dire need of surgical care. Haunted by Delorme's warnings and overwhelmed by carnage, they stammered expletives and moved on to more agreeable cases. As a result, droves of wounded languished at railway terminals and on overcrowded roads. Critics came forward. Maurice Barrès was a French journalist and political activist. Together with the Duchesse of Uzès and other prominent citizens, he had backed the extremely charismatic and popular Georges Boulanger in his bid for presidency of the republic in the elections of 1889. Barrès was an avid patriot of France and staunch supporter of France's military efforts in the Great War. But he was shocked at the condition of the wounded, the soldiers who had fought and fell for their country. Although the Ministry of War made some attempts to squelch to the press problems that had arisen on the frontiers that August, Barrès lashed out.[36] Not enough of France's touted physicians and surgeons and not nearly enough hospital beds had been made available, he argued, to serve the massive number of French casualties at the onset of the war:

We sent wounded far back, and subsequently in Paris they were crammed into premises insufficiently aseptic, while we refused to put them in the hospitals of Public Assistance, where large empty rooms and seven or eight thousand beds awaited them.[37]

Gangrène gazeuse—gas gangrene—had made its appearance. Putrid, rotting limbs soon filled hospital beds. Surgeons grappled with a solution. Mortality skyrocketed. Some said more than half of those cases died. Delays getting the injured to surgeons and that outdated practice of ignoring "clean" injuries were the reason. The manure and mud of France's farms and the spinning, slicing artillery fragments made even the smallest of skin punctures a deadly occurrence.[38] Amputations were the only hope; arms and legs were chopped off at a ferocious pace, and even that did not stop some infections as they quickly spread to virgin torsos, literally eating their victim alive. Soon the pallor of death descended like some merciful angel, whisking the poor souls to a better existence. Amputations were swift. "En saucisson" ("like cutting sausage"), it was called, a quick circular amputation as if done by a meat cleaver. The advantages were obvious: rapid, simple, economical. No time then for the careful cutting and paring and cleansing that would be the hallmark of surgery for these wounds in the months to come. "If we cannot be brilliant we would hope for the certainty of saving many lives," was the attitude.[39] Some said almost half of large wounds received amputations those early months.[40] Was it the inattention doctors practiced that caused so much delay and suffering? Was it the sheer number of wounded? Or was it an intoxication with doctrines that had their root in another, different age?

Whatever the reason, change had to occur. Fresh innovation was the key, but it would come from outside the ranks of academia. For one, Maurice Marcille, bored with his paper shuffling, understood the value of motorized transport. Swift access (provided roads were passable) to the front was now within reach of medical teams.[41] Why not send surgeons? Frontline doctors seemed ill prepared or unwilling to operate on these men, at a time when damage from newer weapons was far graver than before. Surgery there could certainly do no harm. Marcille was intrigued by Boulant's surgical automobile. But maybe it was too small, not equipped for long stays. The number of wounded to be cared for would be limited by personnel and supplies. In any event, Boulant's entire surgical truck had been lost. It had mysteriously disappeared from the Charleroi battlefield in August 1914. Some thought it had been captured by the Germans. No trace of it was ever discovered. Now Marcille had a better idea: an entire surgical automobile *ambulance*—an entire field hospital on wheels,

> [A]bundant enough to allow the surgeons to operate, so to speak, almost continually and under excellent conditions, and more, to ensure a sufficient housing of the operated until their evacuation to a hospital further to the rear . . .[42]

His mobile unit (it would be called an *ambulance chirurgicale*) was not just one truck, as Boulant had planned. A string of a dozen or more vans and cars would carry pharmacy supplies, instruments, dressings, sterilization equipment, bedding, blankets, canvas for tents, nurses, and other medical staff. Enough of horse and wagon; Marcille's motorized entourage would zip along at the dizzying speed of ten miles per hour (on good roads). Within sound of gunfire, crews would unload trucks, pitch canvas, fire up generators, and open for business. As Marcille designed it, there was a tent for surgery, space for the sterilizing autoclaves, and tents to hold patients before and after operations. He had even included six Renault motorcars modified to shuttle stretcher patients from battlefield aid stations near the trenches. The entire setup, he reckoned, could house perhaps a hundred wounded. On October 14, 1914, Marcille delivered a prototype, proudly exhibiting it at the Grand Parc for automobiles at Vincennes. The centerpiece—the masterpiece even—was his portable operating room and all its most modern technology. Even the mighty Troussaint seemed impressed—his remarks carefully made, though, "without enthusiasm," according to witnesses like Alfred Mignon. After all, Marcille might just be a young upstart, maybe even a quack. Still, it was a seductive idea. Marcille's unit would be known for its mobility and ability to carry out major surgical operations as close as possible to the "moment du traumatisme" ("moment of trauma"), Troussaint agreed. His support, even "without enthusiasm," carried weight. But Troussaint had to be careful, he knew. His political appointment had strings attached. Positions such as his required close attention to the whims and opinions of that most conservative of Parisian assemblies, the Société nationale de chirurgie. They were far from convinced, the young Marcille a complete unknown. Safety, they maintained, was their chief concern. This "experiment" would have to be carefully and thoroughly evaluated before radically changing battlefield medicine. [43]

And so, the experiment began. On November 9, 1914, trucks and automobiles packed with surgical supplies left the Porte Maillot in Paris's Seventeenth Arrondissement, just a short distance from the Arc de Triomphe. The convoy chugged along at a steady pace of seven miles per hour despite twisting, muddy roads—still faster than horse-drawn conveyance—for three days and nights until they arrived at the courtyard of the Château de Lignereuil, six miles from the Artois front. Dr. Paul Hallopeau, a surgeon colleague of Marcille and son of the famous Parisian dermatologist Henri Hallopeau, was designated operating surgeon, while Marcille busied himself with training his assistants, arranging tables and lights, and preparing instruments. In a two-week span at Lignereuil the Renault motor carriages transported ninety-two gravely wounded men from nearby aid stations and *ambulances*. Seventy of these passed through Hallopeau's operating room. Many, those with gunshot and shrapnel wounds to their limbs, were immediately operated on, opening and exploring tears and bruises and fractures. Dirt, clothing, and metal fragments were dug out; damaged, devitalized flesh and muscle were pared away until the deep cavities were the rosy red of health. Few amputations were needed. Of over two dozen cases only one patient died. Hallopeau even ventured into the abdomen—that soft underbelly long the dread of even the most ambitious surgeons. He was often met by the swirling mess of leaking intestines or pools of exsanguinating blood from shattered livers and spleens. Seldom could he staunch the surge. Many were almost dead on arrival—thanks to quick evacuation from the battlefield. Only two of these cases survived. [44] Yet, early surgery by his automobile team, Marcille had shown, could help prevent later problems, mostly infections like gas gangrene.

But problems surfaced. There was far too little tent space for the crowd of recovering patients. Out of necessity, he commandeered the roomy, adjoining château for his recuperating men. But, like many French manor houses, chambers were expansive, high-ceilinged affairs, poorly heated and distinctly chilly in November. Bandaged and splinted cases languished in haphazard arrangements wrapped in blankets or whatever covering could be found. The great halls echoed with moans and pleas. "Every day the scene became more gloomy," Georges Duhamel, one of Marcille's young doctor assistants, reported. The nearness to battle unnerved everyone, the rolling, distant thunder a constant reminder to men who had fallen victim to those same artillery blasts. Sometimes the windows shook with the sound of cannonading. Yet, Marcille, oblivious to it all, did little to calm anxieties. He raged like a narcissistic tyrant, bullying his doctors and nursing staff, leveling insults and ranting in tantrums. At one point Duhamel claimed Marcille stuffed cotton into the mouth of a patient screaming over his rough handling of a wound. To make matters worse, Hallopeau had been stricken with scarlet fever and evacuated, leaving the unit without competent surgical help. Before long, Tenth Army surgeon *médecin-chef* Edmond Potherat, camped in a nearby village, heard of the uproar and notified General Philippe Pétain who, in short order, paid a surprise visit to Marcille. Predictably, Marcille and his *ambulance* were abruptly recalled to Paris.[45]

From this point forward, Marcille's ingenious mobile hospital ran into trouble. According to historian François Olier, General Paul Chavasse, director of the Service de santé, promptly issued a scathing report of Marcille's unit to the Seventh Directorate . It was a vicious commentary, an *assassinés exécutait* (a deliberate murder [of character]). Not only was Marcille's professional competence called into question but also his honesty and integrity. Chavasse claimed Marcille, with his impetuous location of the hospital so close to enemy artillery, had compromised the safety of his surgical team. The Lignereuil "experiment" was a shambles, Chavasse insisted. Marcille had not fulfilled his purpose. The medical staff lacked training in military surgery, personnel were poorly prepared, and the operative results were not impressive.[46] And there would be more. Another circular, issued February 4, 1915, was even more accusatory. Marcille had lied about his results, it maintained. He had falsified his operative reports. And then directly to character: "Marcille was a bad surgeon; he operated precipitously, before the wounded were sufficiently resuscitated and out of shock . . ."[47] Overall mortality was not 50 percent as Hallopeau had claimed, but near 100 percent, Chavasse implied. In essence, Marcille was proclaimed a charlatan. His career and his mobile *ambulance* were perilously close to the trash heap.

Was it true? Did Hallopeau—with the complicity of Marcille—whitewash his report? Marcille's enigmatic and volatile personality was largely to blame—and his chummy relationship with the affluent of Paris, who made no secret of their admiration for him. All this intrigue and societal pressure rankled academic surgery, especially those embedded in that seemingly impenetrable cocoon of tradition. Yes, in truth, there were problems. Marcille's surgical unit was loosely organized and ill prepared for the rigors of the battlefield. Marcille had little self-control. He was brash and insensitive, acting, at times, "inhuman" toward his patients. Edmond Delorme, for one, would never be a fan. Even after the war he would write that Marcille's "formations" were "too heavy, too bulky, too difficult to handle the roads . . . too expensive." An experienced doctor could provide as much in the conventional horse-drawn ambulances. And there was no provision for housing the wounded, he went on to say, curtly concluding, "It was an operating team and nothing more." Wounded men deserved better. As for Hallopeau, he was an honest man it seems, and nothing ever surfaced to put his facts in question.

Marcille remained indignant—and unrepentant—taking his case to those influential political figures whom he had infused with enthusiasm in the first place. His engaging, effusive personality, charming when he had to be, even perhaps a bit on the manic side, did not fail to bias his well-positioned admirers. In turn, they pressed the Health Directorate to reconsider Chavasse's biting circulars. And, furthermore, before any official determination could be made, Hallopeau and Marcille published their optimistic results—albeit controversial—in the prestigious medical journal *La Presse médicale*. For further emphasis, Hallopeau, a respected member of academic surgery, promptly presented, in person, their experience before the Société de chirurgie. Hallopeau was different from Marcille: professional, polished, and academically persuasive. His fellow surgeons (and the public) became instantly aware of the reported value of immediate surgical care for its soldiers, eclipsing Chavasse's insinuations to the contrary and offering some hope for the terrible neglect of the wounded.

In response to Chavasse's accusations (and Hallopeau's compelling report), a special council, the Commission supérieure consultative de Service de santé, chaired by longtime good Marcille supporter Joseph Reinach, a progressive reformer of injustices, convened. Members included Doctors Delorme, Mignon, and Troussaint. Their report to the minister of war was issued on March 2, 1915. While critical of the shortcomings of Marcille's initial hospital construct (inadequate matériel and housing of patients), the commission overwhelmingly supported his concept of mobility, early surgical intervention, and rapid evacuation. Units should be filled with full technology and equipment, the commission said, set up within a few miles of the front, and staffed by respected, career surgeons—not young, inexperienced doctors who knew little of the surgical arts. Surgical teams should be complete with assistants, nurses, and technicians trained in the rigors of battlefield medicine. In fact, surgery near the front lines was a new imperative. The commission agreed:

> It is necessary to create in each army, at the rate of at least one
> per [army] corps, surgical units for the emergency operative
> treatment of serious injuries. These surgical formations will,
> during the period of static warfare, be added to the groups of
> ambulances and organic army units. [48]

Doyen, no stranger to drama himself, drove the point home later that summer speaking in front of the Senate and Chamber of Deputies on military health matters. He had had enough of inaction by his professional colleagues. "It would be impossible to make a mockery of the public more casually . . . everyone in France knows that the Service de santé has banned interventions up front." These unfortunate men had died by the thousands during their long journey to the hospitals, he went on to say. "In the face of this neglect and misery, praise had been heaped on this same Service de santé for doing nothing." [49]

Damn that Marcille and his crazy ideas! He had stirred up such sentiment. Professional and public support mounted. Troussaint was under pressure to react. He looked for a diplomat, someone trusted by his academic community and the cadres of surgeons now recruited for the national crisis. Delorme? Hardly. Instead, he found his man in *Professeur* Antonin Gosset, newly minted *médecin-major de 1ère classe* (roughly equivalent to colonel and one grade below a general officer). Gosset agreed to take another look at the usefulness of Marcille's mobile *ambulance*—with modifications—in the way Marcille had intended—and maybe with a more even temperament. Troussaint asked Gosset to locate his unit with the Third Army near Verdun under *médecin inspecteur général* Alfred Mignon (inspector general of the Health Service), a known sympathizer with early surgical treatment. Marcille's "experiment" was given new life.

A HIGHER CALLING

Henri Alexandre Alfred Mignon was born in Poitiers, that storied city in the Poitou region of France, on November 22, 1854. Poitiers had a central role in French military history. Nearby, Charles Martel's troops had routed Muslims in 732, the English Black Prince had done the same to French forces in 1356, and the town hosted an ill-fated inquest of the captured Joan of Arc in 1431. Mignon's father, according to the cryptic expression on the birth certificate, was an employee of the new "electric telegraph." But Alfred had different aspirations, more of a military nature. He was accepted into the Service de santé—the military health service—in 1876 and earned his doctorate from the Faculté de médecine of Paris. On assignment to Algiers he developed an interest in surgery, and his deep intellectual curiosity and persistence led him to an associate surgery position at the Val-de-Grâce in 1891. By 1900, his talents were obvious: he had been awarded the respected title of *professeur*. The next eight years would be a time of great productivity—a burgeoning clinical practice, magnificent performances in the operating room, remarkable scientific publications, and above all the growing admiration of a body of students who would always emulate his dedication and high moral character. "The gifts of the teacher will survive in our memories," it would be written of him. But it would be in his later role as *médecin-chef supérieur* (surgeon in chief) for General Philippe Pétain's Second Army, responsible for the defense of Verdun, that would truly define him.[50]

It would be a consummate calling for a principled surgeon such as he; one intent on preservation of life and limb—and quite fitting for a man of noble bearing. Yet Mignon, the diplomat, the polished bureaucrat, would soon clash with the directives of high command on the care of his wounded soldiers.

Mignon knew full well the inadequacies of medical care near the frontline trenches. It had pained him to see the fate of fallen soldiers those early days of the war. The forward *ambulances*, to his dismay, had indeed become chambers of horrors. Those who could easily travel—those "transportable" patients—had already been evacuated. But the others:

> My throat gagged before so many miseries assembled [in the forward ambulances]. Agitated cries were added to the sweet and tranquil delirium of the great traumas to the brain; the vomiting of those with peritonitis mingled with the noisy breathing of those with suffocating chest damage; those already septic burned into one's subconscious. [51]

Yet, despite the human agonies unfolding, it seemed "a certain resistance" had surfaced with some medical chiefs of these surgical *ambulances*. As if many were quite content to pass over the mangled mobs who filled their tents. It all fit with Delorme's invectives on purposeful inattention—*abstention*—to combat wounds. Surgery here was too dangerous, the patients uncomfortably close to enemy guns. Surgeons would be hesitant, nervous, not able to practice the delicate skills necessary on lungs, intestines, even the heart. Yet, such thinking prompted neglect. Mignon simply did not buy it. It was here, he reasoned, that surgery could be of most use, on men freshly injured. It was here where surgeons skilled in the art should be, not treating patients later, when days of neglect had bled bodies white and filled fractured tissue with the poisons of gluttonous bacteria. To add insult to injury, doctors were rarely brought in for planning sessions. Field commanders felt them of little use in plotting strategy and tactics. Casualties seemed almost an afterthought in the grand maneuverings of troops and artillery; once disabled, they became useless debris to be cleaned up by roving camp followers. "We had been kept away from projects in progress as if we had been strangers to the Army," Mignon wrote. And, any questions he did raise with the general staff "were decided by the single word: 'impossible.'" [52]

Mignon had sat on the commission to review Chavasse's report on Marcille's mobile surgical contraption. There were problems, to be sure, but the concept was persuasive. He hoped that Gosset's mobile surgical hospital would be the answer. Officially, his directive was to assess "the usefulness of an improved surgical unit in various situations." So Gosset's truck-laden surgical *ambulance* lumbered in—fifteen vehicles in all—now with seven physicians, thirty-seven nurses, and twenty-seven support workers. Top-heavy camions carried three operating tables instead of two, dozens of cots, heavy autoclaves, and chests filled with clamps, retractors, scissors, saws, knives, and suture; all the accoutrements of a busy surgery clinic. The irascible Marcille was even aboard, not as a surgeon but as an engineer, assisting in setting up. He was strictly forbidden to participate in any patient care. Mignon put the *ambulance* at Sainte-Menehould, a town almost due west of Verdun and directly in the path of evacuating casualties. Unlike Marcille's plan at Lignereuil, Gosset expanded the hospital section to provide shelter, beds, and supplies for his wounded. He designed spacious rooms for examination, operating, and recovery; the true focus of the *ambulance*. [53] Mignon was impressed; finally the ability to care for the injured at once. It was almost an apparition for him:

> It seems to me that my surgical ideal was realized . . . This was really what an operating room is for surgeons . . . In a word, real surgery. And when the operation was finished, so that the description of the operating environment was complete, Gosset took me to the wards. Uniform beds, elegant bunk beds, flattering hospitality. The cause of the automobile surgery unit was won in my eyes. What a nasty dream to have witnessed so much bastard surgery universally practiced since the beginning of the war! [54]

In fifteen days, Gosset's team performed eighty operations. Seven laparotomies even—that most formidable of operations in 1915—were done for abdominal injuries. Gosset, long a student of abdominal surgery, knew that customary treatment—abstention—was almost uniformly fatal. Here at Sainte-Menehould four of the seven patients survived; a remarkable success. Why? Early intervention was the only reasonable answer.

> All these wounds were operated on average eleven hours after the injury. Except in the case of major damage by shrapnel or shock, and not improving despite serum and camphor oil, one must intervene. It is necessary to operate early and quickly, clean the abdomen with ether and give the greatest post-operative care. [55]

Gosset and Mignon agreed. Early surgery seemed to produce wonders. With Gosset's keen eye and foresight, Marcille's preposterous idea had been vindicated. This time, there was no lack of space for patients recovering from surgery. Operations could be done faster and better and the patients moved out quicker. To be sure, Marcille had provided some technical improvements. His tinkering produced sterilizers—the key to keeping instruments clean, sterile, and ready for use—more durable and reliable. Marcille somehow also brightened the operating lamps and warmed the tents, another crucial feature in year-round service. But it was Gosset's good sense and diplomacy that carried the day. He was a man of pleasing features, a gentleman and a motivator. His words of praise and encouragement stirred a confidence in his colleagues and a desire to excel. For doctors and nurses who labored beneath bloodstained aprons, reeking of perspiration and teetering on the verge of collapse, his unflappable nature was an inspiration. And, in turn, his surgeons were simply marvelous; his teams worked their subjects like medieval armorers, straightening, weaving, and tempering human frames as if preparing for the king's inspection. So impressed was Gosset by the performance of this new version of Marcille's automobile *ambulance*—his version—that he lobbied for an even bigger footprint: more operating tables, partitioned rooms for resuscitation, surgery, recovery, and convalescence. He even envisioned an area for infected cases, to contain the spread of contagion (mostly gas gangrene). Gosset was simply in love with it all. To enhance its portability, he would streamline transportation. He specifically outfitted trucks to carry sterilization equipment, the new portable radiology units, and the breadth of operating instruments. His enthusiasm was infectious. Chavasse now was convinced. He would call them *ambulances chirurgicales automobiles* (automotive surgical hospitals)—and soon *auto-chir* for short. Chavasse wanted each army corps to have at least one. Gosset was acclaimed as a pioneer, a superb visionary, in keeping with his impeccable reputation. Maurice Marcille, effectively marginalized, would slip into obscurity.

On May 4, Gosset's new mobile unit was unveiled to the public and touted by the press as a remarkable accomplishment in care of the wounded. Gosset was acclaimed as brilliant, and his name attached to it: *auto-chir* Gosset. Marcille's nemesis, aristocratic surgery, had won out. He was totally ignored and, for lack of a better term, discarded. Production of Gosset's *auto-chirs* soared. A total of twenty-three would be assembled and distributed to army units in the field.[56]

Good riddance to Marcille, some would murmur. Georges Duhamel, bullied by Marcille at Lignereuil, could not have been happier. "The manic could still be satisfied with this victory. But I'm sure he's dying, that he's struggling to open up some new career. Bah! Let him go away over the torrent. He made me suffer enough."[57] And, indeed, Marcille moved on, thumbing his nose at Parisian medicine. With the help of his Russian friends, he was allowed to develop several of his prototype mobile surgical operating units that were donated to the Formations chirurgicales franco-russes (Franco-Russian Surgical Formations) by his complice and supporter, the incomparable Duchesse d'Uzès—all with the consent of the Seventh Directorate. *Le Petit Parisien* described it as an "incomparable gift made to France by our Russian friends."[58]

THE CENTER OF THE UNIVERSE

Verdun had held a certain fascination with Germanic peoples for centuries, a seeming gateway to the West, a pivotal city of the watershed

areas of Alsace and Lorraine—astride the Meuse River and the borders
of Charlemagne's dispersed empire. The fortress had been sacked by
Prussian forces in 1792 during the War of the First Coalition, clearing a
path into eastern France. German writer Johann Goethe had marveled at
the pleasing village surrounded by "meadows and gardens," but delighted
in the bombardments that piecemeal destroyed its beauty.[59] Now, in
1916, columnist Maurice Barrès resurrected the image of Verdun as *le
Thermopyles de la France*—France's Thermopylae. It is here, he contended,
that the enemy must be stopped. His piece in *L'Écho de Paris* of February
26 claimed Germany's Crown Prince Friedrich Wilhelm, in Frankish
fashion, pined for the citadel as its rightful heir.[60] Indeed, he would now
lead General Erich von Falkenhayn's Fifth Army to assemble before the
gates of the city.

And France knew it. Verdun had been the prime focus of defense since
Prussia's intrusion in 1870. The area bristled with cement fortifications
and heavy guns. It had even been given special designation as Région
Fortifiée de Verdun, the Fortified Region of Verdun, or RFV for short.
The RFV encompassed an area on both sides of the Meuse from Avocourt
to the northwest to Saint-Mihiel southeast. It had been a relatively quiet
sector, French commanders lulled into a sense of complacency. So much
so that many of the munitions were moved from the network of forts
around Verdun to more active sectors north and west. Alfred Mignon
became medical director for the RFV and the new Army of Verdun
on February 1, 1916. The village itself was near deserted. Bombardments
in June 1915 had forced inhabitants out; patients in the six hospitals of the
town had been evacuated to Bar-le-Duc, some forty-five miles southwest
of Verdun. But Mignon would not be fooled. The salient was simply too
tempting for Kaiser Wilhelm. If so, his Service de santé would deliver
swift surgical care and orderly evacuation of casualties. Mignon had a
surgical temperament, inclined to action, to decisive feats. A restless man,
given to skepticism but convinced of the surgical nature of battlefield
medicine, he would have the RFV prepared for disaster.

Like Napoleon's famous surgeon, Dominique Larrey, Mignon wanted
his wounded treated as close to gunfire as possible. Gosset's and Marcille's
mobile unit had made that possible. He formed a new doctrine around

it: first, aggressive, early surgical care—stabilize critical patients, stop bleeding, clean dirty wounds—then move the patients out, to hospitals designed for total repair of their injuries. It was Mignon's intent to have skilled, experienced surgeons available to do this work, from frontline *ambulances* to the larger HOEs. Around Verdun the smaller surgical *ambulances* peppered the countryside, within easy reach of truck transport from frontline aid stations. They were found in sleepy towns like Vadelaincourt, Clermont-en-Argonne, and Revigny. Even here would be skilled surgical care for critical cases. This would be the first place for surgery: stop hemorrhage, splint fractures, clean wounds of mud and grime. Further down the road, about six miles or so, were the HOEs. Two large HOEs serviced the RFV, one positioned at Baleycourt, about six miles southwest of Verdun, and the other at Petit Monthairon, twelve miles almost due south. Baleycourt would be key, receiving patients from forward *ambulances* on both sides of the Meuse. At Baleycourt he would set up *Auto-chir* No. 3. At Petits Monthairon would be *Auto-chir* No. 13. No longer mere holding stations, Mignon transformed HOEs to surgical hospitals. Patients would undergo another round of examination and triage. Surgeons from the nearby Gosset *auto-chirs* poised to descend on anyone in precarious condition: repair lingering wounds leading to sepsis or breathing issues, shore up mangled limbs. Then on the road again, now funneled through the marshalling town of Bar-le-Duc some thirty miles distant, with seven hospitals, one thousand beds, and thirteen surgical teams. After that, Paris.

Mignon was satisfied. All was in place. And now he waited, peering out over the snow-covered undulations of the Verdun countryside in the winter of 1916.

At dawn on a clear, frosty February 21 morning, somewhere between seven and quarter past, it all started. A thunderous bombardment by 1,200 German guns, some monstrous in size, showered French positions along the northern borders of the salient. The commotion was so violent that it could be felt in the Vosges over ninety miles away. Shells excavated sectors of turf and moved on, crumbling forests and pulverizing anything in their path. Men clung to the earth, "stunned by noise, drunk with smoke, suffocated by gas . . . Steel flakes whistled in their

ears, earth, stones, timbers were hurled at them indiscriminately." Each
man sensed obliteration, each man prayed for silence.[61] Suddenly, once
again, Verdun had become, in the words of Maurice Barrès, "the center
of the universe . . . where we will recognize the best of humanity."[62]

Hell on earth had arrived. For the next three hundred days Verdun
and its pretty landscapes turned into a microcosm of the First World War.
"Verdun has literally become a place of horror," historian Louis Madelin
remembered as a lieutenant in Pétain's Second Army.[63] Mignon observed
that "the primary characteristic of the battle of Verdun is its conduct on
the same theater of operations of a remarkable 'smallness.'"[64] Prodigious
use of artillery, incessant infantry charges, slaughter, and retreat, ground
gained and lost, produced enormous death, suffering, and casualties, with
almost no strategic gain. Visiting American reporters were aghast at the
carnage. "Words cannot describe the desolation . . . dead horses and mules
lie and rot by the roadside where they fell. Here and there are the wrecks
of motor cars, torn by shell fragments."[65] The French would not budge,
no matter the cost. Clemenceau was determined to take a stand here. It
indeed had become Thermopylae. Barrès would later write:

> *"Il ne passeront pas!"* ["They will not pass!"] This is the motto
> spoken at all the stations for the wounded about to be evacu-
> ated. It is the last cry, the slogan, the prophecy, the entreaty
> of the valiant who have fallen on the field of honor.[66]

Mignon's system, elaborate as it was, felt the strain. The HOE at
Baleycourt had received 725 wounded by February 22, then 1,075 on
the twenty-third, 1,350 on the twenty-fourth, 1,700 on the twenty-fifth,
and 1,850 on the twenty-sixth. But, with German long-range cannon, it
was much too close. The barrages were so extreme, and artillery shells so
enormous that soon projectiles began falling almost next door:

> The rumor spread that the wounded were panicking, that they
> were coming out of their beds and asking to be taken [away]. . .
> One must have lived the scene which unfolded to understand
> what was poignant—the sight of the mutilated just the day

before, sometimes that very day, which, scarcely out of the carnage, [they] believed it again would plunge them into it and begged that they be removed from the threatening danger.[67]

On February 28, Mignon made the decision. Evacuate Baleycourt, the key hospital in his network. Tents and housing were taken down, patients were transferred to the hospital complexes at Vadelaincourt farther to the south. Heavy traffic, poor roads, and winter mud made the whole affair laborious. Routes out were hopelessly clogged with an endless stream of bogged-down camions, cars, and foot traffic. Vadelaincourt itself soon filled with swarms of bandaged soldiers and countless litters, of doctors and nurses and those myriad surgical assistants. Patients were laid anywhere—hallways, basements, alleyways, and tents. Mignon demanded action. Expand. Around-the-clock construction added beds and rooms. Annexes were built for additional space, now housing *Auto-Chir* No. 3, just arrived from Baleycourt. The roads in and out were paved. Triage improved so that those who needed surgery most urgently were identified and taken first. Soon the hospital complex at Clermont-en-Argonne was evacuated. Same problem: German artillery had bombed the railway station and cut the railway lines. Shells began falling near the hospital. All patients and staff were moved a few miles south to Froidos. A new *auto-chir* arrived, No. 12. Mignon positioned it close by.

Now all the villages and hamlets surrounding Verdun would swell with a steady influx of refugees, soldiers, and the innumerable victims of the slaughter. Vadelaincourt and Froidos would become hubs of surgical activity. From February 22 to June 15, hospitals around Vadelaincourt took in almost eleven thousand wounded, most of them by artillery blasts. One in ten were grave injuries to chest or abdomen, and many needed serious attention and harrowing surgery. Three surgical teams worked day and night there. "Death descended everywhere," Mignon said, "The ranks of the brave health care workers, the only emissaries of human feeling in the midst of continual carnage, have been a bright spot." Mignon's *auto-chirs* soon became the darlings of the press, touted as medical marvels—salvation for French casualties. Teams at the front were now equipped with the finest of instruments and the most comfortable of accommodations, rivaling those of the grand hospitals of the interior.[68] Mignon loved his autochirs, eventually placing four around Verdun, at Froidos, Petit Monthairon, and Chaumont-sur-Aire, all just outside the range of German artillery. And he kept sixteen mobile surgical teams, *groupes complémentaire chirurgicales*, ready to rotate and relieve crews at forward ambulances—*chirurgiens à l'avant* was the cry, "surgeons to the front." Verdun would be their proving ground.

In fact, all the eyes of the world were on Verdun. It was central to French defense and key to German victory. As for the meat grinder it had become, by March Mignon had systematized care of the countless numbers of casualties and funneled them to hospitals according to Commander Philippe Pétain's new combat sectors. In desperation, Pétain had assigned army *groupements* to the region around Verdun on both sides of the Meuse. Haggard French poilus, blue trench coats and pithy Adrian helmets now the color of the mud that engulfed them, sank into their subterranean trenches and fortifications and inhabited bombed-out vestiges of villages long bereft of human activity. Shells flew back and forth like hailstorms, and troops charged and retreated, littering the moonscape with human debris. In each of these sectors Mignon assembled his forward surgical ambulances that, in turn, sent their patients to HOEs at Vadelaincourt, Froidos, or Petits Monthairon and from there farther back to Bar-le-Duc, Revigny, and beyond. It was the only way so many casualties could be managed:

> The Service de santé presented three echelons of surgical formations: one at the front (division and corps ambulances) for the critical wounded, another a distance out of reach of artillery for serious casualties, and a third about 100 to 200 km from the lines for the wounded whose operation could be delayed by a dozen hours.[69]

This was the monotonous pattern of medical care at Verdun—day after day after day. First encounters were at *postes de secours*—battalion aid posts—makeshift arrangements, often in dilapidated houses, cellars, tunnels, or caves with scant lighting, heat, and sanitation, artillery always a threat. These were dreary places and the men who manned them dreary as well. In dark recesses stolen from families, war riddled with calamity; calloused doctors—hardened by too much misery—unshaven, unbathed, reeking in sweat, bent over stretchers bearing forms caked in brown slurry and soiled by thickened blood who might be thought dead were it not for a twitch of finger or fading moan. First aid amidst flickering candlelight was brief, almost reluctant, such was often the proximity of death. Little inclined were these jaded medics to forego prudence and assault severed arteries and roughened bowels leaking vitality. Instead, they waited for dusk and the brave brancardiers who shouldered their sinking victims aboard camions that would chug away in search of Mignon's hospitals, not that far from the dank catacombs of aid stations where these haggard medics fitfully hunkered.

It was a relief to get the casualties away from the din of battle. The surgical *ambulances* were a godsend. Now well lit, and better equipped, doctors with knife, saw, and skill assailed the bloodletting of combat, pulled away bodily detritus as if so much cluttered basement trash, and forestalled the inevitability of death, which loomed over each man. Keep the patient alive, stabilize, immobilize. Then transport to the HOEs, with their *auto-chirs*, and, then to the haven of Bar-le-Duc far distant.

In those forward *ambulances* surgeons had the greatest challenges. Men were often in dire condition. Mignon saw it firsthand:

> Most of these wounded arrive at the ambulance in full shock. The loss of blood which they have undergone, the attrition of the tissues the violence of the blow, the multiplicity of the wounds inhibit the nervous system and leave the man pale, annihilated, sometimes subconscious, and in cardiogenic hypotension. And the fatigue of the road is added to the effects of the projectile![70]

In many cases, surgery was lifesaving. In one such *ambulance* in the village of Brocourt, just fifteen miles from the trenches, only sixty-one of almost one thousand casualties died. Others were not so fortunate. *Ambulance* 1/21, only eight miles from the front, lost one-fourth of their admissions.[71] It was simply a matter of luck and the voracity of shelling in any given sector.

◆

The stress on surgeons was indescribable. Georges Duhamel, now with a frontline *ambulance* near Verdun, recalled that, "confronted by the overwhelming flood of work to be done, the surgeon . . . had to meditate deeply, and make a decision as to the sacrifice which would ensure life, or give some hope of life." The chorus of wounded rose in gusts, he remembered, moaning, rattling, choking, "hoping for an impossible repose."[72] All the while, of course, under bombardment as ferocious as the gales of hurricane gusts.

Yet, make no mistake. When they stood over their subjects, now painlessly asleep, these same surgeons were filled with vigor, as if the fatigue of past cases left as surely as driven by spikes of whiskey. They were intoxicated with their skill and boldness in slicing through human hide and into cavities that held nothing pretty to lesser men but to them the exquisite slaughter of weaponry. Coils of intestines belching the green of bilious digestion and coated with the beautiful crimson of dribbled blood excited them as much as the sight of seductive women. With supreme enthusiasm they toiled, hands sliding soundlessly over chaotic viscera. Fingers pinched and clicked silver instruments that, as projections of a guileless intensity, weaved and stitched in minute movements that pushed time and tiredness into the realms of irrelevance. It was a passion as holy as blessed sacraments and as total as transubstantiation. They had become possessed of their art and their calling. Only after wards cleared of desperate victims would they return to ordinary sanity and fall exasperated onto their sweat-laden bunks.

The fury of Verdun eventually subsided, but not until well into 1917. The country was stripped of beauty and littered with dead. Quaint villages had been erased. Numbers of wounded soared beyond belief. No one knows for sure but perhaps over 250,000 on each side. But in all the carnage Alfred Mignon had reversed conventional wisdom and revolutionized battlefield medicine. In the words of Vincent Viet, "Verdun constituted a decisive 'surgical experience,' marked by the replacement of the expectant surgery of the beginning of the war by an active, immediate and preventive surgery for infection."[73] Furthermore, Mignon had insisted: "It was necessary to operate quickly and carefully, and, obviously, subordinate the length of the evacuation route to the degree of gravity of the wound." Long gone would be the days of benign neglect for those devastating wounds—shredded tissue, maimed limbs, and perforated viscera. Mobile surgical units and teams had proved their worth and would be a mainstay into the future.

As for Alfred Mignon, he would not pass easily into retirement. After the war and for eight years hence, 1920–1928, he traveled between Paris and Tours, where he would comb over documents and compile chronicles of the Great War and his experiences in the Verdun sector. His works would be published in four volumes and detail down to the finest measure the medical care under his supervision.[74] His companions were his memories and the preoccupation of reconstructing the past, events that impregnated their significance deep in him. Only afterward, in that small apartment, in his twilight years, when all had been scrutinized and assembled, might loneliness have found its mark. Yet his biographers would remember him well. "He was more than a skillful surgeon, more than an admirable teacher, more than a fine writer: [he was] a man of high conscience, an example to emulate, a trophy to honor."[75] And he had set forth principles of battlefield surgery that would soon be mimicked by Americans and their allies and carried far into the future, even to the present day.[76] The massive firepower of modern munitions demanded it. Echeloned and early surgical intervention coupled with smooth, expeditious evacuation would become mainstays of care. Delays were costly to life and limb and seemed to escalate disabling complications. Think of the portable surgical hospitals of the South Pacific and the auxiliary surgical groups of the European Theater in World War II. Consider the Mobile Army Surgical Hospitals of Korea and the Antenne Chirurgicale Mobile of France's ill-fated war in Indochina. Even the forward surgical teams of Iraq and Afghanistan. These were direct descendants of the surgical teams of Marcille and Gosset and Mignon's battlefield blueprints. They had shaped the future of combat care. Surgeons would be among the vanguard, in harm's way, at the edge of action, all for the salvage of those heroes who demand nothing less. Latter day epidemiologists Gilbert Beebe and Michael DeBakey sized it up after compiling the results of casualty care during the Second World War: "A fundamental determinant of mortality among the wounded is the speed with which they are given medical care, particularly first aid, resuscitation, and initial surgery."[77] That conclusion is nothing more than a sterling endorsement of those Great War pioneers who ignored convention and launched the mobile surgical units that are commonplace today.

And what of that pioneer Maurice Marcille, the catalyst for such a metamorphosis? He eventually was elected into the Société nationale de chirurgie in 1920, the same organization that chastised him in 1915. But his rebellious nature did not keep him long in Paris. The loss of one of his daughters forced him into an early retirement in his Loire Valley homestead, where he devoted much time to gardening, lost in the sadness of grief. Some years later, he again surfaced in Paris, this time to research the effects of chemical warfare. The war had made quite an impression on him. He died quietly in 1941 in the Loiret, finally recognized in posterity for his novel automobile surgical *ambulance*. "He was one of those who foresaw events of the last war," his eulogizer wrote. "He leaves us the memory of an ardent, honest, and good man."[78]

THREE

Deep Mischief Lurking:
The Unraveling of Traumatic Shock

"Shock has long been one of the great mysteries in surgery."
—Walter B. Cannon, 1919[1]

SEIZURES AND COMMOTIONS

Oh, the blood that must spill for man to hate man. It is a badge of war, a badge of bravery, Stephen Crane's *Red Badge of Courage*. Blood sport. As ancient as prehistory, weapons have sharpened to pierce, slice, and finally propel into the soft underbelly of humanity. Let out blood and victims hesitate, falter, and collapse. Victory is then declared, one over the other. And the violence wrought on man, the malevolence—or panic—to strike and strike, until a stunned opponent stumbles pale and trembling to the ground. What destruction here must be redeemed? What vitality sapped must be restored. This is a story of resurrection, of revitalization from death in motion.

Hemorrhage, epochs have called it: the streaming of blood from opened flesh. It has been the faithful companion to military combat since antiquity. In Homer's *Iliad*, the Achaean hero Eurypylus sought the attention of companion Patroclus in removing an impaled arrow from his thigh upon which "black blood gushed", and poor Harpalion, after being skewered by an arrow in his buttock, collapsed "like a worm on the ground," and "black blood streamed and drenched the earth."[2] The gush of blood signaled the opening trumpets of death's inexorable chorus. Bloodspill and lethality were linked in the slashing and crushing wounds of ancient warfare just as were bashed brains, decapitations, or disembowelments. As blood pooled on the ground, the demise of the fallen warrior was almost assured. And, if signs of life were still present at battle's end, a swift coup de grâce was the parting solution. It was the task of the victors to dispatch the fallen, almost an act of mercy. Not until centuries later would moaning survivors be hauled off the battlefield and brought to the attention of traveling surgeons—however imperfect their art. And it would be some of these hacked victims, alive but gray and languid, who would so perplex those healers as they watched a spiraling course of waning consciousness, diminishing pulse, and eventual death.[3] There was little to be done and even less inclination to waste time on these unfortunate cases. Surgery, then, was a practical skill, many practitioners barely literate and certainly not disposed to the lofty empiricism of academic physicians.

That is, until the advent of firearms and the ability to wound at a distance. Only then would men fall from shot and lay within the ranks of the salvageable. It was from these wounded men that the 18th-century French military surgeon Henri Le Dran recorded his observations. He may have been the first to show a curiosity for such pictures of distress. Based on his experiences, Le Dran, in 1738, provided a classic description of those who teetered on the brink of impending doom:

> Mais quand même un blessé ne seroit pas pléthorique, il suffit que le saisissement et la commotion qui accompagnent souvent les playes d'armes à feu suspende pour quelques momens l'ordre oéconomique. [But even if an injury would not be plethoric, it suffices that the seizure and the commotion which often accompanies the wounds of firearms suspend for a few moments the economic order.][4]

Saisissement and *commotion*: *saisissement* in older French meant "a seizing, a laying hold of, a possession," and *commotion* "a tumult or uproar." Le Dran was fully aware that such a traumatic event brought about an excitation in behavior as if the blow itself—a striking musket ball perhaps—had provoked an internal energy to be released.

A mysterious author, an Englishman it seems, by the name of J. S. Surgeon (also known as John Sparrow) translated Le Dran's text two years later and boldly submitted a name for this condition, introduced into the medical lexicon forevermore. He would call it "shock":

> With regard to the Accidents that supervened, they could only
> be occasioned by the universal Shock of the whole Machine,
> which Shocks frequently require the most earnest Attention
> of the Surgeons.[5]

The surreptitious Sparrow argued that shock was caused by an impact so forceful that the body recoils as if jarred to its very foundation. It fell to the British military surgeon George Guthrie to popularize Sparrow's shock. This sudden *commotion*, Guthrie reasoned, could be considered a "constitutional alarm," writing that "a peculiar constitutional alarm ensues" after injury with a severe blow (he cited cannon or grapeshot or shell) then later added the word "shock" as a descriptor. Often blood has been spilled; perhaps even an arm or a leg carried off. Guthrie saw what Le Dran had described. There is a "peculiar anxiety, alarm and loss of animal and organic powers," he wrote, "a deadly paleness overspreads the countenance . . . the heart almost ceases to act." Guthrie went on to say that the "general affection" was not dependent on the shock alone but blamed the whole matter on the nervous system.[6] Was this the source of Le Dran's *commotion*?

Others felt the same. Surgeon and anatomist Astley Cooper called it "shock to the nervous system." Disruptive forces such as external blows—his so-named "irritations"—could unbalance the "beautiful harmony" of organs and tissues, mediated, Cooper thought, through the rich network of nerve fibers running in and out of the spinal cord and up and down from the brain itself.[7] A prevailing "sympathy" of the nervous system throughout the body was at the heart of its role in producing the altered states seen in shock. Although hemorrhage could initiate the syndrome, it did not seem to be the entire explanation.

The American Civil War (1861–65) provided Philadelphian surgeon Samuel Gross with plenty of shock cases. He, too, was perplexed by the internal derangements that he was sure were at the heart of this malady, as if some "vital power" were depressed by a catastrophic concussion, seemingly paralyzing the entire circulatory system:

> There is a form of shock which has been, not inaptly, called insidious . . . The person although severely injured, congratulates himself upon having made an excellent escape . . . But a more careful examination soon serves to show that *deep mischief is lurking in the system; that the machinery of life has been rudely unhinged* [all italics mine], and that the whole system is profoundly shocked; in a word, that the nervous fluid has been exhausted, and that there is not enough power in the constitution to reproduce and maintain it.[8]

A contemporary of Gross's, the famous John Collins Warren Jr. of Boston, noticed the indifference of those in shock—almost a state of suspended animation—commenting that often the patient "is strangely apathetic, and seems to realize but imperfectly the full meaning of the questions put to him . . . the pulse, however, does not respond; it grows feebler, and finally disappears, and 'this momentary pause in the act of death' is soon followed by the grim reality."[9]

But then the late 19th century was a time of marvels. Physiology and experimental medicine ruled the lecture halls and laboratories of European science. The master experimentalist French physiologist Claude Bernard had introduced his *milieu intérieur*, that tendency of organisms to maintain equipoise. Any external threat would be met with an active neural network—action and reaction. Any menacing change prompted a reactionary motor response—nerve fibers designed to galvanize—so as to restore balance. So as to restore constancy:

The phenomena of life are not the spontaneous manifestations of an interior vital principle: they are . . . the result of a
conflict between living matter and external conditions. Life
results constantly from the reciprocal relationship of these two
factors, both in the manifestations of sensibility [*sensibilité*]
and motion [*motilité*], which is usually considered to be of the
highest order . . . [10]

Was this "shock," then, a grave unbalance that, unless rectified,
disturbed the *milieu intérieur*? And did the *milieu*, so unhinged, then
struggle to reset through an internal and undefinable will to survive?
Was this, as Bernard suspected, the manifestation of a policing nervous
system in disarray, an environment of humors and vapors so lawless now
that the harmony of life itself was jeopardized?

Yet what to make of all this for those more pragmatic? What of the
bloodletting so characteristic of battlefield trauma? Could Bernard and
his theories explain that? British surgeon William Savory had an opinion.
While shock, he considered, was still a result of a nervous system in
turmoil, "excessive hemorrhage, even if gradual, will produce a state of
extreme exhaustion and debility."[11] To be sure, the portrayal of such
victims gives the impression of exhaustion, of a person totally devoid of
vigor, of will, of fortitude. "Eyes dull . . . The gaze stares indifferently
and into the distance . . . No limbs move spontaneously . . . The pulse is
barely perceptible . . . The respirations appear irregular," so noted Prussian
surgeon Herman Fischer.[12] It was as if circulation, depleted by bleeding,
slowed and diminished, and the life-humors it carried faded away.

But, still, it must be a nerve network—that which sensed and
responded, that which controlled all internal function—traumatized
and in shambles.

Yes, surely a derangement of the nervous system, which, stunned by
force of injury, let slip its regulation of heart, blood vessels, and even
respiratory mechanisms. Others felt so as well. British surgeon Charles
Mansell-Moullin had already determined that the most conspicuous
finding in shock was "an extreme diminution in arterial tension." Fingers on the wrist, the groin, the neck would tell the tale. The pulse,

he felt, weakened precipitously. He argued that the nerve centers were responsible. An inherent property of these centers, he claimed, was an outpouring of a blocking influence on ganglia that controlled the entire vascular system. Ganglia, those discrete nodes of nervous activity apart from the spinal cord, were aggregates of nerve cells that modified and amplified impulses generated by the spinal reflex arc.[13] In fact, American Harvey Cushing maintained that hindering propagation of sensory-type impulses with cocaine—essentially poisoning the ganglia—would interrupt this nervous reflex arc and prevent any fading of blood circulation.[14]

How could it be proven? How could blood circulation be measured? In 1896 an Italian physician by the name of Scipione Riva-Rocci offered a device he called his sphygmomanometer, a method of measuring blood flow by way of determining arterial pressure. His apparatus he had modified from models developed by predecessors. Some years earlier, the German physiologist Karl von Vierordt had showcased an instrument "that manometrically measures the force necessary to prevent the progression of the pulse," using a column of mercury. The height to which mercury was pushed by the pulse was determined to correlate with the arterial tension.[15] In 1881 Austrian Karl von Basch took Vierordt's principles of pulse compression to restructure a cumbersome yet portable instrument that squeezed and, also by mercury column, measured return of the pulse at the wrist. Riva-Rocci's design, though, was different. He used a cuff (he called it a "sleeve") around the upper arm that had an inflatable inner bladder. By inflating the cuff with air, "we will be in the best conditions to exercise a gradual and progressive compression on the whole circumference of the limb." It was simple, portable, and squeezed the entire circumference of the upper arm—uniform compression of the brachial artery. Readings of systolic blood pressure in millimeters of mercury—that pressure at which the pulse at the wrist reappeared—were accurate and reproducible.[16] In 1897, two Englishmen, Leonard Hill and Harold Barnard, further refined the Riva-Rocci sphygmomanometer by broadening the "armlet" and introducing a pressure gauge, which allowed for measurement not only of systolic but also diastolic blood pressure—the pressure at which the heart rests between beats—and is very similar to the sphygmomanometers in use today.[17]

Certainly, American surgeon George Crile was intrigued. An Ohioan farm boy, his elementary education was a one-room schoolhouse near Chili, Ohio. Yet early on there was an intensity about him, and a fascination with biology and animal husbandry. A local physician had seen his enthusiasm and urged that he pursue a medical career. But there was little money for such education. No mind. Crile literally willed his way through schooling. Part-time teaching in Plainfield, Ohio, earned his tuition for college and, while studying medicine, he served as principal for that same Plainfield elementary school. Even with all that extracurricular activity, Crile achieved the highest honors in medicine and began work as a house officer at the new University Hospital in Cleveland.[18] Those bedside experiences would be eye-openers. Early in his training, Crile watched an acquaintance die following amputation of both his legs. Blood loss and that peculiar malady called shock took hold, and Crile was powerless to stop it. The stark appearance of the poor fellow, his pallor, his sweaty skin, the sunken eyes, the rapid pulse, all etched indelible memories in Crile's mind. Such happenings strike deep in the soul of scientists and fuel an unquenchable desire to find and fix. It would be his mission to uncover an explanation for that awful, morbid event.[19] Physiology, anatomy, pathology consumed him; surely, there lay the answers. He worked in the laboratory, studied in New York, and traveled to Europe, somehow hoping to unravel the riddle of his new adversary. It was a surgical disease, he knew, and surgery would be his chosen profession. Yet, to be sure, images of his friend would surface with each coming victim of shock on the bloody fields of France. "What can I do," "what could I have done," were haunting words that stalked every surgeon, no less Crile, who undoubtedly listened to the same troubling voices as they ricocheted through his mind.[20]

He battled back with determination. A decade into the new 20th century, Crile had come up with his kinetic theory of shock. "Shock is the result of the excessive conversion of potential into kinetic energy in response to adequate stimuli." These discharges of energy, he theorized, when prolonged lead to "exhaustion," or his conception of "shock."[21] And what did he think was the mediator of all this excitation? It was, as Claude Bernard had proposed, the nervous system. Skin and special senses, "ceptors" Crile called them, when stimulated, triggered an out-burst of energy. His solution? Remove as much stimulation as possible to avoid startling those tender sensory nerves. He would give it the name *anoci*-association—a state of almost suspended animation.

But he did not totally discount the role of the circulatory system in all this. Blood and the oxygen it carried were life-sustaining elements. Since very often hemorrhage played an obvious role, Crile felt it imperative to measure blood flow and how it behaved during those times of "shock." But how? At first, he designed animal experiments using a self-made mercury manometer. It was primitive, unwieldy, and ill-suited to labora-tory work. Then he learned of Riva-Rocci's sphygmomanometer from his friend Harvey Cushing of Baltimore. Using the Riva-Rocci device, he ran animal experiments on the effects of various vasoactive agents. Crile was taken with Riva-Rocci's contraption. It displayed the up and down changes of arterial tension—and hence circulation—as he gave his drugs. Satisfied that blood pressure was key, he brought his sphygmomanomoter into the operating room and began measuring blood pressures during surgery.[22] As any surgeon was aware, there was such a thing as "surgical shock." Inexplicably, some patients would seem to fail on the operating table or in recovering—weak pulse, pasty appearance. Was it the same as traumatic shock? Measurements in those patients with his sphygmo-manometer showed a low blood pressure. "The essential phenomenon is a diminution of the blood-pressure," he wrote in 1903. Not convinced it was solely due to blood loss, he thought maybe fatigue of the heart or blood vessels, or even the nervous system (vasomotor centers), was the cause. Yet, in his mind, all was not "shock." In fact, he felt "shock" was not solely from blood loss. Instead, he blamed "shock" on exhaustion of the nerve centers controlling blood vessel tension (his vasomotor cen-ters). Once exhaustion set in, artery tone diminished and blood pressure dropped. Patients, deprived of blood flow and oxygen, understandably weakened and began to fade. He called the sudden fall in blood pressure from massive blood loss "collapse." In contrast to "shock," with his idea of "collapse" the obvious solution was blood or fluid infusions, whereas in "shock" stimulants to the nervous system might work better. In fact, Crile suggested his anoci-association was central to treatment. Monitoring of circulation through blood pressure measurements, though, was key. "In many instances the control of the blood-pressure is the control of life itself," he asserted. [23]

Extremes of violence were not often seen in civilian life. Yes, automobile collisions had furnished a new wave of broken bodies, but not yet the epidemic they would become. Those forces so jarring as to batter, mangle, and bleed victims into traumatic shock could only be found in open warfare. The Great War and all its malignancy rushed to the forefront and would provide shocked cases in abundance. It would give scientists plenty of subjects to study. Surgeon Edward Archibald, recently returned from the horrors of France, was aghast at the violence. In numbing sentences, he reported before the American Surgical Association in 1917 that shock was

> seen to an extent unparalleled in the experience of any surgeon at home. The very frequency of it, and the terrible nature of it, were impressive, and, not less so, our inability to rescue such patients when the degree of shock was really serious. [24]

The western front was fertile ground indeed for surgeons and scientists. So much of medicine changed as a result, and one change came with zealous attempts to salvage men broken and bleeding. Here would be the answers to the shock question, doctors believed. Theories ran rampant: a "nervous" temperament, cold, fatigue, hunger, mangling trauma, fractures, and hemorrhage. Hemorrhage: the frontlines were soaked in it. Still, hemorrhage alone was not always the explanation. [25] Crile's blood and saline infusions did not always help, surgeons discovered. Yet, at first, blood transfusions were experimental, given hesitantly, cautiously. There was little chance of infusing blood in as fast as it was pouring out, not in the early days. Men died in the meantime or were simply too near death to spend such time and effort on.

In Cleveland, Crile impatiently paced. He brimmed with curiosity on the shock question and saw the European war as a gigantic opportunity. Through his contacts, he got wind of a call for volunteers. In Paris, an American military hospital—it was now called the Ambulance

Américaine—had been set up and needed surgeons. This American field hospital was not new to Paris. Something similar had gone up in the aftermath of the Franco-Prussian War of 1870 and 1871.

In those days, French forces had been badly beaten and Paris turned into a bedlam of internecine violence. Rebellious Communards, incensed by the foolish capitulation and humiliating armistice settled by the government of Napoleon III, provoked a wanton slaughter of thousands of Parisians, most of whom were defenseless and caught in a bloodthirsty gambit to overthrow equally brutal forces of the National Assembly in a bid for revolutionary supremacy—even restoration of the monarchy.[26] "The carnival of blood—or, as it became known, *la Semaine Sanglante* ('Bloody Week')—began on Sunday, May 21 . . . the carnage was horrific even for a city that had witnessed the murderous excesses of the French Revolution," so British author Ross King portrayed the scene.[27] As many as 25,000 Communards were massacred by government troops who stormed the boulevards, upending barricades, burning buildings, and ravaging simple neighborhoods. Wounded poured from tenements and alleyways, cut down by shellfire and snipers. There were not enough hospital beds and not enough doctors. In response, members of the American International Sanitary Committee, set up soon after war began "for the purpose of being a direct agent of American charity in behalf of the victims of war," assembled a field hospital with tents and makeshift barracks in the heart of Paris.[28] And now, in 1914, Americans in Paris wanted to do it again: to organize an American hospital they would call *Ambulance Américaine*. The French government, eager for any medical assistance, agreed. They found a boys' high school, the Lycée Pasteur, in the affluent neighborhood of Neuilly-sur-Seine, as a suitable site.

The first wounded entered in late August. By the time of the Marne battles patients were streaming in, filling every one of the hospital's 450 beds. Overseeing this human sea of devastation were only two surgeons; their workload was impossible. In somewhat of a panic, Ambassador Myron Herrick called out to George Crile for aid. Would he, in fact, be willing to bring a team to staff one of the hospital's three services? Crile quickly agreed. He even pledged to organize rotating teams of American surgeons. Privately, like many inquisitive researchers surveying expanses

of human misery, he wondered if this would become his human laboratory to study shock:

> The research to be carried out is that of observing the effects of
> fear and exhaustion on the human body . . . In my laboratory
> . . . there is almost no opportunity for the study of human
> material. In Europe such opportunities are now abundant.
> They may never again be available on such a scale.[29]

Crile's Lakeside (Cleveland) unit arrived early January 1915. A
few days later, his team was busy operating. The condition of his war-
weary patients stunned him. "The hospital was filled with every sort
of wound," Crile recalled. Some who were brought in from outlying
villages had been injured nine days before and had received no treatment and no food or water. "They had reached a stage of uncondi-
tional exhaustion and desired only to be left alone," Crile wrote. "No
investigator would dream of subjecting animals without anesthesia to
a tithe of injuries that were inflicted in battle by normal young men
upon each other."[30] His remedy? Nothing to any avail. By the time
they arrived to him, so many cases were almost hopeless. In a report
that appeared in July 1915, after his return to the United States, a
disheartened Crile wrote:

> As for the treatment of shock . . . the best that can be done is to
> give morphia [morphine]. When from three to five thousand
> wounded must be cared for by a few surgeons only, it is idle to
> think of any treatment—many of the wounded cannot secure
> a drink of water even.[31]

"Morphia," that divine narcotic, seemed uncannily close to his idea
of anoci-association—freedom from pain, suffering, and stress. His colleague Alexis Carrel had even found that morphine seemed to revive men
in shock, raising their blood pressure—all in sync with Crile's theory of
an overloaded and frazzled sensory nervous system.[32] As for his work at
the Ambulance Américaine, the torrent of patients slowed after Germans

retreated from the Marne. He saw few cases of shock; they were corralled nearer the front now, where many of them would die from ignorance. [33]

So, Crile was left to speculate. How best to raise a sinking blood pressure? What role would agents like adrenaline, digitalis, strychnine, nitroglycerin, atropine—stimulants and antagonists—play? Would intravenous fluids help? How much to give? Some patients, he had heard, dramatically improved after infusions. In Crile's dog experiments, quantities of saline solution increased cardiac activity and output from the heart, although edema of the tissues occurred with high volumes of fluid. Saline by itself was probably not the solution, he felt. [34] Then, how about blood transfusions?

THE MIRACLE OF RESURRECTION

Long before he went to France, George Crile and his wife, Grace, had witnessed a miracle, as if the biblical Lazarus had once again come to life.

What was, literally, miraculous for dying patients was the dramatic effect of whole blood transfusion. Richard Lower had tried it in 1667, transfusing twelve ounces of sheep's blood into a human via "pipes and quills" with no apparent ill effect. [35] A century and a half later James Blundell resuscitated bled dogs near death with transfused blood from another animal and showed the dramatic effect of these fresh transfusions in restoring pulse, respiration, and "sensibility." In short, life was replenished. [36] Intrigued by the possibilities, Crile had begun experiments on transfusion in his laboratory in 1898. In the course of reviving dogs with whole blood infusions, he realized that transfusions alone could restore circulatory equipoise far better than other stimulants and seemed to override any effects of shock. [37] It was all quite intriguing. But what cemented his hunch was an occasion with a young Russian man, bleeding from hemorrhage following kidney surgery. On an August night in 1906, George and Grace had been hurriedly summoned from a dinner party to Saint Alexis Hospital in Cleveland. He arrived in full formal attire and none too soon. The patient, Crile saw, was in trouble. His pulse was weak, respirations shallow, lips blue. The man was in shock and perilously close to death. In desperation, Crile decided to try a blood exchange. The young man's brother agreed to donate. That evening, in the operating room laying side by side, Crile sewed donor radial artery to recipient vein and let blood pour across. Crile's wife, Grace, was in attendance. She recalled, "I stood at the foot of the operating table and witnessed the miracle of resurrection." Nothing could have been more dramatic. The patient shortly awoke, regained his senses, and flaunted a "rosy glow" to his cheeks. His liveliness was so buoyant he seemed "like a man intoxicated." Without immediately realizing it, however, the bewildered Crile almost bled the poor donor to death, who had more difficulty recovering than his grateful brother.[38]

It was all quite remarkable. The surgery was painstaking and delicate, demanding patience, time, and extreme surgical skill. Fine silk suture, the width of a human hair, brought paper-thin artery and vein together. In his 1909 book, *Hemorrhage and Transfusion*, Crile described other cases. Volume and rate of blood exchange were barely controllable, and the chief danger was over-transfusion, overloading the heart—and, at the same time, bleeding donors to the point of shock themselves. There was another patient, this time a father-to-son transfusion. The boy was bleeding from a mangled leg. Again, father and son lay side by side. Crile connected father's radial artery to son's forearm vein. And again, success. But another case ended in failure, a mother-to-son transfusion. The boy had been crushed and was hemorrhaging into his abdomen (a ruptured spleen, as it turned out). Mother's blood was not enough—or too late; the son died. There was so much promise, but Crile knew that preparation, surgery, and transfusion were time-consuming and not meant for rapidly bleeding victims. Nevertheless, to Crile it was a milestone in treatment of shock: "in uncomplicated hemorrhage . . . transfusion is a specific remedy."[39] Others were not so easily swayed. An editorial in the *British Medical Journal* on October 12, 1907, spoke harshly of it. While experimental results in animals were encouraging, the authors said, Crile presented no convincing evidence that blood transfusions in humans had much redeeming value:

Excellent results were certainly obtained in some cases of shock, but in the treatment of this condition, and, indeed, of all others in which intravascular infusion of some kind is clearly indicated, surgeons, we imagine, will find no good reason given here for abandoning the safe and simple method of saline injection.[40]

In truth, exchanges from donor artery to recipient vein were dangerous. In almost a blink of an eye, who knew how much blood had flowed from one to the other? There had to be a better way. In 1913, Edward Lindeman at Bellevue Hospital in New York worked out a method of syringe transfusion, the donor and recipient veins cannulated with hollow needles and blood drawn via a syringe from the donor, then passed immediately to attendants who quickly infused the amount into the recipient vein.[41] Back and forth it went until the recipient was replenished or the donor near syncope. Even easier, a two-way stopcock was used to avoid passing syringes back and forth. Fill the syringe from the donor, turn the stopcock, and infuse the blood. At the onset of war in 1914, this was the method available for transfusing wounded soldiers. French surgeon Émile Jeanbrau gave the first blood transfusion in the French Army that October to a soldier who had undergone a thigh amputation. The donor was a fellow soldier recovering from a light wound. It all went perfectly. Jeanbrau would go on to perform fifty transfusions himself by the end of 1914.[42]

George Crile returned to the United States on February 8. In all his enthusiasm for blood transfer, there was mention of not a one in his autobiography while at Neuilly-sur-Seine. Altogether, he had made little headway in treating shock and even less with his miracles of blood transfusions. Anyway, exchanging blood was still an elaborate process, not meant yet for the hemorrhaging patients fresh from the battlefield. And there were so many. Clearly, busy surgeons could not take the time in field hospitals to set it all up. They were rushed as it was doing quick amputations or simple *débridements*. Maybe, as Jeanbrau had shown, blood could be given later, to men so anemic in their recuperation that transfusions might hasten recovery. But that would not be frontline work.

So it was a sober Crile who left France. War and the vast numbers of wounded—far too many for his inquisitive mind to digest—had made an impression. All in all, the inhumanity bedazzled him. Visits to the front lines visibly moved him. Naked landscapes were littered with thousands of unburied, decaying dead, and the "weary, bedraggled survivors mingled their own filthy bodies . . . with that of their decomposing comrades."[43]

On April 1, 1915, the entire Lakeside unit vacated the Ambulance Américaine. Now, according to Crile's rotational plan, it was Harvard's turn. Harvey Cushing and his teams from the new Peter Bent Brigham Hospital in Boston had arrived. Among them was surgeon Beth Vincent, an enthusiast himself of blood transfusions. Vincent had performed at least one transfusion in his civilian practice, using that same tedious connection of donor and recipient blood vessels to shunt blood across.[44] He was anxious to try it in Paris and wasted no time. Vincent gave a transfusion on April 10, "which went beautifully and which is quite the talk of the hospital." He performed another one in May, this time at Alexis Carrel's research hospital at Compiègne. As spectacular as it might have seemed, the only comment from Carrel's team was: "It was greatly appreciated."[45]

There would be other pioneers in transfusion therapy. Canada, as part of the United Kingdom, had entered the war against Germany in 1914. She quickly mobilized her army, and by September 1914 the Second Canadian Division was already marching through Paris. Sometime later, as part of Canada's expeditionary force, two physicians, Bruce Robertson and Edward Archibald, finally joined the troops. They were strangers to each other, but both had a keen interest in blood as restoration from hemorrhagic, traumatic shock.

The newly commissioned Major Bruce Robertson received his medical degree from the University of Toronto in 1909. His upbringing had been one of affluence; he attended all the proper schools, but wealth could not dissuade the hands of fate. He suffered the loss of his father in 1904. It was a critical time for a young man of privilege, navigating the wilderness of upper crust adulthood where parental fostering was so beneficial. The unfairness may have robbed Robertson of a measure of fortitude, although his resolve to excel remained unchanged. Mentoring fell to his uncle, a prominent citizen of the city of Toronto. After graduating medical school, Bruce Robertson traveled to New York City for his internship. While at Bellevue Hospital, training in orthopedic surgery and pediatrics, he spent time studying Edward Lindeman's elaborate technique of blood transfusion.[46] He finally mastered the syringe exchange technique, and returned to Toronto in 1913 to work at the Hospital for Sick Children, on which his uncle sat as chairman of the board. Robertson volunteered for military service at the outbreak of war in 1914. It would be over a year before he set foot on French soil, September 1915. There he was to be assigned to the Canadian No. 2 Casualty Clearing Station.[47] As was typical for field hospitals, casualty clearing stations, being primarily surgical units, positioned for offensive operations or in areas of heavy combat. This changed over time. No. 2 Casualty Clearing Station was no exception. For the eager Robertson, though, finding its current location proved impossible. Instead, Robertson ended up at No. 14 General Hospital at Wimereux, on the coast near Boulogne.[48] Still, he was keen to try his new skills of blood transfusion. Battlefield casualties seemed the ideal patients, he reckoned, and blood the perfect solution for traumatic shock.

Yet, at Wimereux he saw a different casualty. Absent were the soldiers rushed in hemorrhaging to death. They had either died or been revived long before reaching General Hospital No. 14. The men he now met were horribly mangled, to be sure, but not in the throes of fatal bleeding. Most had been cut, repaired, stitched, casted, and bandaged but now lingered, vexed by insidious infections and a peculiar failure of healing that so often drained vitality from wasting bodies. Their gaunt eyes and blank stares were testaments to waning constitutions. Still, Robertson wondered, could blood be that magic elixir to pump vigor into lackluster façades? The young major wasted no time and found four willing candidates. For each man a donor volunteered and Lindeman's setup arranged. From donor to recipient syringe after syringe instilled rich red blood. Each received the equivalent of one to two units (400–900 ml). Two out of the four eventually recovered. Robertson was encouraged. He had managed the elaborate technique flawlessly. Even in wartime, he had shown, transfusion was feasible. "Transfused blood is the best substitute for blood lost in acute hemorrhages . . . the addition of salt solution to the circulation [in shock states] is at best only a temporary measure and merely makes up for the loss of fluid," he had written while in Canada. [49]

Still, how would he truly know unless faced with men literally bleeding to death? For that he needed to be much closer to the front, in those hollows where the wounded first arrived, where hemorrhage had not stopped, where shock was unfolding before his eyes. These were the men whom blood might save. In fact, the elusive Casualty Clearing Station No. 2 provided the experience. Robertson chased it down at a place called Remy Siding, in the Ypres sector of Belgium. As "Surgeon Specialist," he was to spend the next two years repairing the thousands of gravely wounded men generated by pounding artillery duels and pointless infantry charges. Sixteen-hour days in surgery and precious little sleep were the norm. Blood transfusions were a luxury too few could receive. Yet by November of 1917, in all the human misery, Robertson had found the time to transfuse thirty-six hemorrhaging patients. In most, it was still that time-consuming, awkward method of Lindeman, syringe after syringe, sometimes injecting up to 1,200 ml. In a few, he had used the new preserved blood, treated with citrate to prevent clotting and run right into the vein through a needle. He was sure he had saved twenty or more men. "In the cases of severe primary haemorrhage [sic] accompanied by shock, blood transfusion frequently produces an immediate and almost incredible improvement," he wrote. His colleagues were impressed. In the War Diary of Casualty Clearing Station No. 2 in July 1917, there was a notation: "as one of the chief and early advocates of Blood Transfusion he [Robertson] has so popularized this method of resuscitation that it has become one of first importance in CCS [Casualty Clearing Station] work." [50] Word spread beyond. Both Canadian and British physicians, even Consulting Surgeon Major General Anthony Bowlby, visited his hospital to watch his transfusion technique. He was one of the medical celebrities of the war, a champion for a righteous cause, a pacesetter in modern medicine.

But the work was exhausting and becoming dangerous. There seemed to be no letup in wounded, and surgery was too often punctuated by the blasts of incoming cannon fire. The entire staff was jittery and, at times, delicate operations had to be put off, considered foolhardy with the jarring of exploding shells. In a more personal sense, there was likely not a man or woman who did not feel the nearness of obliteration. By August 1917 Robertson was done in. He was near collapse and furloughed to England:

> The strain on [Dr. Robertson] was very great and I suppose it was his intense concentration on his job that enabled him to carry on for such a long time . . . It was abeled [sic] what he and his staff did there under the most terrible conditions.[51]

The grinding war in all its carnage had taken a toll. A man of gentle sentiments, the dizzying brutality eclipsed him. Robertson could restore hemorrhaging men, but his own emotional hemoglobin leaked unchecked. He simply did not have the will to return to the field. In February 1918, Robertson returned to Canada but continued hospital work on convalescing soldiers, now fully aware of the folly of warfare that completely overshadowed his scientific curiosity.

But he had accomplished much. His use of transfusions near the front lines on bleeding men revolutionized treatment. He had truly introduced resuscitation as an active process for a sagging physiology. Whatever shock might be, its antidote lay in the hidden powers of red blood cells and plasma. His tireless efforts to transfer blood from donor to needy recipient saved lives, and numbers of Canadian and British surgeons were witnesses. In fact, his fame extended beyond Europe. On the Macedonian front, fellow Canadians Alexander Primrose and Stanley Ryerson filled some of their wounded with blood as well:

> We have reason to believe that all the elements of transfused blood function in the recipient. If such be the case it is undoubtedly the ideal therapeutic measure in haemorrhage, and in cases where there is shock *plus* haemorrhage.[52]

So impressive were Robertson's results that Surgeon General Sir George Makins, no pushover for flimflam, felt blood transfusion for hemorrhaging casualties should be standard procedures for British surgeons:

The main advance in treatment has consisted in a return to the practice of transfusion of "whole blood" which has in great measure displaced the unsatisfactory saline infusion. For the popularization of this method we are mainly indebted to our Canadian colleagues in France [specifically mentioning Robertson].[53]

Robertson's enthusiasm was indeed infectious. Even in dingy aid stations even closer to the front, some had tried transfusions. Canadian doctor Norman Guiou was one. He used the cumbersome syringe method, transferring blood from donor to recipient, on two patients in shock just behind the trenches. One patient died, but the other fellow—leg mangled, barely conscious, and lips "lead-blue"—literally came to life with 800 ml of fresh donor blood. "After the operation [transfusion] the patient's neck and face were definitely red and his cheeks warm to the touch," Guiou described. The soldier was given tea and café au lait, placed on a heated stretcher, surrounded by hot-water bottles, and sent off to a clearing station—quite alive. Guiou had carried out the whole affair, he boasted, under conditions dark, noisy, and barely clean.[54]

The other Canadian who ended up in France was Edward Archibald. Archibald, too, was a product of aristocracy. His ancestors were hardy stock, immigrating from Northern Ireland in the 17th century and favoring the cause of the American Revolution. He had been schooled in Canada but, as was the practice of the day for the well-heeled, toured the major academic centers of Britain, France, and Germany. With such impeccable credentials, he returned to his native Canada and a faculty position at McGill University. He was one of those surgeons with an insatiable curiosity about deranged physiology, eager to examine and explore, eager to find answers. Some later said, "he was first and always . . . the experimentalist."[55] In particular, shock intrigued Archibald. Was it a simple matter of blood loss or was there more? He was aware that a mainstay of treatment must be replenishment of a drained vascular system. He was familiar with Crile's transfusion practices, having visited him in Cleveland just after the war began. By June 1915 Archibald was in France and, like Robertson, in a rear-area general hospital. He, too, saw the soldiers struggling, dwindling. Their spent bodies, plagued by uncontrolled infections, were exhausted, minds equally so, barely wanting to live. This was a form of shock, he concluded, just as lethal as gushing hemorrhage:

> I have become gradually impressed with the belief that shock kills more often than pure hemorrhage; and that, even when a considerable amount of blood is found in the [abdominal] cavity the later death, if it occurs, is often more directly the result of the shock than that of the loss of blood.[56]

Yes, shock was more than blood loss. Yet, Archibald reasoned that the vital faculties of blood might still have a restorative effect, that they just might be remedies for the mysterious shock syndrome.

And so he tried. From the menagerie of ghastly wounds, he selected four men for transfusion. Blood seemed to immediately revive the men, restoring color and improving blood pressure. While the effect was temporary and at least one died from gas gangrene, Archibald claimed success. The "immediate return of colour in the face of the blanched patient,"[57] the brief but real vitality they felt, was enough reward.

Like Robertson, Archibald, too, wanted to be closer to the front. In the spring of 1916, he transferred to No. 1 Casualty Clearing Station. Just like Robertson had, Archibald now saw more patients arriving so soon that they were still hemorrhaging: wounds of arms, legs, belly, and chest provided the source. Here, too, he saw, for the first time, the special "moribund wards," where hopeless cases were stashed until death overcame them. These were men, who, as surgeon Georges Duhamel had seen at Verdun, "had passed beyond human aid, and awaited, numb and unconscious, the crowning mercy of death." Even worse, there were men who, in better times, with hours of labor, could be saved, but now the sheer numbers of wounded forbade such indulgence. Surges of combat flooded field hospitals with casualties, far too many for fatigued doctors to revive. Surgeons toiled, "choosing among the heaps of wounded, and tending two while twenty more poured in."[58] Howard Somervell, one of those beleaguered surgeons, remembered vividly:

> We surgeons were hard at it in the operating-theatre . . .
> occasionally we made a brief look around to select from the
> thousands of patients those few fortunate ones whose life or
> limbs we had time to save. It was terrible business. Even now I
> am haunted by the touching look of the young, bright, anxious
> eyes, as we passed along the rows of sufferers . . . Abdominal
> cases and others requiring long operations simply had to be
> left to die.[59]

Which one, with the efforts of their razor-sharp knives, would have
life? Which ones with the slicing of skin and muscle, the scooping
of blood and grass and dirt, would awake, clear their eyes, and talk of
home? And which ones, bellies like boards, mouths aghast, mumbling
crazy thoughts, would be opened to disgorge blood and bowel juice,
feces and gore, and, hours later, be placed in burlap bags and buried?
These were the ones at whom surgeons smiled and simply walked past.
In their wake, they were "sedated, washed, fed, given to drink, com-
forted by female nurses, shielded from the fact of their approaching
death."[60] These were the moribund ones.

Archibald was no ordinary surgeon. He was drawn to such cases.
The shock of trauma, that brutal power that is so unhinged mechanisms of vitality, possessed them.[61] Exhausted, listless, they lay on
stretchers, racing, thready pulses, gasping breaths, cold, clammy flesh,
tottering on this side of paradise. These were the sad souls who, in
brief moments of clarity, called for mothers or girlfriends or reached
weakly for a nurse's arm. The specter of death filled each of their
minds with immediacy. For some the cause was clear: intestines lolling
through gaping belly rents, limbs smashed and dangling—or missing
altogether—scalps torn, skulls crushed. Some, shellfire had so altered
that resemblance to humanity was a matter of faith. For others, just
the gray of approaching death colored their fate, the bloodletting done
internally, only tiny skin punctures as witness. This was his ward;
this was his laboratory. Here indeed was the ebb of Bernard's *milieu
intérieur*, the energy collapse preached by Crile.[62] Here must hold the
secret of traumatic shock.

Would it be found in the marvels of blood? Yet, for use at a moment's notice, there was hardly enough. For all the wonders of Crile's and Lindeman's transfusion clumsiness, time was the enemy. Blood had to be quickly taken and just as quickly instilled. If not, that invariable agglutination occurred rendering precious blood a useless, jellied muddle. Sodium citrate provided the solution. Citrate was an anticoagulant. When added, blood would not clot. The mechanism was straightforward. Citrate binds calcium in the blood. Without calcium, blood remains liquid—and for long periods of time. The first use of citrated blood for human transfusion actually predated the Great War. In March 1914, the Belgian physician Albert Hustin successfully gave human-to-human transfusions using citrated blood, after experiments in dogs failed to show any ill effects or to alter the properties of the blood.[63] And from the laboratories of the Rockefeller Institute, scientists Peyton Rous and Joseph Turner showed that blood stored in citrate could be preserved at least fourteen days with immediate function on transfusion.[64] The implications were staggering. Blood could be taken from volunteers, stored (*banked* might be a better term), and used later, without the anxiety of urgently finding donors. Robertson had used it on occasion, but for some reason still preferred the syringe transfer method. Archibald had given citrated blood to his four patients. In each case the men responded, more alert, a fuller pulse, a definite improvement, albeit temporary. Clearly, then, the preserved blood acted like blood, with all the properties as if it had come directly from a donor vein.[65]

Archibald was called back to Montreal in April 1916. Funds had run out. His posting as surgeon specialist for No. 1 Casualty Clearing Station was filled by his assistant, Walter McLean. Like Crile, Archibald felt he had made little headway. He was no closer to an explanation of the shock syndrome or to how to remedy it. "I feel rather hopeless over the treatment of these shock cases . . . We know so little of shock beyond a certain point," he later wrote.[66] His young assistant, McLean, had learned techniques of transfusion from him, and, more to the point, shared a sympathy for the wretched inhabitants of the "moribund" tents. McLean set about improving their lot: rehydration—if only with saline solutions—warming, water to drink if they were able. He even tried blood transfusions on some in hopes they would be better prepared for surgery. All his efforts sadly came to an abrupt end. A freak aerial bombardment on November 9, 1917, caught him in the open. He did not survive. No one at No. 1 Casualty Clearing Station remained to take his place. Nevertheless, the Canadians had left a legacy. Blood transfusions, particularly with citrated, stored blood, were a practicality. They had proven to be a crucial step in reversing hemorrhagic shock.[67]

By now blood transfusion had become a beacon of salvation, a crimson Siren, and all worthy journeymen flocked to her.[68] Next was Oswald Hope Robertson, a native of England but a naturalized United States citizen. This new Robertson had a keen interest in transfusion medicine. He, too, witnessed the spell that blood cast for shock victims. But, for broader use, an understanding of blood and its components was critical.

Certain principles were inviolate. One was the subject of human blood types. The Austrian Karl Landsteiner had first worked out blood typing—so-called ABO compatibility—in 1900. Typing was essential of course; failure to match donor and recipient blood destroyed transfused red blood cells, often with fatal consequences. Antigens on the surface of red blood cells could provoke a violent immune response in the recipient blood if not compatible. Hematologists at Mount Sinai Hospital in New York were the first to use blood typing for human transfusion in 1907, but it took several years for surgeons to be convinced it was necessary. It all had certainly been fascinating for Robertson. While in medical school at Harvard, he began working in the laboratories of the famed hematologist Homer Wright. The study of blood fascinated him. This led to collaboration with the brilliant researcher Peyton Rous at the Rockefeller Institute from 1915 to 1917. Rous had recently gained notoriety for developing a rapid agglutination test to determine Landsteiner's donor-recipient blood compatibility.[69] In 1917, Robertson returned to Boston and came under the influence of another Harvard hematologist, Roger Lee. Lee had also done work in agglutination and blood storage and quickly became a mentor to Robertson.

With declaration of war by the United States in April 1917, university surgical teams were swiftly mobilized for deployment. One of those was Harvey Cushing's Harvard unit. Surgeons were well aware of the numbers of casualties generated by the war and the likely need for volumes of stored blood. Lee named Robertson to the team as it prepared to sail for Europe. Their task was to set up a blood bank of citrated blood and prepare speedy typing for ABO compatibility. Both Lee and Roberston were in France by June.[70] In fact, Robertson managed to set up the first blood bank in France. Most of the blood flowed not from eager American recruits but from the veins of willing French citizens. With those batches, he began transfusing American and British soldiers. It was indeed just as Grace Crile had described: a miracle of resurrection. He saw an astonishing number immediately rebound from their shock. "An attempt was made to choose only those cases who would probably die without transfusion and yet who had a chance of recovery if given blood," he later wrote. Many would certainly have come from Archibald's moribund tents. Of the twenty men he transfused, over half left his hospital "in good condition."[71] But frontline service was hazardous. For Robertson it almost proved his undoing. In that last desperate German offensive during the summer of 1918, he barely escaped, but his coveted blood bank did not. Advancing Germans and their artillery completely destroyed it.[72]

The Army Medical Department also tagged Cleveland's Lakeside unit for deployment. On May 18, 1917, George Crile and his team returned to France. Surgeon General William Gorgas had specifically picked him to head the medical effort for the American Expeditionary Force. In fact, Crile's team was the first contingent of the American Expeditionary Force to set foot on the continent. They took over Base Hospital No. 4 at Rouen in the busy Flanders sector. The restless Crile could not sit still. While his unit was setting up, he again toured the front lines. Preparations were underway for the big offensive that summer, but the bleak battlefields still chewing up men were familiar specters for Crile. Casualty clearing stations found no letup in wounded, and the moribund tents of Archibald were still packed with hopeless cases.[73] Crile shared with Archibald a fascination with these casualties. He propositioned Sir Anthony Bowlby to turn moribund tents into resuscitation wards—to turn death into life. Here he could find his bleeding, fading shock victims to revitalize.[74] Here was his human laboratory. The energetic Crile wasted no time suffusing British casualties with his transfusions—and took credit to boot. In fact, it was he, Crile claimed, who brought blood transfusions to the British (an assertion Bruce Robertson and Edward Archibald might have disputed). By May of 1918, blood transfusions had become so commonplace that Crile bragged, "think of it! Transfusion is now such a routine procedure that today's order of the day carries a recommendation . . . that the C.O. [Commanding Officer] of each hospital give a donor of blood for transfusion a certificate granting leave for one day."[75]

In fact, the British felt the same. Shock soon dominated battlefield medicine. Artillery was opening wounds from which blood poured and men, not blown to bits at once, watched their black blood soak the earth, little different than in Homeric times. So worried were doctors that, in Great Britain, the Medical Research Committee, formed to address pressing health issues for the military, focused on traumatic shock. So many factors besides hemorrhage seemed to contribute: cold weather, fatigue, evacuation delays, even rough handling of men carried from the trenches.[76]

Scientists and clinicians from the Allied nations weighed in. One of them would be an American, Walter Cannon. Cannon was a member of the Harvard faculty. He completed his undergraduate and medical education at Harvard and straightaway took a position on the faculty in the physiology laboratory. His phenomenal capacity for research and experimentation quickly pegged him as a rising star.[77] He had turned down an offer to go to France with Cushing in 1915. Vital work in Boston, he said, was the reason. His wife was more circumspect. "In some ways he is tempted," she wrote, "but I think he fears the horror of the thing would so overcome him that he would be useless."[78] Cannon refused a second invitation from the Rockefeller Institute the following year, this time to join Alexis Carrel's group at Compiègne. But, after war was declared in 1917, to his surprise he was offered a position as chairman of the committee on physiology for the National Research Council. Cannon the scientist could no longer refuse. By then, war had generated such heaps of suffering that there must be attempts to bring order to disorder, to provide relief from unmitigated misery.

His obsession? Shock it was to be, that bane of the battlefield. He actually knew little about it. What he did know was that numbers of men were dying because of it and, unquestionably, numbers of Americans would soon be included in that group. In typical Cannon fashion, he threw himself into the subject, talking to colleagues and spending endless nights awake, studying. Compelled by an overriding desire to unravel complexities so long hidden under the guise of nervous exhaustion or toxins or simple bloodletting, Cannon launched into a frenzy of inquiry on the manner and undulations of traumatic shock. His wife said he could hardly eat or sleep, so enraptured was he with his work. Cannon explored blood pressure, the sphygmomanometer, transfusions, adrenaline, and all the battlefield experiences of Allied surgeons on the Western Front. But, Cannon also knew that this was not just his usual laboratory challenge, and he could not grasp this complex syndrome fully from afar. He needed to *see* the human condition—to examine, feel, interrogate. He needed to go to France. And so, Cannon signed up with Cushing's detachment as a special investigator. His deep concern was whether he could experiment on humans. "You will," a friend said, "when you know that you are their only hope."[79]

Cannon's first stop was England. His reputation had preceded him. Walter Fletcher, head of the Medical Research Committee, eagerly awaited him and right off persuaded him to join his team of British doctors studying shock near the front lines. But his first experience at Base Hospital No. 5 at Camiers, near the coast, was a long way from the front—and it was disappointing. Truly critical patients—those bleeding acutely and in shock—were lacking and laboratory equipment for basic research was nonexistent. He pleaded for a closer assignment that landed him at Casualty Clearing Station No. 33 near Béthune, in northeastern France. It was an eye-opener for the scientist. "Their wounds were appalling," he wrote. Blood was everywhere, he found, on clothes, in jellied clumps on the floor, and mixed with mud to coat flesh. "Hands used to stop the bleeding were streaked and blotched with blood. It had streamed over their tunics and trousers," he went on.[80] Cannon did menial tasks, bandaging, assisting in surgery, record keeping, but beyond his intellectual curiosities, he finally felt valued. "I got into action where there was need," he wrote his wife. "It has been an immense reassurance of self-respect."[81] In the process, though, he did countless blood pressure measurements, finding, as others had, that low blood pressure was a hallmark of traumatic shock. In many, hemorrhage was obvious—*exemia*, Cannon called it. Rapid heart rate, clammy skin, and sinking blood pressure were typical findings. Compounded by some type of nervous system reaction, Cannon wondered? Maybe. Maybe fear, fatigue, and pain played a role. There were other men, gravely wounded, who had lost little blood but had the same sickly look. Were there still other factors involved? Cannon wondered about "toxin" released from damaged tissue. Not simply nervous system exhaustion as Crile had insisted. It was all still mystifying.

Others had reported something similar. William Porter, another Harvard physiologist sent to France by the Rockefeller Institute to study traumatic shock, had claimed that surgeons at Carrel's hospital in Compiègne noticed shock came on mostly after wounds of the great bones or after multiple shrapnel wounds. In fact, Porter witnessed such a case himself at La Panne. A bad thigh fracture and open wound had mandated surgery. During the operation, Porter measured the blood pressure. At first, it was normal, but then a sudden and unexpected plunge. His patient became deathly pale. Porter and the surgeons feared the fellow was literally bleeding into his veins—that the abdominal veins opened up and arterial blood poured in, where it stagnated. The heart had little left to pump, and the patient could die. Surgeons stopped the operation, elevated the patient's legs, and gave adrenaline. Life resumed. Could it be, he surmised that fat-laden marrow released by shattered bones somehow flooded the circulation and poisoned the nervous system? There was no easy answer. That debate would rage for decades.[82]

Or could there be a spectrum of traumatic shock? At one extreme a type with massive blood loss starting soon after wounding. Hemorrhage was the key factor. At the other end, beginning later, a variety brought on by pain, thirst, fatigue, broken bones, and macerated tissue—even the jostling of stretcher carries could contribute. Maybe this was a different form with other bodily reactions—toxins and the like—the cause. Cannon knew well that no one could provide the proof.[83]

Armed with an array of clinical information, Cannon returned to England to continue his research into shock. He teamed up with the renowned British physiologist William Bayliss. There, work centered on the acid-base balance in the blood of shock victims. Perhaps the acid nature of blood in these cases was the cause of low blood pressure. Cannon thought not. It was a consequence but not a cause.[84] The etiology remained obscure. What was for sure was the almost immediate improvement of these patients with some type of intravenous fluid—blood preferable, but even saline or other protein-rich infusions helped.[85]

To his surprise, Cannon had become something of a celebrity with traumatic shock. The Red Cross Medical Research Society, a forum for exchange of the war experiences of French, British, and American physicians, soon elected him president. In March 1918 he returned to France where he was appointed director of the American Expeditionary Force Central Medical Laboratory in Dijon. It was here that he instructed medical officers on the nature and treatment of shock to prepare them for casualties in upcoming combat operations. Yet Cannon's interest in shock paled in comparison to the pathetic sights and sounds of the shock wards he visited. Their complements of sickening wounds and plaintive moans stirred unforgettable memories. Such recollections seemed to consume him when writing his autobiography years later. These pitiful men plagued all doctors and scientists who spent time in dingy field hospitals surrounded by so many bloodied forms. It completely took over their recollections and surely flavored their interpretations of even the hardest, most objective of clinical measurements.

And for traumatic shock, what made the greatest impression was what Crile and his wife saw years before: the absolutely astonishing revival that occurred with transfusion of blood. This is what bleeding men needed. Was it enough? What about those boys who Crile and Cannon saw not bleeding but languishing pale, drawn, and weak; those with crushed arms or legs or shattered bones? And those, too, with dropping blood pressures and feeble pulses. This was shock as well. Could those cases be revived? Did fright, fatigue, pain, and bruised and battered tissue play a role? Was it more than simple hemorrhage? In these wasting men, the life force of Bernard and Crile and

Cannon was also dwindling away, but not just in blood. And so would continue the enigma of traumatic shock.

Still, it was World War I that brought the complexities of traumatic shock front and center. These desperate soldiers, laid low in muddy trenches and no-man's-land, had, in their sad way, contributed to the foundation of our understanding of hemorrhage and the effects of massive injuries. They led us to solutions, albeit imperfect ones, but solutions nevertheless. Of course, some mysteries of shock remain. Yet, World War I saw the first breakthroughs. Blood preservation, blood storage, and means of rapid infusion were the opening salvos for not all victims of shock, but for a good majority. It was truly, for many, the miracle of the resurrection, the first "gift of life." It would be a mainstay of battlefield medicine, nay, medicine in general, for centuries to come.[86]

FOUR

"The Most Atrocious of Ills"[1]: The Great War and the Scourge of Gas Gangrene

"We are powerless to prevent gas-gangrene, for it is impossible to sterilize the wounds."
—Alexis Carrel, 1914

The gangrenous. Redemption came at an agonizing pace for those stricken with the putrid ailment of slow decomposition. French soil and time had rendered battle's ragged etchings so. One could smell them at once upon entering a ward: that sickening sweet odor of rotting meat. Unwrap a dirty dressing and then behold, flesh as if dead for days—blistered blue and purple. Raging under swollen skin, the pain fired like electricity, driving victims insane. Until, that is, angels of death arrived and then an eerie calm, a blank stare, and, shortly, a lifeless corpse. The mumblings of prayers preceded them—to no avail. Prayers for the living? Incantations over the wounds infested with manured dirt? It would take far more than prayers to salvage these poor souls. Rigid science. Painstaking probing. Infallible curiosity. There, that would be the redemption. God helps those who help themselves.

GANGRÈNE FOUDROYANTE

Jules Germain François Maisonneuve had studied under the talented Parisian surgeon Guillaume Dupuytren, whose practice in Paris was titanic and expertise unparalleled, particularly in maladies of the limbs and all the ramifications of tendon and bone wounds. In urban life, with the crowded streets and steady stream of horse-driven conveyances, it was not infrequent that a pedestrian fell or slipped into the path of oncoming wagons. Crush injuries to limbs were often presented to doctors in a complex disarray of torn flesh, bleeding muscle, and fragmented bone. Outcome was often unfavorable, the amputation knife the final arbitrator of survival or death.

As a result, Maisonneuve's knowledge of those injuries to the extremities was extensive, his experience unparalleled. However, in 1853, he encountered two patients who alarmed him with the viciousness of their ailments, and he felt compelled to alert his colleagues. The first case was a healthy young man of twenty-eight years brought to him with a leg crushed under the weight of a falling cart. Within hours, putrefaction had seized the limb, now swollen with a sickening, crackling, crunching feel, the feel of tiny pockets of air in the tissues—what Maisonneuve would term "emphysema."[2] Deep incisions of the affected limb by his scalpel liberated bubbles of gas and, to Maisonneuve's surprise, the veins themselves now contained such vapors. Despite his surgical paring, the gentleman was dead by morning. It must be, Maisonneuve thought, that those tiny fumes incubated a deadly toxin. A second case followed, this time a man of thirty, his right arm mashed by a wagon wheel. Overnight the limb, up to the shoulder, was gangrenous, the skin a purplish discoloration and raised by underlying giant blisters—*bullae*, they were called. Fearing that the only hope lay in amputation, Maisonneuve took to this pitiful patient at once with the knife, not even waiting on his saw, and to his dismay, once again noticed froths of gas escape the veins. Indeed, examination of the severed member showed streaks of air throughout the muscles. However, the amputation must have been lifesaving, for the individual recovered and since "enjoys perfect health." Based on these two grave circumstances, Maisonneuve labeled such rampant putrefaction

abeled foudroyante (fulminant or lightning gangrene[3]), to emphasize the
suddenness of onset, the rapidity of progression, and the inevitability of
outcome if not at once and with radical purpose addressed. As to the
somewhat vexing cause, Maisonneuve went on to say that brutal injury

> [H]as, by the violence of its action, produced a deep disorga-
> nization of tissues . . . crushed by contusion . . . [that] putre-
> fies under the influence of heat and humidity from the air;
> their prompt decomposition then gives rise to the formation
> of putrid gases which seep into the cellular interstices, and
> their deleterious contact extinguishes the vital forces in parts
> already struck by stupor as a result of the concussion. All these
> causes together give the fermentation putrid a terrible activity;
> so it does not take long to encompass in its destructive move-
> ment even completely healthy parts . . .[4]

Yet, Maisonneuve was not the first to witness such maladies. In 1846,
Alfred Velpeau described cases where gangrenous limbs resulting from
injury were amputated, but the rotting process soon appeared in the
stump; the so-called tissue emphysema followed, and the patient shortly
expired. "Surgeons were dismayed to see gangrene appear on the stump,
to continue to spread up to the trunk, to finally stop with the life of the
patient."[5] Of course, gangrene itself was no stranger to the battlefield.
Wounds with fractures and muscle injury and gunshots often turned
putrid—swollen, discolored, sickening in their odor. The great Napoleon
Bonaparte's own surgeon, Dominique Larrey, recognized the perplexing
face of gangrenous toxemia, where the putrefaction marched relentlessly
onward, from one limb to another, reaching the trunk and infecting the
organs of life. Such perfidy soon produces a "pallor of the face, an anguish,
a delirium, and, if the contagion continues, soon a prompt death." There
is the characteristic rotting like spoiled meat, absence of any pus—that
signature finding of possible recovery—early affectations of the senses
(the poor victims were absolutely frantic in their impending doom), and
a high likelihood of death.[6] But Larrey failed to mention those peculiar
air pockets foaming below the skin. Was this the same phenomenon?

Yes, gangrene was the plague of wounded troops. Over the centuries battlefields seemed to spawn crops of young men with smelly, decaying legs and arms jamming field hospitals and, with their ailing features, provide ample experience for overtaxed surgeons at the ready with knife and saw. There was no doubt about the report of Eugène Romain Salleron writing of his encounters during the Crimean War while at l'Hôpital militaire de Dolma-Bagtché in Constantinople. In 1858, Salleron described over six dozen cases of an unchecked and quickly fatal form of gangrene accompanied by those characteristic crackling sounds when tissue was pressed (he referred to it as *abeled instantanée*). Physical appearances were particularly notable: a gloomy, fearful patient who, when questioned, felt a deep, throbbing, aching pain in the affected leg, even after amputation. After a short time, a "sudden terror" gripped the individuals. The pulse accelerated, breathing quickened, and the tissue crepitance advanced almost under watch. In most cases, large muscle groups were affected: those of the calf, thigh, or shoulder. The limb had invariably been injured—a musket ball, a piece of shrapnel, a crushing fracture. There were characteristic changes of the skin with blistering and an engorged tenseness—the appendage suffused with rancid fluid and gas and decomposition—that, in turn, produced a marbling surface discoloration. After amputation, when that was undertaken, the discarded member showed tiny bubbles of gas tracking through the subcutaneous tissue and deep into the muscle fibers, the muscles themselves now pale, discolored, "like washed macerated flesh." Within arteries and veins could be seen bubbles of gas, just as Maisonneuve had reported years before. The wound exuded a unique odor—that sickly smell of rancid flesh. Sadly, patients often had to watch the decay advance, helpless to stop it. They were conscious until the end, terror-stricken at the approaching doom.[7] Salleron, too, was astonished at the suddenness of onset and the unyielding progression, as if "the emphysematous gangrene began like a lightning flash [*éclat foudroyant*] that precipitously broke the spirit of life without possible repair."[8]

And he finished with the ominous conclusion:

Whichever name it is considered appropriate to give to the morbid phenomena which I call gangrene with emphysema or gangrenous emphysema, the fact remains to preserve in all its pathological significance that salvation is impossible, manifestations lightening in onset, and incurability absolute.[9]

In contrast, few such reports surfaced during the American Civil War in either the Union or Confederate armies. There was much talk of gangrene and the mortification, putrefaction, and dwindling vigor seen in hospital settings (it was called then "hospital gangrene"), but little mention of a rapidly fatal version. Clearly, infections plagued any number of patients and pus could be found deep in muscle layers, but nothing resembling Salleron's fatal illness was encountered, and, particularly, no gas formation was ever mentioned either before or after death. Instead, a different rotting affected the wounded. It was the close bedding of hospitalized patients—frequently clustered in cramped, stuffy wards—that seemed to give rise to a smoldering, lazy, purulent decay that, over weeks or months, gradually sucked life and vigor from its victim and often caused a withering death from inanition.[10] Yes, on rare occasion, there were reports of far graver occurrences, those more suggestive of the European *éclat foudroyant*. But these were hidden in the memoirs of individual surgeons and not in official recordings of medical histories. One such case was a narrative by Confederate surgeon Joseph Jones. His case of a particular Southern soldier stabbed in the scrotum was eerily reminiscent of European experiences:

> The marks of inflammation and disorganization progressed most rapidly on the uninjured side . . . and the left thigh, groin, and lower portion of the abdomen on this side soon presented a swollen green, purplish, grayish, and in parts blackish look, as if the parts were undergoing rapid decomposition . . . When I plunged my lancet into this elevated purplish and greenish putrid-looking mass . . . a dark greenish and purplish, horribly offensive matter, mixed with numerous bubbles of air, poured out in large quantity . . . Death closed this distressing case in less than seven days after the reception of the wound.[11]

The fiendish nature of this patient's demise certainly shared features with Maisonneuve's and Salleron's sad victims. And the expelled gas no doubt reflected the same pervasive bedlam. Yet the fetid, melting muscle tissue, so characteristic of this event, seemed lacking. Nevertheless, it was likely the same. One can imagine, in those filthy, unsanitary military camps of the day, that genitalia frequently went unwashed, and expelled diarrhea dried on the buttocks of men rarely inclined to clean themselves. As the Confederate surgeon Julian Chisolm had pointed out in 1864, major impediments to vigor in field camps were "continued exposure and fatigue, bad and insufficient food, salt meat, indifferent clothing, want of cleanliness, poor shelter . . . [and] infected tents and camps."[12] Were these the disgusting conditions that cloaked soldiers and, once driven deep inside by the tip of a bayonet or conical Minié balls, mixed with ill-health and were the source of a process that seemed to bring about internal rotting? It appeared so closely tied to hygiene and fecal matter and even the earth itself.

So few cases were seen, though, that it remained a dreadful but anecdotal occurrence.

At least in humans. Veterinarians were well-versed in such disorders. They knew about a similar sickness—on a much grander scale—that swept through herds of livestock. Anthrax was a centuries-old affliction that affected livestock in the fields and farms of Europe, felling countless sheep and cattle with dire economic consequences. The disease struck quickly, causing hemorrhages, convulsions, and rapid death. When examined even shortly after death, the tissues of infected animals contained gas pockets and areas of slimy, decomposing muscle. It would fall to two brilliant microbiologists of the era to begin to unravel the mysteries of this disease that literally devoured its host alive. The Frenchman Louis Pasteur was already almost a Parisian luminary. He had taken control of the prestigious École normale supérieure, the most selective graduate school in Paris. There Pasteur had completely revamped the standards of scientific effort. Personally, his work on the germ theory and the process of fermentation was groundbreaking and exposed the previously invisible world of busy microorganisms. This was the new field of bacteriology. Pasteur had firmly established that bacteria were the agents of fermentation and putrefaction—the decomposition of living matter. In fact, he had recently demonstrated that certain bacteria were adverse to oxygen—the pivotal molecule of life—and seemed to remain alive only in the *absence* of it. For that observation, Pasteur had labeled these types of bacteria *anaerobes* ("without oxygen").[13] In fact, ordinarily the presence of oxygen was lethal to these microbes. Could some of these peculiar anaerobes be involved with the decomposition of tissue in animals struck down with anthrax?

Peering into his dimly lit microscope at the congregated miniature life-forms—these animalcules named by Antonie van Leeuwenhoek in 1677[14]—Pasteur uncovered the causative agent to be a rod-shaped and spore-forming bacterium that he labeled *Vibrion septique*. *Vibrion* (from the Latin verb *vibrāre*, "to vibrate") was a kind of bacteria with a squiggly, wormlike appearance and a propensity, when seen under the microscope, to move or shake. Earlier work by the Italian Filippo Pacini had associated this comma-shaped microbe to cholera epidemics—and in the *Gazzetta Medica Italiana* he named the restless comma-shaped microbe "Vibrio cholerae."[15] For his wormy bacterium—so reminiscent of Pacini's—Pasteur added the species s*eptique* ("septic") because this bacterium caused an early and fatal outcome. They were found in abundance in tissue of animals dying from anthrax, and, when injected into guinea pigs, produced the same stormy illness: muscles literally liquefying ("seat of the most intense inflammation") and gaseous miasmas seeping through. These microorganisms, Pasteur found, were capable of putrefying living tissue. Their anaerobic biology—one that excludes oxygen—proved ideal for conditions of scant blood flow. Without blood there was no oxygen, and without oxygen these bacteria could flourish. Even more remarkable, oxygen proved not so much lethal as transformative. The squirming, wiggling rod forms changed into inanimate spherical spores, dormant but still viable, as if in hibernation. They could exist for years in this state. Pasteur had heard of the "cursed fields" of Beauce—that expanse of farmland southwest of Paris. In this region, anthrax was endemic.[16] As it turned out, he found, lolling in the buried carcasses afflicted with anthrax, those same spores. The spores were then carried by earthworms to the surface. Here they mixed with the soil and contaminated the minor cuts and scrapes of grazing farm animals. Once amidst living juices, the spores blossomed into their bacterial form, now not so averse to oxygen, a metamorphosis Pasteur would call by a new term: facultative anaerobes. And then the infection began, seeding tissues and bloodstream and quickly felling the beast.[17]

In 1877, Pasteur wrote about his new *Vibrion septique*. In some respects, anthrax resembled the violent bubbling disease seen in humans.[18] But now he was not alone. The bright German physician and bacteriologist Robert Koch, twenty years Pasteur's junior, had just set up practice in the town of Wöllstein in present-day Poland. He, too, was aware of the major impact on farmers caused by anthrax. Koch had already learned of Pasteur's work with bacteria and their ability to cause putrefaction. Convinced that germs were a direct cause of many diseases, he set out to confirm or refute Pasteur's findings on anthrax. Koch was a gifted scientist and had already begun to grow bacteria in a laboratory adjacent to his clinic. While his experiments were rather primitive in design, his laboratory techniques for isolating bacteria were ingenious and enabled him to determine the entire life cycle of what he believed was the bacterium of anthrax. In a larger sense, his work seemed to verify Pasteur's conclusions as well. In fact, Pasteur's publications, while critical of Koch's novel experimental methods, were professional and even respectful. Yet, for reasons not entirely clear, the labor of the two men, while seemingly complementary, would spark intense animosity. Some would claim it was simple jealousy; Koch rankled at Pasteur's fame. In any event, the malevolence of academic rivalry had shown its pernicious face.

It may have been that Pasteur was not sure Koch had proven that his bacillus was the cause of anthrax. Koch, perhaps chafing at the skepticism of the famous Pasteur, may have reacted indignantly. For his part, Koch was not at all sure Pasteur's culture techniques were adequate. Perhaps he was not cultivating pure clusters of bacteria—in which case his results were worthless. Pasteur bristled at such accusations. Exasperated, Pasteur finally had enough. He retorted:

> You do not acknowledge that you are mistaken . . . Your pamphlet [critical of Pasteur's anthrax work] contains a great

> many passages in which the impertinence of error . . . is really
> carried too far . . . However violent your attacks, Monsieur,
> they will not prevent me from succeeding. [19]

Or, maybe it was a deeper issue. Koch had served in the Franco-Prussian war of 1870–71, as had three of his brothers. He had come away from his service with bitter sentiments against the French. Pasteur, on the other hand, had been too old to serve but still harbored resentment for Prussian militarism, as did many Frenchmen of the time. In any event, their relationship deteriorated to a series of back-and-forth polemics that accomplished very little in resolving their scientific (or nationalistic) differences. Yet, despite the sniping that occurred over the next decades—and it turned quite bitter—each man made substantial contributions to the understanding of the oxygen-independent, spore-forming microorganism so lethal for livestock. [20] Even more to the point, their work opened the door to an understanding of these peculiar spore-forming bacteria in general: their unique ability to lay dormant almost indefinitely, but once placed into the right environment, to morph into active, moving forms that seep insidiously through living flesh.

A decade later, in 1892, American microbiologist William Welch at the Johns Hopkins Hospital in Baltimore, made his own discoveries. Welch, a descendant of New England Irish physicians, was sympathetic to German science. An education at Yale forged his intellectual intensity and an appreciation for the logic of the classics. In fact, Latin and Greek had so absorbed him, he at first envisioned a life of study and teaching. But medicine exerted an invisible pull, as if his heredity forbade any other profession. After graduation from the College of Physicians in New York, one of the premier medical schools of the country, Welch headed to Germany in 1876. At that time, German centers of biologic experimentation led the world with breakthroughs in physiologic chemistry and pathology and attracted the brightest of American talent. His travels landed him in the laboratories of Carl Ludwig, one of the leading physiologists of the day, where he learned the intricacies of experimental physiology. He later teamed with the great Julius Cohnheim in Breslau and delved into the mysterious world of microscopic pathology. Welch was taken by Cohnheim's passionate curiosity about the invisible frontiers his powerful lenses opened, and, in turn, fell in rapture with the logic of it all, how damage to minuscule cells could wreak havoc on the equanimity of mankind. "Pathology and even practical medicine have entered upon a new era since Cohnheim's discoveries in the process of inflammation," he wrote his father, referring to that common bodily reaction to so many noxious agents in nature. It was on his return to New York that Welch found six discarded microscopes and began his own love affair with bacteria. Their habitats in drinking water and diarrhea and their intimate association with diseases captivated him and became a major focus of his professional life. Later, in 1885, he returned to Europe and to the laboratories of Carl Ludwig. This time, though, he also visited the irascible Robert Koch in Berlin, attracted to the bacteriologist's rigid methodology and incessant obsession with detail.[21]

It was later, after returning to Baltimore, that Welch stumbled onto the causative agent of those sickening postmortem vapors found in blood vessels of certain recently deceased individuals. It was such an early finding that Welch was confident it was not standard bodily decomposition. Microscopic rods called bacilli were seen. He labeled his new microbe *Bacillus aerogenes capsulatus*, an anaerobic nonmotile bacterium, like Pasteur's and Koch's, capable of spore formation. These microbes, Welch observed, were also able to grow rapidly and produce gas bubbles when cultured on agar, milk, and bouillon media. After injection into rabbits they reproduced swiftly and excreted their gaseous metabolites throughout the body, often within hours of inoculation. While incapable of development in the presence of oxygenated blood, Welch's bacilli flourished without it. "If . . . the bacilli should find access to dead tissue, old fibrinous clots, cavities such as the intestines or uterus . . . there they might grow . . . and with it the bacilli might enter the circulation," Welch concluded.[22]

At the same time, the German bacteriologist Eugen Fraenkel described four cases eerily similar to Maisonneuve's. Fraenkel had been working at the Eppendorf Krankenhaus in Hamburg since 1874. He originally trained as an ophthalmologist but was drawn to the tragedy of deadly and contagious cholera epidemics affecting Hamburg. It was then that he immersed himself in the new field of bacteriology. Now, Fraenkel brought to light four cases of a gas-producing infections found in the tissues under the skin, sometimes extending deeper, into muscle. He gave these the name *Gasphlegmone* (roughly, "gaseous inflammation").[23] The infection produced massive swelling of flesh, tiny gas bubbles, and giant blisters on the skin surface, and when he cut into them, a rancid, watery fluid emerged. In one patient he found that "the muscles of the quadriceps [thigh muscles] have completely disintegrated and can be rubbed to a pulp." All cases proved lethal, with or without surgery to cut away dead tissue, within days. Fraenkel knew these patients were almost identical to those with the *foudroyant* inflammation of Maisonneuve. The anaerobic bacillus identified by Fraenkel—which he believed to be the offending agent—was clearly different from the usual pus-forming bacteria. And it had marked similarities to the bacillus described by Welch.

Furthermore, Fraenkel was convinced his bacillus resembled those that caused other diseases in livestock similar to anthrax: diseases called malignant edema and *rauschbrand* (blackleg of cattle and sheep).[24] Both conditions displayed those ominous patches of pale, dead muscle and a quick and fatal course. And both conditions frothed telltale gas in the tissues—what others had called tissue emphysema. So Fraenkel named his microbe *Bacillus phlegmones emphysematose*—but it would be forever known as Fraenkel's bacillus. After receiving cultures of the bacillus from Fraenkel, Welch was sure it was identical to his *Bacillus aerogenes capsulatus*.[25] It now seemed these spore-forming bacteria, ubiquitous in soil and intestines of man, could, under favorable conditions—traumatic injury, poor circulation—transform and produce a variety of life-threatening infections, all characterized by gas production. In fact, they acted much like Pasteur's *Vibrion septique*.

Eugen Fraenkel, the Jewish German patriot, would go on to serve as a physician in the German army. He died in 1925, mercifully before he would have witnessed Hitler's Gestapo hunt down and capture his ailing elderly widow and his daughter, both of whom were to die in extermination camps in 1944: Marie, his wife, at Theresienstadt, and Margarethe, his daughter, in the gas chambers of Auschwitz-Birkenau.

Of the other great 19th-century microbiologists, Louis Pasteur died in 1895, Robert Koch in 1910. But their legacy with the bacteria of putrefaction proved fundamental for future understanding. And human gas gangrene infections, although infrequent, continued to rivet the attention of civilian surgeons—such virulence could not be ignored. In 1912 Walter Cramp, a surgeon at New York's busy Bellevue Hospital, reported on twenty-five patients with gas gangrene, a startling disease, he admits, that was little understood, but filled with "much uncertainty and confusion." Yet he was able to identify three principle features: gangrene (tissue decay), emphysema (gas), and "a wild type of infection." But here was the interesting part: Unlike in livestock, when any of the gangrenous infections, such as anthrax, were quickly fatal, in humans this was not the case. Cramp found some infections involved only skin and fatty tissue just below and were more easily treated. In other cases, the disease was much more violent, reaching deeper and rotting muscle. These needed to be dealt with by "prompt and energetic action." His tally for the twenty-five patients seen at Bellevue? Fourteen survived and eleven died, a mortality of 44 percent.[26] In all, Cramp was to collect a total of 187 cases from the literature. And of all these, not one patient with superficial infections died. His conclusion:

> All wounds on which great force has been exerted, and especially those contaminated by soil and dirt-covered objects, should be treated as if infected with gas bacilli. They should be left open where possible and thoroughly irrigated with peroxide.[27]

Peroxide? Hydrogen peroxide; that agent, H2O2, which, under catalytic conditions, liberates oxygen molecules so deadly to certain anaerobic bacteria. It was because, under his microscope, Cramp saw those same sinister rod-shaped, spore-forming bacteria—like the types described by Pasteur and Welch and Fraenkel—sometimes wiggling, taking up Gram's telling stain, in various chains like microscopic linked sausages, or simply in pairs.[28] Were they really the same? Were the clinical syndromes similar? Once again, the inescapable similarities to anthrax and blackleg and malignant edema in cattle and sheep were striking. The liquefying muscle and tissue gas were dominant findings. It seemed the bacteria causing all these were somehow related.[29] Some of his colleagues even contended that one form of bacteria could mutate to another so that they were all interrelated.[30] Was it indeed in common dirt that these bacteria existed, and, if so, surgeons like Cramp wondered if wounds exposed to the earth of farm fields not be ignored but, instead, opened widely and washed out to remove any imbedded germs. Let air and oxygen get into the tissues, Cramp may have speculated.

Yet in the days before August 1914 military surgeons ignored such advice, and these rare occurrences. Infection in wounds was not a major problem. Army physicians were still preoccupied with the spread of camp diseases like dysentery, cholera, and malaria. These were the major threats to marching troops. Yes, gunshot injuries could cause problems. Bullets could certainly drive in dirt and clothing. Yet the prevailing attitude, as the noted German surgeon Ernst von Bergmann (1836–1907) pointed out, considered gunshot wounds basically sterile and, therefore, exempt from meddlesome probing. In those times, rifled bullet wounds often did leave a clean track. There seemed to be little "collateral damage" to muscles, blood vessels, and nerves. "The greatest subcutaneous injury [from gunshot wounds of war] can be far milder than a needle-stick in the finger," Bergmann professed. He instructed battlefield surgeons to hold back. Probe wounds very little, he cautioned, feeling that opening wounds only invited airborne pathogens in and caused pus-laden infections. Instead, Bergmann was a fan of asepsis—the thorough cleansing of skin wounds with antiseptics—and wrapping them in sterile dressings. This, and this alone, would promote healing.[31] His belief was shared by August Hildebrandt, then a surgeon at the prestigious Charité Hospital in Berlin, who, in 1905, had shown that soiled clothing implanted in experimental animals did not provoke infection, even if contaminated with dangerous streptococci. Yes, he conceded, germs on the skin could be driven inside by bullet wounds, but "this risk has always been low as the day-to-day experience has taught the surgeons how rare it is to cause infection."[32] Much more likely, in his opinion, was the implanting of dangerous microbes by the hands of snooping surgeons.

The French felt similarly. That stalwart of French surgery, Edmond Delorme, stuck by the principles that had guided wound care during the Franco-Prussian War. Delorme, mired in traditions of a bygone era, maintained that simple bullet wounds were innocuous. To make his point, he authored the notorious professional regulations in 1910 and again in 1914 mandating minimalist care. In fact, so persuasive was he that he won over the prestigious Société nationale de chirurgie de Paris, a highly influential group in shaping surgical practices. Scrupulous wound exploration and irrigation was time-consuming, he insisted. Gunshot injuries were almost harmless. Besides, throngs of casualties could be cared for much easier if such injuries were simply cleaned, bandaged, and ignored.[33]

CARNAGE

For an anarchist's lucky shots that killed Austrian archduke Franz Ferdinand and his wife, battle was joined in August 1914, by the powers of Europe. The carnage was indescribable. Armies accustomed to the modest fire of German bolt action Mausers and French *fusil* Lebels now faced Maxims and Saint Étienne machine guns spewing four hundred rounds per minute at velocities of almost three thousand feet per second.[34] At impact, the imparted kinetic energy pulverized human tissue. Tactics, far outdistanced by technology, hearkened back to the last war: parade-ground rows of soldiers trotting toward the enemy with reason-blinding bravado, useless bayonets gleaming in the sun. Artillery was prodigious, pounding troops with shells that could weigh tons, exploding overhead and sending sizzling shrapnel into fabric-covered flesh. Men were cut down like wheat. At Charleroi in August, French 75s sprayed the tight German lines from their flanks with enfilading fire. One observer noted:

> Parts of the battlefield . . . presented this unforgettable
> spectacle of thousands of dead standing in several rows sup-
> ported by abutting corpses and placing themselves on top of
> each other, in different inclinations from horizontal up to 60
> degrees.[35]

The clean bullet wounds of a generation earlier gave way to muti-
lating excavations of limbs from high-energy rounds and artillery shell
fragments. To compound the problem evacuation and transport of the
wounded who survived this carnage completely overwhelmed resources.
Injured men lay for hours, sometimes days, in battlefields next to their
rotting, stinking, dead comrades in soil teeming with Welch's spore-
forming rods. Fire from the enemy was sometimes so intense that any
movement was hazardous. Only under the cover of nightfall could a
maimed soldier crawl to a point of safety and await the arrival of evacuation teams—if they ever came. In field hospitals behind the front lines,
there was no room for them, either. Millicent Leveson-Gower, Duchess
of Sutherland, as a volunteer with the Red Cross on the frontiers, recalled
the nightmare of those early days of the war:

> All the evening the wounded and the worn were being rushed
> in. If they had come in tens one would not have minded, but
> the pressure of cases to attend to was exhausting. . . . So many
> of the men were in a state of prostration bordering almost on
> dementia . . . the men had been lying in trenches outside the
> forts. Hundreds of wounded, we believed, were still waiting
> to be brought in, and owing to the German cannonading it
> was impossible to get near them.[36]

On the borders of France and Belgium, during four days of combat
from August 21 to 25, 140,000 Frenchmen fell.[37] At the Marne River, as
British and French forces desperately fought to stop the German advance
on Paris, 85,000 French troops alone were lost, 90 percent of casualties
the result of shell fragments.[38] That icon of French surgery Edmond
Delorme admitted that "there were battles which were almost nothing

but artillery combat." Filthy, torn flesh, macerated muscle, and mutilated limbs dominated in men who made it back. Surgeons were dismayed and ill prepared for the volume and severity of infectious problems that followed. Faced with the carnage now before him, Delorme, like a shepherd amidst his slaughtered sheep, was dumbstruck at the sight and did an about-face, pronouncing, in September 1914, that "shrapnel and shell fragments were vehicles to drive dirt, mud, and clothing into wounds."[39] These injured men were injected with filth, and filth that seeded infection. Their bullet holes and violated flesh could no longer be ignored as harmless matters. To delay was fatal. Yet, many injured had been so neglected for so long that wounds teemed with deadly pathogens. Volunteer American surgeon Harvey Cushing heard after the Marne battle the *ilitar* (French for "wounded") were stuffed into cattle trains and laid out on straw without food or water for two days or longer; their maimed limbs were in frightful shape when finally disembarked.[40]

Ominous reports began to appear describing grisly gas-forming infections—pain, swelling, purplish skin discoloration, giant blisters, and early signs of sepsis—pallid, sunken-eyed victims mumbling incoherently and barely able to hold their head up. Patients died with remarkable alacrity. The whole picture resembled Cramp's civilian series and was given the foreboding label *gas gangrene*. What concerned surgeons was how fast changes came on and how rapidly they progressed. In some cases, despite carving away patches of dead tissue—even amputating affected limbs—the disease spread beyond. One author commented that, after the Battle of the Marne in the autumn of 1914 "there could hardly have been a military hospital where one or more cases of gas gangrene were not observed."[41] Although not required to report such infections early in the war, rough data from German field hospitals suggested approximately 2 percent of their wounded developed some type of gas infection, and with the mounting numbers of casualties, this became a distressing complication for surgeons already swamped with torn limbs, fractures, and human frames peppered with shrapnel.[42]

It was all a nightmare. One alarmed doctor saw that in some of those wounds of arms and legs neglected for twenty-four or forty-eight hours, the pulped muscle, devoid of circulation, gave birth to sprouting anaerobic colonies. Before long, the site would take on a menacing appearance, "a curious half-jellified half-mummified sort of look. Then the whole wounded limb begins to swell up and distend in the most extraordinary fashion, turning, as it does so, first an ashy white and then a greenish color." It was as if the limb was decomposing before his eyes. It would have a sickening, crunching feel when pressed. "The gas and the swelling extend on up over the surface of the body, bloating it." As for the patient, he becomes restless, full of dread. "His face is white and pinched, his lips bluish . . . Small wonder that both surgeon and wounded stood aghast at such a swift and deadly process of destruction when it first began to show its horrid front." The victim would likely be dead in twenty-four hours. [43]

Perfect conditions abounded for this sort of thing. "In the early period of the war . . . everything was in its [gas gangrene's] favour," wrote British major general William G. Macpherson in his medical history of the war. "In the retreat from Mons [August and September 1914] there was no possibility of early surgery. The ambulance trains were defective, evacuation difficult and the journey to base long." [44] Medical personnel soon began to recognize the process, tipped off by a smell that they could not dismiss. A volunteer remembered: "In one case the bullet passed clean through one leg and exploded in the other. Bah! The smell of the gas gangrene—shall we ever forget it?" [45] And volunteer surgeon George Crile, serving with the American hospital in Paris early in the war, lamented that the fever, rapid pulse, delirium, unconsciousness, and death were unassailable. "No specific treatment has yet been found . . . the mastery of this disease is for the future," he remarked in 1915. [46]

But mastery could not wait. A new breed of 20th-century bacteriologists set to work. Michel Weinberg had studied under the great Russian pathologist Élie Metchnikoff at the Pasteur Institute in Paris. [47] Under Metchnikoff's tutelage Weinberg's career in microbiology skyrocketed, and he was appointed *chef de laboratoire* at the Pasteur Institute in 1910. In a patriotic flair, Weinberg joined the military in 1914 and served as aide major, a rank usually given to medical professionals. His reputation allowed a posting at the military hospital in Issy-les-Moulineaux, a Parisian suburb. It was there that he heard about the rampant gas infections on the western front and made it his mission to investigate. He wasted no time. By October 1914 he had his data and delivered a report to officers of the British Expeditionary Force. Weinberg had identified twenty-four cases of some type of gas-forming infection: sixteen cases of gas gangrene and eight cases of what he called gas phlegmon—a sort of gas-infused inflammation. Most of his cases, both gas gangrene and gas phlegmon, had a "constant" presence of the bacilli of Welch, which he now called *Bacillus perfringens*. However, he had discovered other types of bacteria as well: diplococcus, *Bacillus proteus*, staphylococcus, and streptococcus. The wounds were loaded with germs. And they were mostly the type found in the human gut and expelled in feces. In Weinberg's opinion, "the earth of the trenches from which the wounded with gas gangrene most often come, is soiled by human excrement and animal manure." Even the clothing, he was convinced, swarmed with these gut bacteria. Was it Pasteur's same *Vibrion septique*, the culprit in livestock anthrax? Weinstein doubted. Similar, but not the same. Microbiologist Alexander Fleming, working independently with the renowned British scientist Almroth Wright in Boulogne and with the Belgian surgeon Antoine Depage at his seaside *ambulance* in La Panne, agreed.[48] Welch's *Bacillus aerogenes capsulatus* (the *Bacillus perfringens* of Weinberg) literally coated the uniforms of the wounded men and inhabited practically all wounds within seven days (although not always associated with clinical infections).[49]

The mud and dirt of France's farms were the culprit. Soon soldiers' feces, expelled in abundance, and the decomposition of innumerable corpses—bloating, splitting, and rotting—mixed in. The western front had become a cesspool and, like passing livestock, human soldiers in their squalor and muscle-pulping injuries would be unwilling hosts for the life cycles of invisible microbes. Stagnant trench warfare exposed soldiers to a constant contamination of clothing, eating utensils, canteens, and weapons with earthen aggregates of hostile, disease-causing germs. Historians would later reflect on the opening days of war: "men were commonly a couple of months or more without the chance to take off their trousers. They were literally covered from head to foot with clay and earth and mud."[50] Lacerating and macerating shell fragments ripped into limbs with such force that tissues were either torn asunder or minced—ideal foodstuff for anaerobes. Delay and neglect were unwitting catalysts. Wounded lingered for days near the battlefield. Wounds festered. Gangrene commenced. And surgeons provided the neglect—at first either ignorant or overwhelmed—not yet aware of the dangers of pathogens that saturated the battlefields or the power of munitions that tore into their young victims.

GASBRAND

Indeed, bacteriology would become one of the pivotal technologies of World War I. It all stemmed from the ability to peer into the invisible. From his single-lens microscope in 1675, Antonie van Leeuwenhoek's had identified minute *diertjes* (translated from Dutch as animalcules or microbes). In just over two centuries, the elaborate laboratories of Pasteur and Koch discovered invisible creatures responsible for such enigmatic ailments as cholera and diphtheria. Diseases now had causes, not just upset humors or deranged ethers. And now the onset of war brought into play the gigantic laboratory of the battlefield. Not a few German physicians looked upon the utter butchery as a massive bacteriologic experiment.[51] Here was a chance to unravel the mysteries of infection, the bane of surgery and the festering demon of wounds. Of all pestilence in those early days, though, none was more enigmatic than gas gangrene. Germans had recognized its virulence as well. Gas infections stunned their medical professionals. These rancid ailments were inundating the *Kriegslazaretten*—field hospitals—in all manner of appearances. The common denominator was creeping gas in the tissues and swollen, discolored skin. They were called any number of names: *Gasbrand, Gasgangrän, Gasphlegmone*, or *emphysema malignum*. "Infections so virulent," it was said, "that they progress rapidly from the point of infection and lead to sepsis in spite of the widest incision." Amputation was the only hope, and the earlier the better. Doctors were bewildered. By March 1915 some were expressing deep concern about the lethality of it all. Alexander von Rothe, former assistant surgeon at the Charité in Berlin, was one of them:

Above all, the *gasphlegmone* [my italics] shows an absolutely malignant picture. It progresses not only locally in a few hours, deep to the fascia, along vascular and nerve sheaths, or superficial under the skin, but also causes a tremendous reduction of the general condition at high temperatures. If you have seen the whole picture of the disease only once, it will not be forgotten. It is so characteristic.[52]

After all, Germans lived and fought in the same mud and manure as their enemies. Fraenkel's stubborn little spores patiently waited for them, too, until summoned aloft on spinning shrapnel to inhabit the interstices of freshly battered muscle. Among gardens of barbed wire wounded Germans also languished listless and half-alive in the same no-man's-land— sometimes for days—longing for stretcher bearers to find courage and snatch them away. They, too, were carried, their limbs the appearance of a long-dead corpse's, to haggard surgeons almost asleep on their feet.

Fearful of the spreading process, surgeons opted for extreme measures. Advisory surgeon for the German Tenth Corps Walther Kausch quickly understood the lightning nature of *Gasphlegmone* and the need for "urgent amputation." Even then, he acknowledged, *Gasphlegmone* cases of the *foudroyant* variety "kill despite immediate radical operation." Fellow surgeons, too, agreed that those at risk were ones who lingered on the filthy battlefields with neglected wounds, often in heat, rain, or cold. Some had spent up to four days half-buried in manured earth before help arrived.[53] At a meeting of German military surgeons in Brussels in 1915 Hermann Kümmell, surgeon-in-chief at the Allgemeinen Krankenhaus in Hamburg, brought results of over 200 cases of *gasphlegmone*. Almost one-third had died. He, too, recognized the preponderance of Welch's bacillus—in Germany referred to as *Herr* Fräenkel's bacillus (Fraenkel's *Bacillus phlegmones emphysematose*, and maybe identical to Weinberg's *Bacillus perfringens*)—and assumed this microscopic invader was the cause.[54] Others were sure, as Weinberg had found, that many of these infections were a mixed bag of disease-causing bacteria—and not just anaerobes. Hermann Coenen, an understudy of Ernst von Bergmann in Berlin prior to the war, even considered that the presence of "putrid pathogens" or common streptococci acted as catalysts for Fraenkel's bacillus—in the most extreme cases—as it attacked muscle compartments and contributed to the "tremendous speed" of progression of *Gasphlegmone*.[55]

It was bizarre and unpredictable. Just as Cramp had shown years before, not all cases were fatal. Some gas infections remained confined to a small area or quickly responded to surgical therapy. In their attack, surgeons made bold strokes through skin and fat, opening concealed injuries to air, allowing oxygen to suffuse damaged tissues. Recovery often followed. Other infections were deeper, into muscle, turning it from healthy crimson to a cadaveric gray. These were different, a deadly course more likely. What bacteria were causing these? Were they all the same? Was Fraenkel's bacillus the inveterate offender? Austrian surgeon Erwin Payr thought so. He collected a variety that caused edema and a copper discoloration of the skin, but did not seem to penetrate into muscle (he called it *epifascial*). This acted in a benign fashion. Recuperation was the rule if treated by surgical incisions and exposure to air. But there was another, a malignant variety, that arose deep in muscle, turning it into a mousy, chocolate-brown mush, full of gas pockets. Too soon the patient was prostrate, in shock, and headed for the grave. The course was so rapid that therapy was almost useless. Even dismemberment proved futile,[56] the host little more alive than the discarded, decaying limb.

Physicians and scientists alike were baffled. Germany's best academicians could not agree. Even the fastidious Eugen Fraenkel himself admitted confusion in terminology—and etiology. He insisted, though, in his stern fashion, that the diagnosis of classic *Gasbrand* (gas gangrene) be only allowed if his bacillus—the *perfringens* bacillus of Weinberg (and Welch)—could be seen in wounds. In fact, Fraenkel eventually confirmed that his bacillus was found in one third of cases of classic gas gangrene. This bacillus, he was now convinced—and he would never be dissuaded—was the major agent in classic *Gasbrand*. Other types of "gangrene," cases where there was little gas in the tissues and not as much muscle destruction might be caused by different bacteria.[57] Some of his countrymen were still not convinced. In typical ordered German thinking, the learned pathologist Ludwig Aschoff would propose a grouping of the various species of anaerobic bacteria as suggested by the Harvard professor James Simonds in 1915. Simonds had used markers of fermentation as a way to distinguish these bacteria and so group them into three classes. In one of these he categorized the likely culprit in classical gas gangrene (the one found by Welch, Fraenkel, and Weinberg)—in addition to a few others. The anthrax bacillus of Pasteur and Koch was different, he felt, and was put in another category entirely. While the minuscule bacilli of Welch and Fraenkel (and Weinberg) were clearly dangerous in humans, some were not so much.[58]

By their own investigations, the French agreed. Surgeons André Chalier and Roger Glénard insisted that classic gas gangrene "is an anatomo-clinical entity, which should not be confused with any other gangrenous or gaseous infections of wounds of war." To be sure, there were other conditions that caused gas to form in tissues—inflammation from various types of infections or severe trauma. But the hallmark of gas gangrene was rapidly advancing muscle necrosis. "The infection appears to us to be born in the contused, crushed, frayed muscles, and it is from there that it spreads deeper or to the surface according to the cases."

Work in the laboratory seemed to confirm what was being seen on the battlefield. Henri Tissier, a researcher at the Pasteur Institute, had corroborated this. Many wounds festered with a veritable litany of microbes, anaerobic and aerobic species. Experimentally, it could be proven that the virulent gas infections all too often had a mixture of pathogens in addition to the dominant anaerobic varieties. "The aerobes play a capital role," he said. Furthermore:

> In order to reproduce in the guinea-pig fortunes similar to those presented by our wounded, it is necessary not only to inoculate crushed tissue, but also to employ cultures of our anaerobe and aerobic mixtures, to reproduce in a word, what is goes into the wounds of war . . . B. *perfringens* and enterococcus mixtures killed the guinea pig in three days; [*Bacillus perfringens*] with staphylococcus in 24 days; and [*Bacillus perfringens*] with true streptococcus in 15 hours.[59]

Within twenty-four hours the contaminated wound was swarming with bacteria of all types, Tissier found. But eventually, the dreaded *Bacillus perfringens* predominated. Yet it seemed particularly potent in the presence of other bacteria, notably the streptococci, as if their aid and abetment was instrumental in lethality. These tiny round streptococcal bacteria wept a toxin that dissolved blood vessels and allowed the wiggling *perfringens* access to the blood. It was there that the poison they produced paralyzed small arteries and weakened the heart until its limp pumping was to no avail and blood simply stagnated, nutrient oxygen hanging impotently on red blood cells unable to deliver. It was then that death began.

This was the condition that produced those typical symptoms and signs in humans: severe, unrelenting pain; swollen, purplish discoloration of the skin; the characteristic but rank odor from the wound; and the air pockets giving that crunching sensation when pressed upon—*crepitation gazeuse*—from gas streaking through the tissues. The course was all too familiar: a rapid illness producing pallid features, rapid breathing, and an appearance that speaks of impending doom. Doctors and nurses stood helpless, almost able to see the advancing menace marching up arms or legs and taking over the entire body. Death followed within a day or two, sometimes sooner, the pulse diminishing, the heart weakening, and all vitality fleeing.[60]

RUTHLESS SURGERY

More and more cases accumulated in those first months of the war. These were sorry creatures, their limbs the bloated pictures of decomposing cadavers. The only hope for the stricken? "Get the wounded as soon as possible, within the first ten hours if possible, into the hands of a surgeon." Delay in doing so was as much of a danger as the bacillus itself.[61]

Surgery must be quick and uncompromising. German surgeons described it as *unbarmherzig*, "ruthless." After watching rampant gas infections spread from leg to trunk, one sobered practitioner advised: "with such experiences of the most rapid propagation, there is only one possibility left, that is, in every case of *gasphlegmone* [classic gas gangrene], to carry out amputation each time."[62] And the master surgeon Delorme, now dismayed by this new warfare, in a pragmatic if not wordy postwar treatise, instructed surgeons faced with cases of gas gangrene, "who have been witnesses of the state of shock or depression of the wounded with massive gangrenes, who know the hopelessness of the septicemia, the operative act must be, in these cases, precipitate and summary." In other words, amputate early and radically.[63] In some limbs so removed the dead muscle tissue was still full of grass, dirt, and straw, attesting to the violence of the weapons.

Even then, recovery was not assured. For some reason and at some point the bacillus even attacked healthy muscle. Toxins spewing from the bacteria literally digested *any* tissue. Under the microscope, muscle fibers from amputated limbs could be seen in various stages of deterioration, and the minuscule rods spreading throughout like torrents of speckled invaders. For that reason, amputated stumps were left open and watched. All looked nervously for signs of advancing gangrene.[64] Nurses knew the sequence and the futility of treatment:

> Rochard died to-day. He had gas gangrene. His thigh, from knee to buttock, was torn out by a piece of German shell. It was an interesting case, because the infection had developed so quickly. He had been placed under treatment immediately too, reaching the hospital from the trenches about six hours after he had been wounded. To have a thigh torn off, and to reach first-class surgical care within six hours, is practically immediate. Still gas gangrene had developed . . .[65]

But who to amputate? Many wounds of legs and arms healed without delay. How could anyone tell which soldier would be stricken with the deadly gangrene? Small skin breaks from tiny shell fragments might harbor massive muscle injury. Weapons were so much more deadly—speeding, spinning bullets or shell splinters absolutely demolished human tissue and bone. Clothing, dirt, and grass driven inside might not be apparent when the soldier was first examined. Some cases, laying unattended for hours or days, were obvious. They already had the smell and stigma of gangrene—that sweetly sickening stench. For them the choice was clear. Cut and likely amputate. For others options were less decisive: watch and worry, or amputate. Surgeons who had seen the ravages of gas gangrene took no chances. Amputations abounded. During the course of the war, 41,000 British alone would return home with missing limbs. [66]

On occasion, cooler heads prevailed. Certainly, these wounds could not be ignored. The precepts of Delorme in 1914—those calling for *abstention*—had to be discarded. Even Delorme recognized that. But to amputate so many? French Fifth Army surgeon René Lemaitre had a better idea. Unable to tell by examination which wounds were dangerous, he switched to a series of bold, deep incisions, a technique called *ilitaries* by the French, in which the knife sliced through skin, subcutaneous tissue, fascia, and into the deep muscle layers of a traumatized limb. Once opened up he looked and felt and smelled. Any dead tissue he removed. Pieces of garments, bullets, shell fragments, loose bone chips, blood clots, and dirt he pulled out. The wounds were washed out and left gaping. He then applied his bandages. For the four thousand cases he treated this way fewer than forty needed a later amputation, he claimed. In more obvious cases, those smashed and barely attached limbs, he fell on them with scalpel and saw, as quick to lop off as any surgeon.

While Lemaitre's selectivity had appeal, it was a time-consuming process. And the surgery itself, the cutting and probing and cleansing, was backbreaking. The numbers of wounded men staggered surgeons who often worked to the point of collapse. Cases filled their operating spaces, emptied, then filled again. Georges Duhamel, a surgeon around Verdun in 1916, operated in a haze on one pitiful creature after another:

> Many men came to us with one or several limbs torn off completely, and they came still living . . . Some had not one but thirty or forty wounds and even more. Sometimes there was not even enough time to wash and undress men before operating. Surgery would be done through caked mud and dirt and vermin. [67]

Yet, Lemaitre's *ilitaries* gained popularity. Surgeons could agree it was better than amputation. The pleas of men about to lose an arm or leg depleted their equanimity. A revolution in wound care had begun.

◆

French surgeon Alexis Carrel would propel it forward. An imposing figure, Carrel was a man of forceful attention. His close-set eyes peered below a skeptic's brow; a countenance analytic, intolerant of frivolous traits, his address to the camera one of probing intensity. He was an analyst through and through. Carrel had already achieved international notoriety for his work in suturing blood vessels together. This had been a major stumbling block in the far-fetched idea of organ transplantation. Carrel remedied that hurdle with his clever techniques of connecting small arteries and veins.[68] In fact, it had earned him the Nobel Prize in Physiology or Medicine in 1912.[69] Fame notwithstanding, he had become disenchanted with his native France long before. At about the same time as his groundbreaking article on vascular anastomosis was published, he was caught up in a controversy of a different nature, one quite unworldly and seemingly the antithesis of science. After witnessing and testifying to the cure of Marie Bailly from tuberculous peritonitis at Lourdes in 1902, he seemed to have a spiritual transformation. Miracles, he had said before, were distinctly unscientific. "Physiologic laws oppose miracles," he wrote, adding, "to the scientific mind a miracle is an absurdity." But, privately, Lourdes had made him a believer. Prayer indeed can hasten recovery, he had seen. "The only condition indispensable to the occurrence of the phenomenon [miracle] is prayer," he averred. His report on Maire Bailly, which appeared in the local paper *Le Nouvelliste de Lyon* in early June 1902, was incriminating. He freely admitted he had no ready explanation for the sudden improvement of this patient, also witnessed by two other physicians. About the Bailly affair, Carrel was originally quoted as saying:

> Alas, medical science is not infallible and we would have been
> naïve to ask it for more than it can admit, that is to say, in

> contradiction. It [science] is stunned in the presence of such
> cures and we understand its amazement.[70]

Suspecting that such statements would jeopardize his academic potential, he tried to retract his comments, but it was too late. *Le Nouvelliste* would have none of it, quoting again Carrel's comments above. Carrel now took on the mantle of a "Lourdes sympathizer" and lost favor with academia. It seemed attempts to distance himself from Catholicism only fueled the scandal that he was more inclined to clerical apologism than the prevailing positivist sentiment now rampant among the scientific elite of the Third Republic. Such metaphysical nonsense as absurd reports like Carrel's was anathema to organized academia. Anticlericalism marginalized and effectively banished him from university appointments. Indignantly, Carrel fled his homeland to Canada and, finally, to the United States. New York and the Rockefeller Institute were his ultimate destinations, arriving in 1906. He did not escape criticism from his countrymen, however. Animosity at his defection still prevailed and would hound him in all his accomplishments. After mastering the art of vascular suturing, Carrel's work at the institute switched to the healing of wounds—the reparative effort of the body disrupted. He had already generated a number of research studies on the subject.[71] Was it the miraculous events of Lourdes that pulled him in? "The miracle is chiefly characterized by an extreme acceleration of the process of organ repair," he wrote later. Perhaps he could never really clear his mind of the marvelous happenings bestowed on the soulful masses trudging to Lourdes.[72]

And then war erupted. For Carrel and his newfound interest, the timing was impeccable. Tugs of mother country and scientific curiosity meshed and took him swiftly overseas. For one so concerned with the restoration of ravaged tissue and the healing power of diminutive inflammatory cells and oxygen and nutrients, and the dastardly effects bacteria wrought, it was a human laboratory. Were it not for the horrid tragedies that abounded, France's holocaust would be a biologist's playground.

Carrel volunteered for the French Medical Corps. Assigned to duty near his hometown of Lyon, he was shocked by what he then saw. "The slaughter at the beginning of the war, the gravity of the wounds, the serious infections which ensued, the suppurations amplified by the heat, the delay of transport, [leading to] multiple amputations and deaths . . . care was deficient and the Service de santé was overwhelmed."[73] What bothered him most was the absolute rancor of gas gangrene. "We are powerless to prevent gas-gangrene, for it is impossible to sterilize the wounds." He was determined to find a treatment—and to set up his battlefield laboratory. Carrel wanted scientists, technology, and physicians within reach of the front, all talking, sharing, and collaborating. "The solution [to wound healing] will be found only by the combined labors of trained men working together to this end," he maintained.[74] A system of care applied to every patient was the answer. There must be standardization. Success in dealing with wound infections, Carrel had said, "may be due partly to the skill of our surgeons and nurses. I want to be sure that the treatment in an ordinary hospital is efficient. A surgical method is practical only when it can succeed in the hands of unskilled and ignorant doctors."[75] Treatment of wounds at the front in shanty hospitals should be the same as in the academic halls of Paris.

Carrel turned to his friends at the Rockefeller Institute. In 1915, a bookish British chemist by the name of Henry Drysdale Dakin developed a solution of sodium hypochlorite buffered with boric acid that, when applied to organic substances, formed chloramines and became a potent antiseptic agent, particularly against skin flora like staphylococci and streptococci. It even killed the now-infamous *Bacillus perfringens*.[76] Dakin had been working in the private laboratories of New York pathologist and socialite Christian Herter. Herter himself was an acquaintance of John Rockefeller Jr. and had set up research laboratories in his own home. After Herter's premature death in 1910 at age forty-five, Dakin was kept as head of this laboratory and would eventually marry Herter's widow, Susan Dows Herter, in 1916.[77] It was this connection with the Rockefellers that enabled Dakin to travel to France at the onset of the war and link up with pioneering surgeon Théodore Tuffier at the Hôpital Beaujon in Paris. It was in Paris that Dakin finished his work on antiseptics. As it turned out, Tuffier knew Carrel, having worked with him in 1914, also at the Rockefeller Institute, on cardiac valves.[78]

Carrel had developed a deep respect for the tall, slender surgeon whose piercing eyes and pointed goatee gave the impression of fin de siècle elegance. More importantly, Carrel respected Tuffier's intelligence and true scientific acumen, not influenced by simple tradition or presumption. Tuffier also shared Carrel's concern about infection in the wounded, and the common belief that some better form of therapy was necessary if the horrible gangrene seen in field hospitals was to be averted. It was Tuffier who brought the two—Carrel and Dakin—together to begin their work on wound care. Carrel thrived with the synergy, impressed immediately by the imposing, dark-complexioned, and mustachioed Dakin, who began work at once sifting through possible candidates for antisepsis.

In collaboration, Tuffier supported Carrel in his quest for a specialized research hospital to investigate better forms of surgery and antisepsis.[79] In February 1915 Carrel managed to convince his Rockefeller connections, the capitalists James Hazen Hyde and Henry James, to equip his own hospital for research on the outskirts of Paris. With Tuffier's ability to cut through French bureaucracy, Carrel found the Rond Royal at Compiègne, a former resort hotel on the edge of the scenic Forêt de Compiègne ("nothing could be more peaceful and lovely than a well-groomed French forest in the early spring," the American surgeon Harvey Cushing would later comment[80]). The French government approved, and the Rockefeller Foundation supplied $20,000. Carrel's hotel-cum-hospital, crystal chandeliers, painted ceilings and all, was renamed Hôpital temporaire no. 21.[81] It was only nine miles from the front. With accomplice Henry Dakin in tow, Carrel assembled other members of his team: chemist Marcel Daufresne and surgeons Georges Dehelly and J. Dumas. Doors opened in early March but not before he had procured thirty-five topflight nurses from the famed École d'infirmières de la Source in Lausanne, Switzerland.[82] There would be no shortage of infected cases. Wards were soon lined by beds whose occupants were tethered to rubber tubing with hanging bottles of Dakin's disinfectant bathing their wounds.

By that October, he already had enough data to present his findings to the Académie de médecine, that official paragon of scientific worthiness. His technique would be radically different. "The trust in use of iodine and the *emballage* [packaging] of wounded is fading," Carrel claimed. "Experience has shown that shrapnel wounds, mines, torpedoes, and grenades are all infected, and that the applications of iodine do not prevent gaseous gangrene, septicemia, or endless suppuration." His treatment would be different: First, a careful examination, then exploratory surgery like Lemaitre had championed, then washings with Dakin's new hypochlorite antiseptic solution. In fact, after making those broad, deep cuts—*débridements*—Carrel then laid rubber tubing directly inside the gaping crevasses and dripped through Dakin's solution around the clock. When infections were no longer a threat, after a few days, the tubing was removed and the skin sutured together.[83]

Not everyone was convinced. A ranging debate took place the following January at the meeting of the Société de chirurgie in Paris. It was partially political. Carrel's decamp to America and failure to acknowledge his French heritage when accepting the Nobel Prize in 1912 had not been forgotten. And in any event, some were not so sure that his elaborate method held much promise. One such critic was a respected Parisian surgeon by the name of Edouard Quénu, who argued that:

> The improvement in the evolution of wound [care] . . . does not depend on the use of this or that antiseptic, it is due to the precociousness of debridement and cleaning, it is due to this fact that the wounds are six or seven hours from their injury to the ambulance where they find a good surgeon who is current on war surgery, who explores the wounds, opens them and removes the projectiles as soon as possible. [84]

Carrel, not one to be easily dismissed, had an immediate response. "The men who criticized us so severely have taken the trouble neither to examine our methods nor to check our results," he indignantly retorted. Carrel was a perfectionist who had little time for ignorance and incompetence. His technique was a meticulous, careful plumbing of tubing into the depths of the wound and a religious infusion of his precisely formulated Dakin's solution. All must be applied exactly. It was his method, and a method even unskilled doctors could use. The key was adhering to the minutest of details and doing it the same way every time—standardization of care. If not, shame on the imbecility and pomposity of maverick practitioners. He had no time for them:

> The deplorable results obtained in several hospitals by surgeons who believed they were using our methods, but, who, in reality, were altering them according to their fancy, make clear the necessity for observing exactly the directions . . .[85]

There was one disciple who was convinced—and who could follow directions. The Belgian surgeon Antoine Depage had set up an expansive military hospital near the seaside at La Panne in West Flanders, financed by the generosity of Belgian King Albert and Queen Elisabeth. Depage was a cornerstone of Belgian surgery. In fact, he was instrumental in forming the Société belge de chirurgie (Belgian Surgical Society) in 1901 and running hospitals near Constantinople during the Balkan War of 1912. It was there that he began to understand wound care and the importance of thorough and careful surgical exploration of injuries. Later, as president of the Société Internationale de Chirurgie in 1914, his address *"Les enseignements de la chirurgie de guerre"* ("Instructions on the surgery of war") detailed difficulties surgeons encountered near the front lines, where, typically, few resources were found to effectively clean wounds. The results were too often disastrous infections. After his Balkan War experience he made it his mission to somehow improve care for these fresh injuries.[86] Socially, it seemed the distinguished Depage and his wife had also developed a personal friendship with King Albert and the queen. Such acquaintances had deep pockets that Depage did not hesitate to exploit. The result was a sprawling hospital complex named Ambulance de l'Océan. When Depage heard of Carrel's method, he was intrigued. He had already witnessed the horror of gaseous infections among his Belgian patients. Amputation could be curative but was also disagreeable—and irreversible. There must, he felt, be a kinder approach. Like Lemaitre, he was fond of *débridement*, that surgical art of examining and selectively paring away damaged tissue. Then, learning of Carrel's and Dakin's concoction, he began flooding the opened tissues, destroying any bacteria left behind.[87] It all worked so well that the likes of Carrel, Dakin, and Depage spread the word across France's battlefields like modern-day apostles. Thorough *débridement*, open wounds, and delayed closure of skin became standard treatment of war injuries, not only during the Great War, but World War II, Korea, Vietnam, and all future conflicts.

For Depage, he, too, would suffer the evils of war. His wife, Marie, returning from a visit to the United States to promote Belgian relief, drowned with the sinking of RMS *Lusitania* by a German submarine off the coast of Ireland on May 7, 1915.

Across no-man's-land the Germans, too, searched for solutions to deadly infections. *Feldlazaretten* steadily filled with hapless men harboring wretched wounds, fertile flesh for *Gasinfektion* (gas infection). Like the French, doctors were too eager to amputate, only to find most limbs were free of the gas menace. Treatment had to change, but festering anaerobic germs inhabiting deep muscle layers needed purging. Their experience with the Carrel-Dakin method had been hopeful. Few physicians felt there was anything better than Dakin's antiseptic. Comments like those of field surgeon Georg Ahreiner were commonplace: "this much is certain, that the Dakin's solution of all available wound care products fulfills the biological requirements [of antisepsis] and through its vitalistic properties that are associated with the not to be underestimated conservation of tissue."[88]

German ingenuity contrived other provocative methods. A popular treatment of gas gangrene—their *Gasinfektion*—was the so-called hyperemic protocol of August Bier. Bier had become an accomplished surgeon in Berlin and, as personal house physician, had attended the likes of Kaiser Wilhelm II and family members of Nicholas II of Russia. Prior to coming to Berlin, he had been professor of surgery at the University of Kiel. It was there that he developed an interest in the restorative powers of inflammation. This led to the development of his hyperemic protocol in 1903. In Bier's reasoning, inflammation ushered in an increase in blood flow (hyperemia) that brought nature's restorative elements into play, one of which was to fight infection. Why not produce this artificially, then? He would call it *Hyperämie als Heilmittel* (hyperemia as a treatment). The principle was to stimulate more blood flowing into the wound to mimic inflammation. Would this not deliver all the same bacteria-fighting agents as inflammation did? He increased circulation by use of elastic bandages or bands (*Stauung-Hyperämie*), cupping, or even hot air.[89] In some instances, Bier recommended the use of cataplasms: poultices pasted on the skin to instill heat and boost blood flow. His favorite was the use of linseed flour mixed with warm water applied to the wound. What was the result? Bier claimed that his patients who had *Hyperämie* treatments did better. With a combination of surgery and *Hyperämie* a mere fraction of patients died, compared to over half who had surgery only.[90]

Some military surgeons embraced Bier's curious method. One of the more vocal ones was Anton Thies, who used a modified Bier technique. He applied intermittent compression to the injured limb in rhythmic cycles of sixty and ninety seconds on and off to stimulate hyperemia. He called it *rhythmischen Stauung* (rhythmic compression).[91] Like Bier, Thies did not abandon surgery. And he did not believe every discolored limb concealed gas gangrene. For those cases where the limb was swollen, tense, and bluish, surgery was essential. Muscle was likely infected and dead. But for the others, ones with a less offensive brawny edema, he applied his rhythmic compressions. Overall, Thies was pleased. "I am convinced that this method of treatment [cyclical compression] is of great importance in the fight against *gasphlegmone*," he later wrote.[92]

And, as the war progressed, there was the popularity of antisera— serum containing agents of destruction (we now know them as antibodies) for the harmful products of certain bacteria. Tetanus, called lockjaw, was another dreadful infection striking wounded soldiers early in the war. The condition, caused by a different soil-borne anaerobic bacterium, the tetanus bacillus, was perpetrated by a toxin from the bacteria, a substance so vile as to possess its victim; almost always fatal and extremely painful to endure. Three in four afflicted would perish. In some hospitals on the western front all died. Muscle spasms seized the patient, arching backs in otherworldly contortions and literally locking the jaw to prohibit eating, drinking, or even talking. Through clenched features, patients would shriek in agony until the merciful end. Two students of Robert Koch,

Emil von Behring and Kitasato Shibasaburo, developed an antitoxin serum from horses inoculated with the deadly poison. They had stumbled onto the principles of immunology, that molecules could be fashioned to specifically attack invading venoms, what Kitasato would call *diese giftfeindliche Wirkung* (these antitoxin effects). "The properties of destroying tetanus toxin are absent in the blood of animals that are not immune to tetanus," Behring and Kitasato had found. It was this neutralizing substance that chemist Paul Ehrlich named *Antikörper* (antibody) in 1891. As for the tetanus antitoxin, it had been a miracle agent, routinely given to injured soldiers and essentially ridding the hospitals of this ugly disease. [93]

Could not the same principle be applied to the bacillus of gas gangrene? By 1917, Americans Carroll Bull and Ida Pritchett at the Rockefeller Institute had determined that the fatal consequences of infection with *B. perfringens* lay in its poisonous agents dribbled into the bloodstream. There was some optimism that, at least experimentally, animals could be protected against the bacteria after receiving the toxins themselves—similar to Behring's process of immunization for tetanus toxin. They were now *immune*. Something similar had happened in Germany. In 1916, Oberarzt (Senior Physician) Franz Klose, working at the Kaiser Wilhelm Academy in Berlin, isolated a toxin he considered responsible for the lethal effects of invasion by Fraenkel's bacillus (of course, meaning *B. perfringens*): "it was pleasing to present a toxin of the Fraenkel's gas bacillus, the absorption of which is said to be the main cause of the deaths of experimental animals and humans," he wrote in a brief essay in April. [94] His preliminary work was so convincing that the huge German laboratories of Farbwerke Hoechst began manufacturing a bactericidal antitoxin from horse serum to combat gas gangrene. The antisera was then to be distributed on a large scale to field units. However, production lagged and only a small amount was ever sent. Even then, its effect was unpredictable and not very consistent. More work was needed. [95] Still, results were far from convincing. Even though Klose was a believer, he had to temper his remarks when presenting what scientific data he had:

Thus, I believe that with a polyvalent, antitoxic-bactericidal *gasodem* [gas gangrene] serum, the surgeon is given an effective weapon in the fight against the anaerobic wound infection caused by the *gasodem* bacilli; its use, but only in conjunction with professional surgical measures, will let us finally to master this war disease.[96]

Rockefeller researchers Bull and Pritchett remained unconvinced. They could not duplicate Klose's results and wondered about his research methods. In their hands, antisera to *B. perfringens* toxin had only modest success. At the Pasteur Institute in Paris, Weinberg felt antisera had only a limited role in treating gas gangrene. By 1918, understanding of gaseous gangrenous infections pointed, in many cases, to what was called a polymicrobial environment. More than one type of bacterium interacted to produce the extensive skin and muscle rotting and eventual toxic course so characteristic. One vaccine against one bacterium might or might not work. Only in selected situations, and if given early, before much toxin was released into the bloodstream, did scientists see a benefit in preventing life-threatening illnesses.[97]

METAMORPHOSIS

There were to be many nightmares of the Great War. Gas gangrene was certainly one of them. The infection was so sudden, so dramatic, and so lethal that it soon became a demoralizing problem. Men would be segregated into separate hospital wards for fear of contagion as if the Black Death were upon them. Those wards would reek of smelly putrefaction. Doctors and nurses entered with trepidation. The soldiers themselves dreaded the possibility. Daily, they would question caregivers about their injuries, fearful the creeping rot had appeared. German Oberstabsarzt Carl Franz felt that, in the early days of the war, "the frequency . . . was so great in places that gas gangrene had been described as the crisis of military hospitals." In terms of its psychological impact on soldiers and surgeons, indeed it may have been. Yet, despite its graphic nature and lethality, the infection itself had an inflated importance. The numbers of afflicted men were surprisingly low. In raw figures, for the French, of the 2,052,984 wounded, 10,337 are recorded as having developed gas gangrene, 3 percent of all infectious complications. The Germans, too, reported gas infections as an infrequent happening. Franz, in his compilation of wound infections following the war, published that, regardless of theater of combat, individual accounts generally totaled less than 0.5 percent of all wounded (to be exact, 0.24–0.34 percent from Northern France, Austria-Galicia and Russia, and Serbia). Even German field hospitals on average encountered no more than a fraction of one percent of wounded who developed gas-forming infections.[98] Once infected, though, the death rate skyrocketed. For the French over half of these cases died.[99]

Yet, gas gangrene led to a revolution in the way war wounds would be treated. A coming together of scientists and surgeons brought an understanding of cause and a rationale for therapy. Disorganized as those first months were, disjointed as research efforts might have been in the chaos of modern war, the eventual discourse among laboratories and field hospitals resulted in a combination of techniques that, if done in a timely manner, could completely abrogate the occurrence of gas gangrene.

Those early efforts of Pasteur and Koch in bringing to light the destructive force of invisible microbes, the doggedness of Welch and Fraenkel, and the ingenuity of Carrel and Depage proved to be catalysts in shaping modern treatment of battle injuries. In fact, some portrayed Alexis Carrel's work as a miracle of science—as surely mystical as the marvels of Lourdes. Perhaps not so supernatural but rather the consequences of brilliant minds and masterful detective work. In the words of historian Dennis Shanks:

> Medical science was progressing, and got drawn into the maelstrom of World War I. Medical laboratories . . . were deployed with the armies. Top research physicians joined the war as uniformed specialist consultants. World War I marked a key transition towards scientific medicine.[100]

Without doubt, modern weaponry stimulated change. Destructive forces not hitherto encountered forced surgeons to reassess treatment paradigms: old models rooted in wars of the previous century gave way to new templates that would carry battlefield surgeons into the next century. Fundamental in this metamorphosis was the treatment of the myriad injuries to arms and legs, so common and survivable on battlefields, but so disastrous if neglected. The energy imparted now from exploding artillery and blistering bullets inflicted horrible damage on fragile human tissue. Stricken in inconceivable numbers over hundreds of square miles of battlefield, wounded soldiers were operated on by thousands of surgeons. Only a handful understood the complexities of gas gangrene. This in itself was the wonder of Carrel's work, that treatment could be simple and standardized in such a way that any surgeon could master the art. New strategies unfolded, no longer simply the constructs of empiricism alone. Now they were wedded to the foundations of laboratory science and the wisdom of assembled clinical evidence. The famous New York surgeon and academician Lewis Pilcher reflected on these changes in his presidential address before the American Surgical Association at war's end:

> It is most notable that steadily from the beginning to the close of the conflict in every line of effort, better and better results were being secured and more successful responses to the emergent needs of wounded men were being made.[101]

Battlegrounds of the western front would remain Pasteur's cursed fields, but the bacteria residing within would now be recognized as the shadowy agent of this human decay called gas gangrene. Thanks to the scientific work of the likes of Pasteur and Welch and Fraenkel, the ingenuity of Carrel and Dakin, and the standardized practices hammered into ranks of ordinary military surgeons, the limbs and lives of those victims in the trenches and strung across the pocketed landscapes of Belgium and France would immeasurably benefit from the modern machinery of medicine. Even the later advent of antibiotics that could directly kill microbes such as these would not replace the quick and meticulous cutting away of infected tissue and the restoration of life-giving blood flow to that which remained. This was still the key to survival for countless numbers of soldiers (and, in more tranquil times, civilians) subject to the horrendous trauma of gunfire and the other accidental menaces of urban and rural life. Truly, the rudiments of wound care had been reckoned in the filthy trenches of the Great War.

FIVE

"Gas, Gas, Gas!"

"Get back, you bastards!" "Gas turning on us"
"Keep your heads, you men!" "Back like hell, boys!" . . .
"What's happening?" "Gas!" "Back!" "Come on!"
—British Soldier-Poet Robert Graves, 1929

In his final report of America's war effort in Europe in 1919, General John Pershing, commander in chief of the American Expeditionary Forces, cited three major developments of the World War: aviation, armored tanks, and chemical weapons. The horrid chemical gas attacks had captured everyone's attention, though. "Whether or not gas will be employed in future wars is a matter of conjecture," he wrote, "but the effect is so deadly to the unprepared that we can never afford to neglect the question."[1]

From the standpoint of psychological effectiveness—if not the sheer agony of its victims—the chemical agents were the most frightening offensive weapons used, even though they actually produced a minority of casualties. Fear of suffocating from noxious fumes, the fumbling to find and put on the awkward, hot, claustrophic gas mask, and the apprehension of fighting oncoming enemy troops in this confining gear made it more of a psychological weapon than a physical one. Nevertheless, if not prepared, troops could, in fact, die a ghastly asphyxiating death, literally drowning in their secretions, or feel blinded and blistered by the effects of oily mustard gas. This new form of warfare, thrust on the scene in 1915, demanded a quick Allied response at all levels: governments, industries, and medical professions.[2] It was a crisis of the first magnitude that threatened to revolutionize warfare.

As the 19th century drew to a close, the evils of war magnified with development of new weapons and, even more important, by a willingness of state power to exert violence on soldiers and civilians alike. During the brief but violent Franco-Prussian War of 1870–71, the city of Paris and its civilian population had come under indiscriminate bombardment, resulting in the death of hundreds of Parisians. With the fall of Paris and its German occupation, Prussian retribution accelerated. Their targets were "non-conventional" (irregular) militia called *francs-tireurs* (snipers). Pogroms rounded up innocent populations, at times bordering on genocide. In their defense, Germany claimed that, with the defeat of the French Army, this was now a guerilla war where combatants were indistinguishable from civilians. Was this to be the face of "new" war: the bloodthirsty killing of troops and civilians alike? Was it to be a form of ethnic cleansing much like medieval hordes ransacking and slaughtering populations of conquered foes?

The Franco-Prussian War put neighboring countries on alert. An uneasy peace settled in, but nations bristled with new weapons of destruction, each striving for superiority in a 19th-century arms race. In an attempt to defuse tension, Russian Czar Alexander II convened a conference in Brussels in 1874 to discuss, of all things, proper behavior during times of war. There had already been a conference in 1868—also convened at Russian invitation—in Saint Petersburg, Russia, to "humanize" warfare. One of the items resolved was the ban on explosive small-arms bullets, a first step in condemning certain types of weapons. At the 1874 Brussels meeting, the international delegates who attended displayed surprising benevolence by forging restrictions on state power. Violence to civilians was a strict violation of their "new" order of warfare. Total war and reprisals against innocents were condemned. The Brussels Declaration of 1874, as it would be called, comprised fifty-six articles outlining expected behavior of belligerents, combatants, and noncombatants; means of injury, sieges, and bombardments; and the treatment of prisoners of war and the sick and wounded.[3] All hoped it would be the foundation for international humanitarian law as the world headed for the 20th century, as if, somehow, war could now be construed as civilized.

Then, in a move tailored to embellish the humanitarian works of his grandfather, Alexander II's grandson, Nicholas II, convened another session in May 1899, inviting participants of the 1868 and 1874 meetings. This would be known as the First Hague Peace Conference. Encouraged by the two previous conventions, Nicholas hoped further progress would be made in promoting placid coexistence and limiting unbridled weapons development. Could there, in fact, even be "rules of war"? While many attendees frittered away their time in flirtatious self-absorption, important items were brought up: submarines, projectiles launched from kites and balloons, dumdum bullets, and "asphyxiating gases." In particular, chemical agents prompted a heated debate. Inhuman, deplorable agents, diplomats maintained—abolish them. Hogwash, the American delegate, Navy Captain Alfred Thayer Mahan retorted. Poison gases were no more abhorrent than submarine warfare, the silent killing of innocent seafarers by torpedoes that could sink merchant vessels in minutes. Besides, Mahan pointed out (perhaps too prematurely) chemical weapons were not even available yet. Mahan, in all his eloquence, was voted down. Bombs from balloons, dumdum bullets, and poisonous gases were forbidden (submarines were not). Germany, France, and Austria-Hungary said as much. The United States eventually agreed.[4]

But war would ever be far from humane. Diplomats in all their noble talk were pushed aside by militants more intent on conquest than diplomacy. August of 1914 saw to that. And then industrialized weaponry—unfettered and unabashed by humanitarian concerns—would be unleashed. German U-boats would sink sickening numbers of civilian ships. The prohibition of explosive bullets did nothing to affect the devastation of huge high-explosive artillery shells or the mass murder inflicted by the rapid-fire machine gun. And as for poisonous gases . . .

In the late afternoon of April 22, 1915, on the Ypres front near Bixschoote, 168 tons of chlorine gas in billowing ashen clouds were released from over 5,700 German cylinders against two French divisions, the Eighty-Seventh Territorials and the Forty-Fifth Algerians, caught in their trenches totally by surprise without any type of mask protection.

French *tirailleurs* (light infantry) climbed out of their dugouts and ditches panic-stricken, coughing, choking, and clutching their throats. For a time, the front lines crumbled, but, despite the fogs of gas, reinforcements were quickly brought forward to shore up defenses. At the same time Germans who had reached the French trench works saw that chlorine fumes had lingered, sinking to the bottom of dugouts, and were fearful of any further advance. Yet they corralled 1,800 bewildered French prisoners, and 70 machine guns.[5] Frustrated by their blunted initial poison gas attack and with the winds still favorable, Germans let loose a second wave of chlorine, this time against neighboring Canadian troops (Forty-Eighth Royal Highlanders). Once again, the suffocating vapors drove not a few Canadians from their trenches but many held on, using gauze as improvised gas masks and somehow turning the German tide with the loss of only a few hundred yards of turf. Animals were less fortunate. Cattle died at a distance of four thousand to five thousand yards from the front lines.[6]

The price paid by Allied troops to stand their ground in these attacks was heavy. "When we got to the French lines," one German soldier wrote, "the trenches were empty but in a half mile the bodies of French soldiers were everywhere . . . Some had shot themselves. The horses . . . cows, chickens, everything, all were dead."[7]

It was not long before the public took notice. Gas inspired fear among the civilian populations of England. What if the Germans delivered poison gas to the isles, inflicting the asphyxiating substance on the women and children of London? The Allied press was quick to condemn. Disgust even spread to neutral America. From the *New York Tribune*, April 27, 1915:

> The gaseous vapor which the Germans used against the French divisions near Ypres last Thursday, contrary to the rules of The Hague Convention, introduces a new element into warfare. The attack of last Thursday evening was preceded by the rising of a cloud of vapor, greenish gray and iridescent. That vapor settled to the ground like a swamp mist and drifted toward the French trenches on a brisk wind. Its effect on the

French was a violent nausea and faintness, followed by an utter collapse. [8]

It was barbarism, the press bitterly claimed. Totally inhuman and opposed to any laws of chivalry, if indeed that term any longer applied to modern warfare. Hyperbole dominated the British periodicals (as it later turned out). The sights of gassed men were "awful, fighting and gasping for breath," so the propaganda flowed. The *New York Times* reminded its readers of Germany's pledge not to use asphyxiating gases at the Hague Peace Conventions and that "it is still binding on Germany."[9] The slow strangulation of struggling victims was a picture of pure torture, far worse, it seemed, than to be dismembered by shell fragments or cut in half by machine gun bullets.[10] Of course, for Americans there was little reason to doubt the contentions of the Allies.[11] Germany's transatlantic cable had been cut by the British at the onset of war.[12] Her response to accusations of barbarism therefore went largely unheard. Nevertheless, Berlin did respond, and those who were able to listen heard the indignant German claim that, alas, the French actually used poisonous gas first, even bringing forth a memorandum from the French Ministry of War justifying such use (Berlin also touted Mahan's view that gas was not inhumane).[13] Nevertheless, the Ypres experience was, indeed, an ugly affair. American Harvey Cushing, touring field hospitals in Flanders in 1915 witnessed firsthand the effects of gas. He saw gassed men at a casualty clearing station in Bailleul and shuddered at the sight:

> Then we saw many of the severely "gassed" men who had come in this morning—a terrible business—one man, blue as a sailor's serge, simply pouring out with every cough a thick albuminous secretion, and too busy fighting for air to bother much about anything else—a most horrible form of death for a strong man.[14]

It did not escape the scientific literature either. The effect of chlorine vapors was graphically described in publications shortly after the initial attacks around Ypres. The fumes, almost always described as having a greenish hue, caused sudden onset of choking, coughing, gasping for breath, and inability to speak. Soon, if inhalation continued, headaches appeared, the legs became weak, and many affected individuals simply fell to the ground. Chest pain was crushing, victims' tracheas horribly inflamed. For those dying in the first few hours, the patient himself turned a greenish-yellow color, lapsing into a quiet stupor, the agony of breathing lessening until there was none at all. For those who survived the first few hours, some would succumb in the next few days from progressive air hunger—their breathing extremely rapid, sometimes up to sixty times a minute, and shallow—pulmonary tissue destroyed. The patient suffocated for lack of oxygen, his lungs filled with edema fluid until he literally drowned in his own secretions. Asphyxiation was the official term used. And then there were those who survived still longer but eventually died of pneumonia bacteria that invaded the inflamed, naked respiratory architecture—a likely death sentence in days before antibiotics.[15] How deadly was it? Studies done later in May on chlorine-gassed victims showed that of those caught in the thick of the cloud, without protection, almost one quarter would die within thirty-six hours. Not counting the immediate deaths, few died afterward, perhaps five out of a hundred.[16] A terribly toxic weapon? From the standpoint of lethality probably not, but as the mastermind of German chemical weapons Fritz Haber sardonically (but truthfully) said: "all modern means of combat, though they seem to be aimed at the death of the enemy, in truth owe their success only to the vigor with which they momentarily shatter the psychic power of the adversary."[17] It was not hard to get the common soldier to agree. A young British private in the Machine Gun Corps admitted, "I was terrified of gas, to tell you the truth. I was more frightened with gas than I was with shell fire."[18]

Yet, the Allies were hardly blameless in all this. And Ypres was not the first use of poisonous gases in the First World War. If Germany could have explained—and the world could have heard—there was more to the story. At the beginning of the war, the French had a small stock of projectiles called *cartouches suffocantes* (suffocating cartridges)—lachrymogenic agents (commonly now known as *tear gas*) filled with ethyl bromoacetate, a tearing substance that can have deadly effects if inhaled (yes, in violation of that Hague convention). These projectiles were actually fired by rifles and mounted as rifle-grenades. In fact, Parisian police attempted to extract the notorious anarchist gang led by Jules Bonnot from their lair in the suburb of Choisy-le-Roi in April 1912 using such weapons.[19] They were again used early in the war, from a reported stockpile of thirty thousand—and not very effectively—against fortifications on the western front to flush out enemy troops. The French were undeterred and insisted their *cartouches suffocantes* had a place on the battlefield. In a bold circular distributed in February 1915, French minister of war Alexandre Millerand urged the use of both hand grenades and rifle grenades. They were irritants, he claimed, and not meant to kill:

> It will never be necessary to use it in the open country or in high winds. At optimum distribution it takes about one [grenade] per meter to make a trench untenable. Its effectiveness will be especially felt in the attack of covered trenches, blockhouses, shelters and houses.[20]

Germans tried using similar lachrymogenic agents in October at Neuve-Chapelle but the vapors only caused mild irritation and sneezing. There was worse to come. The French had learned that the Germans were developing more dangerous chemical weapons to use in explosive shells or in "unbreathable" gas clouds. They needed to find a way to protect their troops from the German gas. Offense was the best defense, and they opened studies to perfect their own poison gases. Tearing agents were only bothersome. They wanted lethality, like asphyxiation from deadly fumes. In fact, chlorine held promise. But, at the time of the gas attacks at Ypres, they were only in the earliest stages of development.[21]

The Germans were ahead of the game. They had already tried using artillery shells filled with xylyl bromide, another lachrymogenic agent, against Russian troops at Bolimów on the eastern front in January 1915. Over eighteen thousand shells were fired, but it was so cold the liquid could not vaporize, and the whole affair was a stunning failure.[22]

Undeterred, Ypres was next; and it proved a modest success, but showed complete ignorance on both sides. The French had no protection and were caught naked-faced to the fumes. German tactics did not follow through and advantage was lost. But the gas itself had worked. Just as Haber might have predicted, troops lost their composure and will to fight. Many simply dropped their weapons and ran off, coughing and gasping. On the other hand, Germans were leery of the lingering poison fog, and were afraid to run headlong after the fleeing French. Experience on both sides would shortly come.

The incensed French wasted no time in responding. Millerand instructed André Kling, director of the Laboratoire municipal de chimie de la ville de Paris to take the lead in investigating the Ypres incident. There were two parallel priorities: provide protection for troops and mass produce gas of their own. Kling wasted no time. The gas used at Ypres was chlorine, he found. Troops had to be protected by some type of filter over nose and mouth.[23] First attempts were hurried and, at best, primitive. Soldiers were told to soak their socks in urine and wrap them around their face—the urea in urine neutralized the chlorine. This would probably only work if the alternative was death. More practical (and pleasing) means followed. The French adopted a German method of cotton pads (muslin) soaked in thiosulfate to be placed over the face as soon as the gas cloud was detected. Within a month 500,000 of these had been sent to Flanders.[24] But the French were determined to blow some gas of their own. They intensified efforts to develop lethal chemical weapons—no more tear gas—so that by May they had field tested their own brand of chlorine gas. Paul-Louis Weiss, director of mines, had already assembled a commission, and by August chemists, engineers, and military and medical personnel were hard at work.[25] Under the direction of Army Général Paul Ozil, the Service du ilitari chimique was officially established that September and remained active until the end of the war. Ozil's organization had full responsibility to design and produce chemical weapons, the protective gear necessary, and delivery methods such as artillery shells.[26] One year later, they had delivered 230 tons of chlorine gas alone.[27]

Yet, without doubt, top priority was protective gear. Soon work on designing mask respirators covering the entire face took precedent. Mining respirators provided the template. Much of the work had already been done by the Dräger company in Lübeck, Germany, before the war. Bernhard

Dräger, son of the company founder, working in concert with Lübeck surgeon Professor Otto Roth, in 1902 had developed the first anesthetic respirator system to deliver oxygen and chloroform or ether. This morphed into a self-contained breathing apparatus of particular use in submarine and mining disasters. In fact, the self-containing respirator, created with Swiss physician Ernest Guglielminetti, saved numbers of trapped miners in the notorious Courrières mine disaster of 1906, allowing French rescuers, wearing the device, to access the depths of gas-filled chambers. Combining science, technology, and industrial innovation, the Dräger family expanded their footprint, and by the time of the war had the facilities and capabilities to mass produce their respirators, now adopted for use on the western front.[28] By 1915, the Dräger company introduced modifications to address portability and effectiveness against chlorine. Frontline troops, especially the specialized pioneers responsible for the Ypres gas release, were equipped with the Dräger HSS (*Heeres Sauerstoff Schutzapparat*—army oxygen protection apparatus), also known as the Dräger Selbstretter (self-rescuer), or, more colloquially, the *Gummimaske* (rubber mask). The device was elaborate: a system of a breathing apparatus, air circulation through a potash cartridge, and an exhalation channel. Oxygen was also introduced via a separate cylinder. The whole affair was strapped on with headgear, mouthpiece, stopper, straps, and nose plug.[29]

Based on principles put forth by the Drägers, by 1916 the French had perfected their respirator called the M2. The M2 was a cloth mask that covered the entire face. It contained layers of cheesecloth to filter out chemical agents. Two mica (cellophane) eyepieces gave a hazy, distorted view. The whole apparatus supposedly could be worn up to five continuous hours. Almost thirty million were manufactured and distributed to French, British, and American troops. Later models, called ARS masks (*appareil respiration special*), had a cylindrical filter filled with activated charcoal that hung like an amputated elephant trunk and had the same two mica lenses as eyepieces.[30] It was similar to the German mask, the Dräger *Gummimaske*. The British designed one of their own, the "small box respirator" or SBR. This was a three-piece device consisting of a rubberized, tight-fitting mask with eyepieces connected by a hose leading to a canister filled with filters and absorbents. The entire apparatus was fitted into a front-worn haversack.[31] It might have been effective but was not popular with the troops. One had to clip his nose while breathing into a mouthpiece. Troops complained that they were claustrophobic even to the point of breathlessness. If worn for more than a few hours it all became unbearable, and many a man simply removed the mask, preferring to take their chances in the open. Peering through his eyepieces, one British officer felt he had become part of a troglodyte world:

> We gaze at one another like goggle-eyed imbecile frogs. The mask makes you only half a man. You can't think. The air you breathe has been filtered of all save a few chemical substances. A man doesn't live on what passes through the filter—he merely exists. He gets the mentality of a wide-awake vegetable.[32]

No "gas mask" would ever be acceptable—neither the French M2 nor the ARC nor the SBR. All were tight-fitting, close, and humid. The mere act of inhaling and exhaling took on enormous importance so that any other activity was an additional strain on energy and, after a time, sanity. Hand-to-hand combat, even firing a weapon, was almost ridiculous. The temptation was to simply to throw it off, sit down, and wait to be gassed. That was the point of the weapon, of course. If not lethality, then demoralization.

And what should the doctors do with these cases? There was no antidote. There were no remedies. Physicians had an almost impossible task. No number of platitudes or amount of hand-wringing seemed to help. Asphyxiant patients were most troublesome—and most frustrating. Yes, keep them warm and comfortable. Beyond that, a number of treatments were tried that bordered on quackery: subcutaneous oxygen, atropine, ammonia, brandy, caffeine, camphor, morphia, aspirin, strychnine, bloodletting. All to no clear benefit. The only measure of some value, it seemed, particularly in lung cases, was oxygen by inhalation. "We just laid them out in the field, in great long lines," one British frontline physician recalled, knowing there was no amount of hospital space for them. It was easy to tell the gassed. "There was froth coming out through their nostrils and their mouths." He then went on:

We had plenty of oxygen, plenty of rubber tubing. It ran like
an irrigation system. We had tubes running between the files
of men, their heads towards the main tubes, head to head in
two lines . . . we stuffed a fine tube up the nose of every man
and kept the oxygen running . . .[33]

But supplies were limited. Oxygen cylinders were quickly depleted,
larger sizes sucked dry within twenty minutes.[34] If pneumonia set in, the
poor fellows were almost doomed. Georges Duhamel saw one such creature in a forward *ambulance* at Verdun. "His eyes had quite disappeared
under his swollen lids. His clothing was so impregnated with the poison
that we all began to cough and weep, and a penetrating odor of garlic
and citric acid hung about the ward."[35] What to do but watch and wait?
Would the breathing turn to rattling hisses, the skin darken to purple,
the thrashing for air turn manic, the pulse slacken? Would death then
consume its captured prey?

In retaliation for the Ypres gassing, the British released over 5,200
canisters of chlorine gas (almost 150 tons) at German troops around
Loos, Belgium, on September 25, 1915. But a fickle breeze blew it back
on the Tommies and failed to affect German lines. A few whiffs of fumes,
maybe, but mostly the Germans shrugged it off. Unaware, over the top
the Tommies went in usual parade-ground fashion, counting on dead,
gassed Germans in the trenches. No such luck. Germans opened up their
machine guns. It was a massacre. Some British units suffered 60 percent
casualties. It was so pitiful that Germans mercifully withheld fire on the
beaten, retreating men.[36]

Certainly not an auspicious start for the Allied gas campaign.
However, Germans were still enamored with the stuff. They had more
gas attacks in mind, several before the end of 1915—mostly chlorine
clouds released from canisters. But in December they brought in a new
agent—phosgene. Phosgene proved even worse than chlorine. It was
almost odorless but sometimes gave off a mildly pleasing aroma, like
new-mown hay. There was no immediate eye irritation like chlorine
or tear gas so that the victim could inhale quantities before symptoms
appeared—and before he put on his mask. But soon throat and lungs

rebelled. Coughing, sputtering, foaming, and breathlessness took over. The casualty simply collapsed, writhing and gagging. Shortly, if no help arrived, frothy pink sputum came up. Then lips turned blue, the skin cyanotic. The outcome in many cases was suffocation.[37] Germans released tons of it. So much so that in places vegetation turned yellow, farm animals dropped, and even the hearty, ubiquitous trench rat succumbed. One American doctor saw countrysides absolutely blighted:

> Blasting and withering every living thing, grass, leaves, garden crops along the whole of its front to a depth of two or three miles, and killing birds, insects, and small animals, three and even four miles behind the front trenches![38]

Even worse, phosgene had the added disadvantage of seeping through protective masks. It was poorly absorbed by purifying cartridges, or, being odorless, inhaled before troops knew it was in the air. Many were nighttime attacks, so sudden and unexpected that men, despite the availability of respirators, were caught in the open, sleeping, without protection.[39]

It was on December 19, 1915, that the Germans first used phosgene, in that same desolate, war-torn sector of the Ypres salient. More German gas attacks followed the next spring and summer, chlorine and phosgene both. It was a nightmare for the poilu. The French Thirty-Fourth Division trench newspaper *Le Filon* described the sense of impending doom brought on by gas clouds:

> With the clouds, death envelops us, impregnating our clothes and bedding, killing everything living around us, everything that breathed. Little birds fell into the trenches, cats and dogs, our companions in misfortune, lay down at our feet and did not awake.[40]

Summer of 1916 saw new tactics: poison gas delivered by artillery. Shells loaded with chemical agents were fired along the broad expanse of the combat zones, their dull thuds in distinct contrast to ear-splitting high explosives. Usually it was a mixture of both, the bang obscuring that telltale soft thump, which liberated toxic vapors. Explosive charges spread the gases even wider. Now, with the "whoosh" of incoming rounds, no one knew what was dropping. Marshalling trenches and artillery units far behind the front lines were favorite targets. All had to don masks. The French were the first to try it, firing off quantities of shells at German positions around Arras in June to silence troublesome artillery batteries. Germans quickly followed. Almost 110,000 gas projectiles fell on French entrenchments near Verdun the night of June 22, 1916. Over 1,600 poilus, mostly artillerymen, were gassed. Germans used a mixture of poisons in their shells: phosgene, diphosgene (another asphyxiate), and agents to induce vomiting that penetrated the fabric of masks. Soldiers became ill, tore off their masks to vomit and inhaled rich mixtures of chlorine and phosgene. The Germans called one of these nauseating gases, diphenyl-chlorarsine, *Maskenbrecher* (mask-breaker). [41]

And so it went now. Back and forth toxic gases were tossed. It became another reality of the battlefield, an almost commonplace terror. The limp puff of gas shells sent bug-eyed soldiers scrambling into their khaki satchels to put on gear and take cover. Even artillerymen were masked, working on the big guns and toting massive shells under the duress of smothering headgear. But what everyone dreaded more was the fright of chemical poisoning. So feared was the threat of suffocation that a type of psychological terror developed. "Gas neurosis," it was called. Even when not really gassed, soldiers felt the symptoms—shortness of breath, cough, lacrimation—and it panicked them. Doctors saw blatant anxiety, gasping for breath, clawing at the throat, attacks of delirium or stupor, stuttering, hyperventilation. All seemed out of proportion to the amount of gas inhaled. [42] Just the threat of a gas attack turned on hysterics in the trenches. British soldier-poet Robert Graves captured such a moment:

> This [suspicion] of gas attacks caused a continued scramble backwards and forwards, to cries of: "Come on!" "Get back, you bastards!" "Gas turning on us" "Keep your heads, you men!" "Back like hell, boys!" . . . "What's happening?" "Gas!"

> "Back!" "Come on!" . . . We were alternately putting on and
> taking off our gas-helmets, which made things worse. [43]

Commanders fired their cannons incessantly, the sickly smell of chlorine or the odorless stifling of phosgene fitting punishment for enemy gunners. The numbers of gas shells grew almost exponentially. Germany, France, England, and the United States would stockpile 6, 5, 2, and 12 percent respectively of their artillery arsenal with gas shells. Eighty-five percent of the casualties produced from chemical agents were caused by artillery gas shells. In fact, toxic gas shells were responsible for more casualties than those filled with high explosives. [44]

On July 12, 1917, Germans, never at a loss for experimentation, sent over a new chemical agent that would transform gas warfare—dichlorodiethyl sulfide. British troops called it mustard gas because the crude material first used by the Germans smelled like mustard or garlic. It would be called "Yellow Cross" by the Germans and "Yperite" by the French. "The introduction of 'mustard gas' (dichloroethylsulfide) was probably the greatest single development of gas warfare," wrote Brigadier General Amos Fries of the United States Chemical Warfare Service. [45] Asphyxiating agents such as chlorine and phosgene had reached their zenith and, thanks to improved masks and troop discipline, their effectiveness was on the decline. Mustard would be different. Once again, the Ypres sector would be the proving ground. Mustard shortly became so popular that it was the principle battle gas of the rest of the war. Actually, mustard was not a gas at all but an atomized liquid dispersed in a fine spray by an explosive charge. It was different than other agents. Mustard had the advantage of penetrating clothing, including rubber and leather. Rather than damage strictly by inhalation, which, of course, it surely could, it settled on skin and other mucosal surfaces and ate away the lining cells to cause blistering. Skin burned and blistered just like the delicate coverings of trachea and bronchi in the lungs and the membranes of eyes. Nothing happened right away. There was no burning or coughing. Soldiers were completely unawares. Only in the course of an hour or two did symptoms develop. Eyes became inflamed, painful, soon swollen shut.

Victims feared blindness. At the same time the irritant, if inhaled, started the same inflammation of respiratory linings. Many times pneumonia followed. Skin soon blistered—like second-degree burns, exquisitely painful.[46] Troubling was the ability of mustard to soak through clothing and to linger for days where it was deposited, unseen on grass, trees, even dirt of the trenches. Around Ypres, for the first few weeks of shelling with mustard gas, over fourteen thousand victims filled British casualty clearing stations, and five hundred died.[47]

Sadly, it brought chemical warfare to new heights of inhumanity. Britain and France scrambled to manufacture the substance, quickly realizing its usefulness and, of course, needing to reestablish battlefield parity. The French chemical weapon industry took on the task with exceptional vigor. Under Général Ozil, thirteen laboratories, led by Charles Moureu, focused on "offensive research." Two of these chemists, André Job and Gabriel Bertrand, developed a new, albeit dangerous, method of manufacturing mustard in November 1917, much faster than the German way. By spring, industrial production began, and daily outputs of mustard-loaded 75 mm artillery shells shortly reached 10,000. By mid-June, French were lobbing mustard all over the western front. British guns followed soon after.[48] By the end of the war, France was producing over five hundred tons of mustard gas per month, faster than the artillery could fire it. Charles Moureu sacrificed no hauteur when he boasted that "[Germany] did not suspect it, and we did not doubt ourselves, what we were capable of. And in truth, our chemical successes are the most brilliant illustration of the miraculous faculties of this nation."[49] Noxious gas vapors soon dominated Allied battlefield strategy and tactics.

Germans were not far behind. High command prepared huge stores of gas shells ready for Kaiserschlacht, their spring offensive of 1918. Almost 6,500 cannon of all calibers delivered a ferocious preinvasion bombardment of five hours' duration on March 21, letting loose over one million rounds. By estimates, one quarter of their projectiles were gas canisters. Against artillery positions, gas shells topped high explosives by a ratio of four to one.[50] Germans had an arsenal from which to select: Green Cross (chlorine, phosgene), Blue Cross (diphenylchlorarsine, an asphyxiate and vomiting agent), and Yellow Cross (mustard). Their tactics were predictable: first, Green Cross shells to paralyze enemy artillery; Blue Cross agents, designed to penetrate gas masks, against machine gun nests; Yellow Cross shells to disable troops beyond front line trenches. [51] For mustard, rear lines and staging areas were the targets, to scatter reinforcements. Mustard shells were also sent to saturate hiding places: woods, villages, billeting areas, even roads—anywhere troops might settle. Germans even mixed gas with high explosives, Green and Blue Cross shells for infantry, and Yellow Cross for artillery. [52] Chemical agents primed every aspect of offensive operations. [53]

The American Expeditionary Force (AEF) arrived in late spring 1918 as unwilling beneficiaries of these new tactics. They would enter combat at a time of maximum German effort to capture territory, and maximum stores of gas weapons. Gone would be the days of static trench warfare. The AEF would witness a war of maneuver and offense, with battle naked and in the open and more dangerous even than past clashes on the western front.

The United States was ill prepared for a European war. The report by the secretary of war in 1917 reflected the woefully inadequate manpower, equipment, sustenance, munitions, and training. Chemical warfare capabilities were even worse. Despite invectives by the secretary of war to the surgeon general of the army, William Gorgas, requiring "the study of defense against gas attack and the preparation of such gas masks and other appliances as can be devised to minimize its effect," nothing had been done—anywhere. [54] There was no official acknowledgment of the development and manufacturing of offensive gas weapons as part of the general stockpile of munitions. In Gorgas's report back to the secretary of war for that same year, gas warfare was not mentioned, either in the procurement of equipment or training of men. Nor were protocols for care of gas victims provided. Not one word about gas.

Thankfully, someone was paying attention—Van Manning, director of the Bureau of Mines. Established in 1908, the bureau had maintained an active interest in noxious and volatile gases in mines, and had already done much work in the development of self-containing breathing devices (gas masks) such as the Dräger-class respirators. As war loomed,

Manning was quite willing to offer what resources and knowledge the Bureau possessed to the government. Eagerly accepting, Washington appointed consulting chemist George Burrell of the bureau as chief investigator of poisonous gases and set up his research laboratories at the American University in Washington, DC.[55]

Research began in April 1917, headed by Manning. He had a number of urgencies: protective gear, protection in trenches and dug-outs, and the manufacture of America's own poison gases. As for gas masks, he chose the British SBR as a template, and began to make his own. Over twenty thousand of those masks would be ready for the first elements of the American Expeditionary Force leaving for Europe. Equally important, thousands of young soldiers needed education and training in gas warfare. That task fell to the Army's Medical Department. Quite unfamiliar with battlefield training in nonmedical issues, the procurement and use of gas masks proceeded in an awkward and halting fashion, yet gave soldiers some degree of acquaintance with the cumbersome devices. Eventually the Army Medical Department would hand over much of their work to the Chemical Warfare Service, organized in May 1918. The Chemical Warfare Service was a new agency, the brainchild of the War Department, and a direct consequence of ever-consuming Allied interest in gas agents. The service now comprehensively covered chemical warfare, branching into divisions for training, research and development, medical care, and production. Anything having to do with gas warfare would fall under its purview.[56]

As poorly prepared as they might have seemed, it was certainly not that the Army was unaware of the promiscuous use of poison gas by both sides in Europe. In fact, they appeared well informed. "The employment of poisonous gases as a means of offensive warfare has made it imperative that medical officers should have some knowledge of the action of various gases that are likely to be met with," so began the War College's *Memorandum on Gas Poisoning in Warfare*, issued to the Medical Department in May 1917, shortly after war was declared. The memorandum discussed the types of gas used by Germany, namely chlorine and phosgene, the symptoms that developed, the treatment necessary, and even the pathological lung changes that occurred after inhalation. Had doctors heard any of this before? It was all scary stuff but possibly the first information shared with American medical officers about chemical agents. Did anyone else understand? The American public was clueless, at least in 1917. Aside from the outcry of protest in Germany's use of chlorine in 1915, citizens—more concerned with neutrality—tried to ignore the viciousness of France's western front. Brazen disregard for international prohibition of such arsenals was condemned, to be sure, but with Allied retaliation (played down in the media) the entire topic had been swept under the rug. Still, Washington and, in particular, Manning were aware. With entry of the United States into the war, defense from gas attacks was a palpable concern. Military preparedness was lacking in so many areas, but the beginnings of a chemical initiative slowly gathered momentum.[57]

And the British were certainly concerned about American preparedness. In October 1917 the chemical adviser for the Third British Army and his selected group of men, as part of the British Military Mission, visited the United States and shared information on chemical munitions and protective equipment. It was imperative, in their opinion, that American troops be properly trained. After all, they knew firsthand the disastrous effects of terrified soldiers under gas attack, and Yanks would likely be on their flanks.[58]

In the interim, to support his expeditionary force, the new American commander, General John Pershing, set up a "Gas Service" in September 1917, under the command of an engineer, Lieutenant Colonel Amos Fries. Fries's Gas Service would bring in the Medical Department, now focusing on the education of medical officers to treat gas casualties. Fries rounded up the Army's version of the British SBR, to be manufactured in quantity in the United States.[59] The Chemical Warfare Service had provided Pershing with the First Gas Regiment, an incorporation of the Thirtieth Engineers as a field unit that would specialize in conducting his chemical warfare.

Yet, by late summer 1917 there were about twelve thousand troops, mostly of the First Infantry Division, the "Big Red One," within thirty miles of the front lines without gas masks or gas training. John Pershing's entire First Infantry Division, four infantry and two (soon to be three) field artillery regiments, bivouacked within harm's way without the slightest notion of chemical warfare. Those twenty thousand masks manufactured in the United States finally arrived in August but were totally unsatisfactory—a major letdown for American ingenuity. With some quick interchange, the decision was made to simply use the British SBR and the French M2 masks as standard issue. One hundred thousand of each were somehow procured in time. And gas training was begun in earnest for Pershing's doughboys at their marshalling site at Gondrecourt, south of Verdun. Major General Robert Bullard, commander of the First Infantry Division, recalled, "Gas was such a deadly and insidious thing that gas training for the protection of the men was carried out almost continuously. It was about the hardest thing for our people to learn."[60] Soldiers were repeatedly schooled and drilled. Mask drills happened daily. Infantry training exercises were conducted with masks on.[61] American boys hated the contrivance. A marine colonel with the Fourth Marine Brigade had his special take on it:

> A gas mask, by the way, is a thing one is anxious to take off at the first opportunity. It is a hot and stifling thing and seems to impede the faculties. The wearer takes in the air through his mouth, after it has been sucked through the purifying chemicals. His nose is not trusted and is clamped shut. Imagine yourself fighting with a clothespin on your nose and a bag over your mouth and you may be able to get some notion of what a gas mask is like.[62]

Still, even after that effort, as men of the Big Red One marched into the line around Ansauville in the Verdun sector at the end of January 1918, large numbers came without their masks. They had either lost them in the march or, in the case of the French M2 mask, got them wet. Their French counterparts were furious. They knew how vital mask discipline was. Panicking American troops, breaking ranks, could crumble the entire line, a disaster in the making. This was especially so in that the Ansauville sector had seen a large number of chemical shellings, mostly with mustard. Masks were replaced, training intensified, gas discipline enforced. Drill, drill, drill. "The enemy employs gas for two purposes," they were told, "to inflict casualties . . . taking advantage of ignorance, bad discipline, faulty training . . . [and] to reduce the fighting efficiency of our forces by compelling them to wear masks."[63]

What happened at Ansauville that February and March was typical of first-time exposure of American units to gas warfare. Unbeknownst to the arriving doughboys, Ansauville had been a quiet sector, but active in gas bombardments. Even more provocative, General Bullard did not wait to be attacked. He was itching to test his men and to try out his artillery. On February 1 he instructed batteries to fire at will with gas shells. And that they did, firing over 250 rounds at German artillery. This obviously rankled the opposing Germans, who were only too willing to reply with the hordes of gas shells at their disposal. They answered with over eight hundred rounds per day, many gas, for the rest of February.[64] It was a blanketing, poisonous artillery duel.

But nothing like the morning of February 26. Cannon of the German Seventy-Eighth Reserve Division opposite the Americans delivered a saturating bombardment launched from mortar-like projectiles, such as the 25-cm, 17-cm, and 7.6-cm *Minenwerfern* (trench mortars), into a wooded segment of the division's position. Gas of such intensity was released that "the suddenness and the violence of the attack, coupled with the overwhelming fumes of the gas, were even more horrifying."[65] Germans said it was mostly phosgene and the nauseating *Maskenbrecher* they hurled at frontline trenches. Artillery units may have gotten some mustard as well. The attack was so sudden that many of the men inhaled fumes before they could adjust their masks. Three died outright, and eight men were crippled from the gas—all had trouble getting their gear in place or keeping it on. A number of others, the figure was twenty-eight, suffered some effect of the gas either because they took their masks off too soon or then ate food impregnated with the gas. Those who died had clearly panicked. One rushed through the trenches shrieking and made no attempt to put on his mask. He died at the dressing station. Another threw himself down and began screaming, pulling at the masks of anyone trying to help. He died shortly afterward. A third man failed to locate his mask, finally putting on a French mask but breathing gas all the time. While being carried away he kept pulling his mask off and inhaling fumes. Restless behavior like this is characteristic of those who lack oxygen. He died, too, at the dressing station.[66] German boys, it seemed, were no wiser. In his classic autobiographical novel *All Quiet on the Western Front*, Erich Remarque, in the fictional person of soldier Paul Bäumer, sees the reckless and irresponsible wastage of young recruits in the face of gas attacks:

> A man would like to spank them, they are so stupid . . . A surprise gas attack carries off a lot of them. They have not yet learned what to do. We found one dug-out full of them, with blue heads and black lips. Some of them in a shell-hole took off their masks too soon . . . they saw others on top without masks, they pulled theirs off too and swallowed enough to scorch their lungs. Their condition is hopeless, they choke to death with hemorrhages and suffocation.[67]

All too often, scenes repeated on both sides. New to the battlefield, young, rookie soldiers panicked in gas attacks. They hunched down in trenches, unaware that chemical vapors, heavier than air, settled nearer the ground so that the relative safety of the parapets (heads-up) was in stark contrast to the floor of the trench, where many soldiers sought protection.

From there on out, almost daily shelling hit artillery batteries with mustard and phosgene. Incoming rounds numbered well into the tens of thousands. In places the gas was so dense that visibility was limited to ten feet. Fortunately, casualties were kept at a minimum with strict adherence to protective measures. Mustard shells fell liberally on artillery batteries to the point that counterbattery fire was most often done with masks in place. Lieutenant Colonel Harry Gilchrist had been appointed director of the Gas Service in France. In his visit to most infantry units and hospitals of the AEF, he took note of the early experiences with mustard gas.

> At first the troops didn't notice the gas and were not uncom-fortable, but in the course of an hour or so, there was marked

inflammation of their eyes. They vomited, and there was erythema of the skin . . . and by the time the gassed cases reached the casualty clearing station, the men were virtually blind . . . [68]

That was the danger of mustard vapors. First order of business at battalion aid stations was to remove clothing, apply SAG paste to mustard burns and wet compresses over the eyes.[69] Little could be done for inhalation injuries, only words of comfort. Frequently, long lines of men, eyes wrapped, were led in a daisy chain, one arm on the shoulder of the man in front, to field hospitals. Usually, at least one had been designated for gas victims.[70] At those hospitals, the same applied. Bathing with soap and water was imperative. In fact, portable bathing units had been set up near the front lines so that contaminated men could quickly be washed. Doctors and nurses were given strict protocols for protection of food and water supplies. Measures were also in place to decontaminate weapons and ammunition—mustard would coat everything. This was especially important among artillery units, as they were the frequent recipient of mustard shells.[71]

American units would suffer disproportionately from gas attacks. Whether it was slack mask discipline, open country battlefields, or the admirable but reckless nature of American tactics, they would shortly endure the saturating effects of German retaliation—and almost ask for it.

The men of America's Second Infantry Division assembled in France in September 1917 on the heels of the Big Red One. Like troops before them, they did not receive their M2 masks or box respirators until almost the end of December 1917. This was an Army division composed of a brigade (two regiments) of U.S. Marines. In March they were moved to "quiet" trenches near Verdun in the French sector. The quietness soon evaporated as AEF commanders were eager to expose their men to trench warfare and combat. Raiding parties and artillery firings shattered the quiet. Germans were more than happy to respond. While occasional gas shells fell, there were no substantial casualties until April 13, when almost two thousand gas canisters were fired at American troops, mostly mustard gas. These Americans, the Germans surmised, had no respect for trench etiquette. What little chivalry existed ended. Yanks would feel the insidious effects of mustard. When enemy shells contained mustard and high explosives there was no way to tell whether mustard vapors had been released until the burning began. Almost three hundred men were evacuated that day with conjunctivitis, infected lungs, and bad blisters, "especially between the legs." The American press soon caught wind of the new mustard gas, inflating its potential, of course, for propaganda purposes. "I hear that the Germans have invented and perhaps are now using in small quantities, a gas that puts out the eyes. The destruction of sight is complete," columnist Charles Grasty reported.[72]

By May, the German offensive was in full swing, and Paris once again, just as in 1914, was in jeopardy. Enemy grenadiers had drawn perilously close to the Marne River and threatened a breakthrough near a town called Château-Thierry. The Second Division rushed from Verdun to plug the line. In front of them lay a German stronghold in the densely forested area known to the French as Bois de Belleau and to the Americans as Belleau Wood. It was to be the task of the Fifth and Sixth Marine Regiments (Fourth Marine Brigade) to clear out those woods and flanking positions on either side. Germans knew it and had heavily fortified the forest. Artillery targeted American marshalling areas just beyond. The marine commander's instructions were crystal clear—take those woods. Marines used little finesse and rushed headlong into the thickets. There was no deception. The Germans knew they were coming and began shelling with gas even before their attack began. The combat in Belleau Wood would be hotly contested and bloody. Heavily forested with dense vegetation, the expanse afforded easy camouflage for both sides so that fighting became very personal, hand-to-hand struggles. Close-quarter grappling and ilitaries were often necessary. Mustard gas was the ideal accompaniment, drifting to soak trees, leaves, and ground, ready to settle on the clothing and skin of passersby. During the night of June 13, a heavy shelling of mustard—perhaps seven thousand rounds—fell on marine positions to the south and east of the woods. The bombardment was described as "drenching" and contaminated a large assembly area for the Sixth Marines, preparing to enter the woods on the southeast edge. Tired, nervous, and always dreading gas attacks, marines might easily panic at the thought of masking to move into areas dripping with mustard—and then, vision compromised, resort to face-hidden small-arms fire. One platoon leader, Lieutenant Clifton Cates, recalled a harrowing few minutes in the midst of a gas shelling the night of June 14:

> I had not gone over twenty feet from my fox hole when I heard a salvo of shells heading our way . . . when they hit with a thud and no detonation my fears were confirmed [gas shells]. Soon I smelled the gas, and I gave the alarm to my men . . . I reached for my gas mask but it wasn't there.[73]

He finally located one of his men who had taken a German mask as a souvenir and wore that. However, in the process he could see the yellow, oily vapors trickling down shrubs, trees, and on the grass. Not so fortunate was Harrison Cale of the Fifth Marines. Thick gas attacks had forced his men to don their mask respirators. It was then that an exploding shell tore his mask off. By the time he found it, Cale had already taken gulps of mustard-laden air. While he was not aware of any harm, he was found staggering about and was led away with several other gassed men, discarding clothing all the way. Nine men in his group died before reaching medical aid. By the time he arrived in Paris, the mustard had blinded him. He did not regain his sight for ten days. Lung damage kept him in the hospital for another eight months.[74]

Numbers of gassed marines were pulled from the fray and led back to safety by buddies, but their absence thinned the ranks of combat troops. The regimental surgeon for the Sixth Marines reported that he had treated 75 to 150 gassed men and that "practically [the] entire battalion [is] physically unfit due to gas."[75] Men were forced to wear their masks continually for five or six hours, as the mustard vapors could be seen everywhere. After two days of continuous gas shelling, the Fourth Marine Brigade had evacuated seven hundred chemical casualties, some of them heavily burned. Colonel Preston Brown, chief of staff, said of the marines' behavior during this time:

> The gas discipline of the men is excellent, and every man had and used his mask. The casualties were largely due to body

burns, caused by clothing saturated with mustard gas. These
were considered unavoidable casualties, when it is recognized
that the troops occupied wooded and thickly grassed positions
which had to be held. [76]

In fact, some men had worn their respirators for eight hours, almost
an intolerable length of time. There was no alternative in this setting of
closed-in, vicious combat. Marines were aggressive to begin with, and
their repeated forays to clean out nests of adversaries contributed to the
high numbers of chemical burns. Yet this strongpoint had to be taken or
the Château-Thierry line would be breached. Pershing knew, their commanders knew, and the marines themselves knew that they could not fail.
For the entire two-week period of June 1–16, the Fifth and Sixth Marines
reported losses of half their normal strength, many from gas attacks. Such
stubbornness and recklessness on the part of the marines, newly nicknamed
Teufel Hunden (Devil Dogs) by their German adversaries, finally cleared the
woods after ten more days of combat and countless rounds of high-explosive
and gas artillery. [77] The official tally of gas casualties for the campaign in
Belleau Wood recorded 1,371 enlisted and officers gassed. [78] By all accounts,
the Second Division took the highest number of casualties of any unit
of the AEF. As one marine private put it in a letter to his mother:

> We never thought much about eating or sleeping, for they
> [Germans] tried to attack almost every night. We were gassed
> so much that we had to wear our masks a good part of the
> time, but we held our ground and never gave an inch, and
> drove back every attack they tried to make. [79]

During the month of June, German artillery fired an estimated
50,000 mustard gas shells on American troops in that sector, with more
than three thousand casualties inflicted. While gas discipline generally
was commendable, some men took their masks off too soon, after one or
two hours, whereas several hours of wearing them were thought necessary to allow mustard droplets to dissipate. Not long enough. Predictably,
mustard burning commenced. Fortunately, deaths were few. [80]

It would be a practice repeated again in the Argonne Forest—that rambling AEF offensive the fall of 1918 against Germany's heavily fortified Hindenburg Line. True to form, Germans blanketed the battlefield with toxic chemicals hoping to impair and remove sizeable numbers of American infantry. Once again, the barrages forced troops to wear their protective gear, all the while advancing against well-camouflaged strongpoints. Soldiers—some new to combat—pressing forward against enemy fire, could not see, could not breathe, and likely could not fight. Casualties, gas and otherwise, soared. And after hours under fire, the temptation was just too great to peel off those clumsy, oppressive masks. The pervasive mustard vapors then did their work, and, before long, daisy chains of blinded doughboys could be seen winding their way to the nearest aid station.

But the AEF leveled equal devastation on their foes. Battlefields became sodden repositories of mustard droplets and phosgene fogs. As American forces advanced through the Argonne, death and decay took precedence over lush forests and fertile countrysides. Yanks were stunned at the destruction they had wrought. Virginian major Jennings Wise with the Blue Ridge (Eightieth) Division remarked: "Upon the fields, along every approach, and in the trenches, still lay the dead. The whole country had been drenched with gas . . . the odor of charred things was everywhere as if the earth were still smoldering." Wise added that "the hot breath of an unseen, evil power was fuming," and was glad for the rain that destroyed "the hot poison in the air." Another young infantryman saw that "the whole earth had been gassed by shells from our artillery." Dead Germans were everywhere, mostly along the banks of roads and streams, hoping to take cover from the deadly fumes.[81]

Still, gas attacks during the major American battles on the Marne, Belleau Wood, and the Meuse-Argonne had stripped the AEF of manpower. Of 224,649 battle casualties admitted to AEF hospitals, 70,521 officers and enlisted (31 percent) were admitted for gas-related injuries. Mustard gas was thought to cause almost 90 percent of those. In other words, over seventy thousand soldiers were effectively removed from the combat ranks. Was it lethal? For the entire period of combat, from 1917–18, 1,221 of the 50,385 battle deaths (2.4 percent) were of gas poisoning, the vast majority after reaching medical care. Only about two hundred men died outright on the battlefield, unimpressive figures when one looks at the aggregate, but that is hardly the story. In comparison, the British lost 180,000 gassed men, the French, 190,000. On the other side, Germans were reported to have lost 53,000 men from gas attacks. However, by far, the AEF suffered proportionately more casualties from gas than other weapons—over one quarter of the hospitalized were from gas exposure, compared to single-digit percentages for Germany, Britain, and France. In the American Army, chemical weapons could have soon become a crippler of combat effectiveness.[82]

World War I provided a peek—nay, a gawk—into the future regarding chemical warfare. Was this total barbarism, or humane attempts to curtail the violence of war? J.B.S. Haldane, son of the famous chemical weapons physiologist John Scott Haldane, the inventor of early gas masks, claimed "that the use of mustard gas in war on the largest possible scale would render it less expensive of life and property, shorter, and more dependent on brains rather than numbers." It would be far less cruel, Haldane argued, than firebombing urban centers with airplanes.[83] After all, no less distinguished figure than American naval historian Alfred Thayer Mahan had argued at the Hague in 1899:

> That it was illogical and not demonstrably humane, to be
> tender about asphyxiating men with gas, when all were pre-
> pared to admit that it was allowable to blow the bottom out of
> an ironclad at midnight, throwing four or five hundred men
> into the sea to be choked by water, with scarcely the remotest
> chance of escape.[84]

Consider this. In his exhaustive review of the effects of gas on armies in World War I, chemical warfare expert Augustin Prentiss pointed out the following facts. In measuring the "humaneness" of any type of warfare, the degree of suffering from gas was less than other weapons, at least with the proper use of mask respirators. Stronger agents like phosgene and chloropicrin, when inhaled in high amounts, caused instant collapse but, according to evidence from the field, with very little agony. Of course, mustard produced painful blistering, but recovery occurred in a week or two in most cases. Overall, suffering with gas was of a shorter duration in those hospitalized (about one half that of other weapons), and the death rate far less than with conventional wounding agents.[85]

Yet, let us keep this in mind: For one thing, all are not in agreement with the cheery perspective of Prentiss. A committee formed in 1993 to look at long-term health risks for veterans exposed to mustard gas found conflicting and confusing information. Their conclusion was more prosaic:

> There is no doubt that the long-term health consequences of exposure to mustard agents or Lewisite can be serious and, in some cases, devastating. This report has demonstrated that complete knowledge of these long-term consequences has been and still is sorely lacking,[86]

And do not forget: The tendency throughout the war was to find stronger and stronger agents that would be more effective in killing and disabling. The potent intercourse of government, industry, and science almost assured that would happen. Use of mustard gas demonstrated clearly the willingness to deploy newer agents that were more effective. It would not have stopped there. In the United States, for example, a little-known doctoral thesis written in 1902 by, of all people, a Catholic priest named Julius Nieuwland, at Catholic University in Washington, DC, demonstrating synthesis of a new compound from arsenic trichloride and aluminum chloride was picked up in 1917 by the director of research for the Chemical Warfare Service, Winford Lewis. He had been tasked to look for an arsenic-based poison gas and found Nieuwland's work. Nieuwland's dichloro(2-chlorovinyl)arsine was trialed on animals and found to be highly lethal whether inhaled or from skin contact. It was named "Lewisite" after its developer. Whether Lewisite would have ever withstood the rigors of combat use was never known. The war ended before it moved to human experiments. Nevertheless, the danger of chemical weapons is the urge to develop more toxic agents that soon might have disastrous consequences on the battlefield and on civilian populations far and above what Prentiss found. This was the pivotal issue arising out of chemical warfare. How ready should nations be to adopt new weaponry? It would be even more important following development of nuclear weapons, which would completely overshadow chemical agents in their lethality. World War I, though, opened the door and exhibited on a massive scale the consequences of the integration of science, engineering, and government in the killing arts.[87]

Following the Armistice in November 1918 much discussion took place among the victorious Allied nations on the wisdom of pursuing chemical weaponry. No decisions could be reached, each nation fearful of sacrificing strategic or tactical advantage by limitation of weapons. It was up to Prentiss, then, to close his treatise with the ominous conclusion:

> It must not be overlooked that in the last analysis there is no sound or logical reason why any nation having the means should be denied the right to defend its soil by the use of chemicals in war, for chemical warfare is not only one of the most effective methods of waging war, but it is also one of the most humane weapons ever devised.[88]

Yes, the inability to limit weapons of mass destruction, a topic that surfaced solely because of this World War, would haunt peacemakers for decades to come. Many would rue the blithe indulgences granted by the likes of Augustin Prentiss. Medical men would face an entirely new dimension of military medicine: the mass prevention and treatment of chemical casualties. The Persian Gulf War of 1990–91 served as a notable example. United States intelligence was convinced Saddam Hussein's Iraqi forces possessed a variety of chemical agents, such as mustard, sarin, and soman, and rather crude delivery systems that, while lacking sophistication, still could send highly lethal agents amidst populations of troops, civilians, and the hospitalized. The United States military mounted an aggressive campaign to familiarize troops on the use of protective mask respirators, clothing, and behavior and stressed the importance of adhering to strict discipline. Soldiers drilled incessantly on the use of their gas masks and adeptness in quickly unpacking and donning the device, realizing just a few whiffs of sarin could be fatal. De rigueur, the mask and its satchel were a constant accompaniment to battle dress. Atropine autoinjectors—the main antidote to nerve gas—were always within reach. Just as in World War I, though, such equipment was particularly odious to soldiers, sailors, airmen, and marines laboring under intense heat and the other necessities of combat (vision, communication, dexterity). Of course, just as in the Great War, the psychological effect of even the threat of chemical agents was demoralizing and hampered adjustment to combat conditions by frontline forces.[89] It seemed almost a replay of admonitions and drills for doughboys of Pershing's AEF. It was now apparent, then, that chemical (and nuclear and biologic) warfare was a reality and must be addressed prior to deploying men and women into harm's way. Similarly, military doctors, faced with the usual exigencies of battlefield crises, now had to prepare for the inevitable surge of chemical casualties, which required an entirely new set of treatment parameters, including decontamination protection of themselves from chemical, biologic, or nuclear contagion—time-consuming procedures that likely would distract from care of other traumatic combat injuries.

Sadly, the danger now extends far beyond the battlefields. Chemical agents, instead of charitably incapacitating troops, would become a preference of territorial tyrants to impose their will on civilian populations that remain totally vulnerable to the effects of any military weapon. Forget the gallantry of the Hague Conventions. Dictators blithely ignore charity. Witness, of course, the millions of Jews and minorities killed in Nazi extermination camps during World War II. Gas would become far less than humane. It would spawn a horrid marriage of science and industry and usher in the nightmares of hell.

SIX

Röntgen's Rays and Petites Curies

"We will try to make ourselves useful."
—Marie Curie to daughter Irène (1914)

Marie Curie was a woman of pleasing features. An alluring face and searching eyes reflected a private sensuality that betrayed her proper scientist's carriage and hinted at a fiery femininity beneath. Lately, though, she had been in utter depression. The death of her husband, Pierre, deprived her of her most capable scientific partner and the object of her deepest affection. Quite unexpectedly, in 1906, after he had stumbled in the streets of Paris, his head was crushed by a passing lorry. He was only forty-seven. The incident drove Marie into the darkest of places, hardly able to immerse in her beloved research, the mysteries of radiation emanating from newfound elements radium and polonium. And then, almost impetuously, she engaged in a torrid love affair with her late husband's close friend, the married Paul Langevin. His enraged and jealous wife discovered them. She had rummaged through her adulterous husband's possessions and found telling love letters—those letters of passion that lovers cannot forsake. Without pity, the scorned woman sent them to the Parisian periodical *L'Œuvre*, where, in merciless candor, they were published. For that, Marie had been castigated by public opinion, and her scientific reputation put on notice, threatening, even, the awarding of her second Nobel Prize.

Curie might have understood, as many ladies of respect did, that in the Belle Epoque only women of firm moral character would be allowed in high society—or taken seriously. Once a whore, always a whore, was the general feeling about indiscriminate sexual liaisons. Nevertheless, discreet dalliances of that nature were a favorite diversion, a hypocrisy silently accepted. Sexual repression and adultery seemed to go hand in hand. Author Edward Berenson pointed out that "strict sexual mores continued to reign within the bourgeoisie only because most French men and women tacitly agreed to keep their transgressions out of sight." Witness the trial and castigation of Madame Henriette Caillaux in 1914, who famously murdered the editor of *Le Figaro* who, she imagined, was to release love letters of her illicit affair with her then still-married husband. An uncontrollable crime of passion, as is the female nature, was the conclusion; but perhaps a better reflection on the intricate weave of virtue and vice in early-20th-century France.[1]

For all that, Madame Curie was a relentless dynamo who had broken the barriers of gender inequities in her adopted country of France. Maria Skłodowska Curie, of Polish birth but French education, already captured two Nobel prizes, one in physics in 1903 and a second in chemistry in 1911—the first woman to do so. She had also been the first female awarded a professorship at the University of Paris. It was a mysterious, radiant force that captivated her, a force emanating from minute substances that excited certain elements impregnated on photographic plates—the so-called phenomenon of phosphorescence. Though, she had not been the first to witness it. The talented physicist Henri Becquerel determined that such energy sprang from the element uranium. Awakened by Becquerel's findings, Marie's analytical mind flirted with the discoveries awaiting her, which could unleash new and powerful forces capable of changing the face of matter itself. Without haste and with the polished expertise of laboratory denizens, she and Pierre launched a whirlwind of activity designed to pin down precisely the origin of such extraordinary invisible energy. Through countless samples of pitchblende, a commonly mined ore, and one that contained minute amounts of uranium, the two isolated other elements emitting far more energy than uranium alone. These she named *polonium* and *radium*. And the energy released, as if from the atom itself, she surmised, she would call *radiation*. For this—the magic of radiation and the first hint of nuclear energy—Marie and Pierre Curie, along with Henri Becquerel, were awarded the Nobel Prize in 1903. Not ten years later, in 1911, she would be selected for her second Nobel Prize, this time in chemistry, for her discovery of polonium and radium.

These invisible rays had been the product of serendipity in late 19th-century Europe. It had all begun in the small laboratory of physicist Professor Wilhelm Conrad Röntgen at the University of Würzburg. It was autumn, 1895. The imposing but mild-mannered scientist had become enthralled with the cathode rays of Johann Hittorf, Heinrich Hertz, and Philipp Lenard. Using an electrified vacuum tube conceived by William Crookes and Hittorf to generate a strong cathode beam, Röntgen set out to investigate this new form of energy, what Crookes himself had called the "fourth state of matter."[2] In particular, Röntgen was intrigued by emissions generated from electric current and the ability of cathode rays to luminesce screens coated with barium platinocyanide. Would they penetrate cardboard? Aluminum? On the afternoon of November 8 he set out to determine. In his basement lab, Röntgen, the inveterate mechanic, tinkered with his own version of the Crookes cathode tube. He added a stronger induction coil, one developed by Heinrich Rühmkorff, to add power to the cathode beam. He then wrapped his Crookes tube in close-fitting black cardboard to block out all ambient light. A piece of the barium platinocyanide paper was placed next to it. The room was now in utter darkness. On activating the cathode rays he found a brilliant fluorescence, indicating that the coated paper was emitting visible light in response to the absorption of some type of invisible energy. And, he concluded, the source of the fluorescence must lie within the vacuum tube. Absolutely dumbfounded by these new ghostly rays, he repeated, and repeated again, his experiments with the cathode rays over the next several days. Röntgen was baffled. They did not behave like the standard cathode beam: magnets would not deflect their course. Nor did they behave like light: prisms wound not scatter their focus. Totally obsessed with his findings, he would forego meals, leisure, sleep, and even conversations with his wife, all to determine the veracity of his experiments. To Bertha, Röntgen could not contain his excitement:

> When at first I made the startling discovery of the penetrating rays, it was such an extraordinary astonishing phenomenon that I had to convince myself repeatedly by doing the same experiment over and over and over again . . .[3]

And then, as he soon scribbled in his urgent *Mittheilung* (communication) to the Physikalische-Medizinischen Gesellschaft of Würzburg, he made the critical observation: "Hält man die Hand zwischen den Entladungsapperat und den Schirm, so sieht man die dunkleren Schatten der Handknochen in dem nur wenig dunklen Schattenbild der Hand" ("If you hold your hand between the discharge device and the screen, you can see the darker shadows of the bones in the [flesh of the] hand, which is only a little dark"). He had even convinced his wife to insert her hand under the Crookes tube, assuring her that it was painless. Indeed, the rays displayed her bones and the hard image of her wedding ring. He would call these new invisible rays *X-rays*. This was a new manner of energy that could penetrate the ordinary barriers to visible light. Yet Röntgen focused not on the spectacular quality of penetration but on the character of these rays. How did they differ from visible light? Were they ultraviolet light? Were they new, longitudinal waves somehow transmitted in the ether?[4]

But the press instantly saw magic. Newspapers in Frankfurt, London, Berlin, carried the "sensational discovery" of Röntgen's rays and their ability to breach objects and literally see inside what cannot be discerned with the naked eye. "Professor Routgen [sic] of Würzburg has discovered a light that, for purposes of photography, will penetrate wood, flesh, and most other organic substances," announced the *London Standard* for January 7, 1896, a mere ten days after Röntgen had submitted his communications.[5] From *Le Petit Parisien* of January 10, 1896: "Un Decouverte Sensationnelle" ("A Sensational Discovery") the front-page article read. "The very distinguished professeur Routgen [as his name was to be misspelled] introduced a new light-conducting agent." On a photographic plate even "we could count all the bones [of the hand], phalanges, joints . . . it is a skeleton and not a living hand, one would say."[6] Such clamor as to this monumental achievement prompted Albert von Kölliker, a trustee of the Physikalische-Medizinischen Gesellschaft of Würzburg (and who, by the way, was one of the first to have his hand radiographed by Röntgen) to call the new ether rays "Röntgen rays."[7]

The scientific community was mad with curiosity. In the year following Röntgen's announcement, exactly 49 books and 1,044 scientific papers were published on the subject of his rays.[8] The prestigious journal *Nature* issued a bulletin on January 26, 1896, that Professor W. C. Röntgen "is reported to have discovered that a number of substances which are opaque to visible rays of light, are transparent to certain waves capable of affecting a photographic plate." Included in their brief communication was a comment on visualizing the bones of a living hand.[9] Was it truly to be believed? Physician Paul Oudin and physicist Toussaint Barthélémy repeated Röntgen's experiments in Paris. Oudin had always dabbled in electricity and high frequency circuits and had been present with Arsène d'Arsonval, Toussaint Barthélémy, and Henri Poincaré when they received Röntgen's iconic radiograph of his wife's hand. They, in turn, had presented the skeletal exhibit to the Académie des sciences on January 20, 1896. All Paris was abuzz at the new invisible rays. Makeshift cathode tubes were fashioned, energy delivered, and photographic demonstrations abounded, some even held in private homes.[10]

Enthusiasts quickly surfaced. In attendance at one of Oudin and Barthélémy's *séances* was a Parisian physician by the name of Antoine Béclère. Béclère began his medical career in infectious diseases, introducing treatment of such afflictions as smallpox with convalescent serum. But these rays of Röntgen infected *him* with unquenchable curiosity. He had been boarding-school friends with Oudin and Barthélémy and happened to attend their demonstration out of curiosity. In amazement, he watched those internal shadows dance before him: fluoroscopy of the beating heart and movements of the diaphragm. Röntgen's device and its mystical powers enthralled him. Béclère is reported to have said after the display, "this appears to me the promised land, I must engage." Recruiting an imaginative mechanical engineer, Béclère developed a small static machine operated by hand that generated enough electricity to make an anticathode blush. The exposed photographic plates were brought home in the evenings to be developed by his wife. By February 1897 he had enough material to put on an anatomic exhibit in Paris with his friends Oudin and Barthélémy showing such detail as movements of the diaphragm, enlarged mediastinal lymph nodes, and lung effusions.[11] By 1898, Béclère had become so proficient that he set up a radiology laboratory at the Hôpital Tenon in Paris, even giving free instructions on this new science.[12]

Word of the wondrous machinery spread like wildfire. Lyonnais physician and photographer Étienne Destot generated his own Röntgen's rays via a Crookes tube donated by a tinkerer in the laboratory of the École supérieure de Paris. With engineering help and his knowledge of anatomy, he soon began developing photographic plates so detailed that they were worthy of exhibition. Following Oudin and Barthélémy's show at the Académie des sciences, Destot presented his own work at the Académie de médecine a week later, including a picture of a needle in a foot. As his experience grew, Destot became something of a prodigy in the new science. In iconoclastic fashion, he took over a florist store on the banks of the Rhone River in Lyon—he called it "the Destot shop"—set up his equipment, and offered to radiograph all comers. Toying with Crookes's cathode-ray tube, Destot was able to refine his technique to show the most intricate of bony trabeculations. So impressive was he that the Hôpital de la Croix-Rousse in Lyon gave space for his clinic of radiology, the first of its kind.[13]

It was now, indeed, the rage in medicine. By March 1896 the Académie des sciences seemed taken with radiation and X-rays. Barthélémy, Destot, and others convinced them that this was no humbug. Displays of the skeletal frame and shadows of viscera opened countless vistas for exploration. Heart and lung outlines, fluid buildups, and tumors were now visible. Localization of foreign material within the human body was of keen interest, and clinicians shortly devised methods to pinpoint such objects using beams in two planes—called the biplanar technique.[14] By April a report appeared describing a revolver bullet hidden in the leg, adroitly fetched with the use of a radiograph.[15] Many more would follow.

Hospitals vied for the Röntgen device. Béclère installed one at Hôpital Saint-Antoine in 1899 where he was now chief of service. He conducted his work in a disused chapel, usually crowded with dozens of observers all standing in the pitch-blackness necessary for radiological illumination. He had even managed to get two units installed in Paris at the Hôpital de la Charité and Hôpital Necker.[16]

Röntgen's invisible rays and their remarkable photographic shadows revolutionized diagnostic medicine. No longer would physicians need to conjecture about internal ailments. Now there was the potential to see through skin and into the depths of human flesh. Thanks to the likes of Destot, refinements in the technique produced shorter exposure times and more focused imaging on photographic plates. Manufacture of the Crookes-Hittorf tubes accelerated as demand for the devices skyrocketed.

For military surgeons, X-rays had their attention. Bullets and shrapnel rifled through skin and muscle, slammed into bone, and shattered the very scaffolding of the human frame. Now fragments, splinters, and loose ends could be aligned, straightened, and encouraged to heal, all using Röntgen's technology. Embedded bullets and shell fragments showed clearly on radiographs. As a threatening source of infection, this unwanted debris often demanded extraction, but blind meddling produced more trauma than the injury itself. With Röntgen's rays, wound exploration could be more focused, more "surgical." During their war in Abyssinia (Ethiopia) in 1896, Italian physicians set up and used the Crookes tube and photographic plates for wounded soldiers brought back to Naples. According to surgeon Giuseppe Alvaro, visualization of bullets using Röntgen's rays was successful in two wounded soldiers with lead fragments lodged in their arms. He felt that the application of this "immortal discovery" was incredible and could easily aid in removal of foreign bodies. "After these positive and undoubtedly successful results, I am pleased and fortunate to present for the first time the search for bullets in the gunshot wounds sustained in war using Rontgen's rays," he reported.[17] Another report surfaced from the brief but violent war between Greece and Turkey (Ottoman Empire) in 1897. The German Red Cross expedition sent to Istanbul led by Professor Hermann Küttner carried with it a rather cumbersome but workable radiology unit using a Crookes tube that was set up at the Yildiz Hospital. The whole procedure "never really let us down," in terms of localizing soft lead bullets from antiquated single-shot Greek Gras rifles. The standard of care, they concluded, now demanded it:

> At the conclusion of our experiences during the war . . . we can make the assertion that we have a new aid in the X-rays, which were so valuable for certain cases in the war that the wounded have an unconditional right to use it. [18]

By the turn of the century, Röntgen's invention had won over hard-to-impress German doctors, who hailed it as a medical triumph of the modern age. Like Küttner, those of military bearing especially cherished the new curiosity:

> In no other medical specialty has the discovery of Roentgen been so beneficial and blessing as in war surgery. This is obvious when you consider that the X-rays celebrated their greatest triumphs when diagnosing bone injuries and recognizing the foreign bodies that entered the human body—*i.e.* in two areas that represent the actual field of work of the war surgeon to have. [19]

Even the United States Army was eager to adapt. During their brief Spanish-American War of 1898 seventeen of Röntgen's machines were in operation, in stateside general hospitals and on board three hospital ships. Radiographs showed the extent of bony fractures, degree of comminution (fragmentation), and, of course, the number and position of lodged missiles. While not yet portable enough to be near the battlefield, X-rays were still a valuable tool for the military surgeon, so said Captain William Borden:

> The use of the Röntgen ray has marked a distinct advance in military surgery. It has favored conservatism and promoted the aseptic healing of bullet wounds made by lodged missiles . . .

[and] it has done away with the necessity for the exploration of wounds by probes or other means.[20]

In fact, Borden became a self-styled radiologic aficionado. He even predicted a lighter-weight device that could be used in field hospitals. In any event, from an official standpoint there was unanimity. Chief surgeon for the United States Sixth Army Corps Nicholas Senn declared: "in the light of our recent experience the X-ray has become an indispensable diagnostic resource to the military surgeon."[21]

Throughout the British Empire, feelings were the same. Major James Battersby, of the Royal Army Medical Corps, who had been in charge of the Röntgen apparatus for the Anglo-Egyptian Nile expedition of 1898–99, felt they were indispensable. "Most of our large military hospitals at home and abroad were now provided with the most efficient x-ray outfits," he boasted. As demonstrated by Bertha Röntgen's wedding ring, the major benefit was in the identification of metallic objects on or in the human frame. Battersby bragged about the British experience during the Battle of Omdurman in 1898. He claimed that of 121 British wounded, X-rays located bullets in 21 where simple examination could not. The major even wanted X-ray machines taken to the battlefield. They would be carried "on the shoulders of four men like an Indian *dhoolie* [covered litter]" using ropes and poles—they were much too heavy for mule transport, he knew.[22]

Portability? Perhaps. Lackeys? Not practical in the modern age. Twentieth-century automobiles provided a better alternative. With the power of nine or ten horses, first-decade vehicles had potential. Could they be used to carry X-ray gadgets closer to the battle? Could enough electrical current be generated to brighten Röntgen's photographic plates? Petrol engines might, with some modification, spin dynamos fast enough to breed the tide of electricity needed. Could these flimsy vehicles and their delicate cargo withstand the rigors of off-road travel? Undecided. All so many daydreams, as it turned out. There was little practical incentive, and those dreams fell flat.

It was probably because a few influential military planners remained skeptical. Commanders on the battlefield had no interest in these cumbersome contrivances. The role of the automobile had yet to be convincing, let alone loaded down with heavy equipment. Some military doctors, too, were unconvinced. It was a technology, they perceived, that was awkward and heavy. Setting up and taking pictures took time and manpower. Wounded needed surgical attention, and most with rifle wounds demanded very little anyway—cleaning and bandaging. Seldom was there need to explore and extract. Röntgen's rays were of little value. Besides, future wars would be brief and fast-paced. X-ray cars and tables and quirky emissions would just get in the way.

So cathode-ray tubes, coils, and plates stood idle in military hospitals, equipment collected dust, and interest waned. By the summer of 1914 doctors familiar with X-rays were relatively scarce. Only 175 could be found in France, and all practiced in hospitals or private clinics. With the outbreak of war that summer, these radiology specialists were assigned elsewhere—aid stations and field hospitals. The few who stayed with their machines were scattered across the country, a total of twenty-one in cities like Paris, Lyon, Bordeaux, Nancy, Rennes, Lille, and Bourges. Those mobile radiology vans were nonexistent still, ailing on the drawing boards of a few die-hard believers.[23]

◆

Marie Curie's frenzied love scandal ruined her. It was over. Paul Langevin had returned to his wife. Marie was alone. She stood on the verge of mental and physical collapse. Only with determination had she sought the haven of her research laboratory. Mathematics, physics, and measurements—even her invisible radiation—were more ordered reality than the emotional turmoil of sexual intimacies. On the eve of War, Marie was at the zenith of her career. By midsummer her new laboratories on the Rue Pierre Curie were almost completed; 800,000 gold francs had been raised by Parisian benefactors. As they went up, Marie spent hours on the scaffolding, imagining work to be done within. Already, the famous professor Claudius Regaud, recruited by Marie, was hard at work in the biological laboratory, finished ahead of the rest. "In that wonderful month of July [1914] the 'temple of the future' in the Rue

Pierre Curie was at last finished," her daughter recalled. Marie was set to move her precious radium and all her workers at once.[24]

But then war erupted. Curie was caught in Paris. Her children, Irène and Ève, though, were vacationing on the coast, far from Paris. "I am dying to come and hug you. [But] I don't have time," she wrote during those first few weeks, "There are moments when I don't know what to do. I want to hold you close so badly."[25] She had tried to reassure them but, after the first week of war, there was little optimism. "[W]hat massacre we are going to see, and what folly to have allowed it to be unchained," she had written in a letter to Irène.[26] Although without her children, Curie could not sit idle. There was that tug of restless energy urging her to contribute, even, at some point, to pull her oldest child with her. "You and I, Irène, we will try to make ourselves useful" (Irène was seventeen at the time, Ève was but nine).[27]

Much of France felt the same. With men off to battle, factories, plants, and mills needed laborers, and women flocked to the opportunity. In fact, the workforce transformed to female legions tooling cannon and rifles, rolling out artillery shells, sewing uniforms, and birthing millions of bullets. Upper classes chose nursing and other volunteer labor. It almost became an obsession. Some socialites even opened their ilitari as hospitals. For Marie Curie, Röntgen's rays held her interest. Of course, she was quite familiar with the machines. Cathode beams had stimulated her interest in radiation in the first place. Now medical reports cemented the value of X-rays for injured men. "It is a wonderful observation," she began in her wartime diary, "that allowed us, for the first time, to explore without aid of surgery, the interior of the human body."[28] But there was no such technology at the front, not that bloody autumn. "[T]he Military Board of Health had no organization of radiology, while the civil organization was also but little developed," she wrote later.[29] And then she saw the throngs of wounded pouring through Paris from the Marne battlefields. "Human suffering is in dire need of relief, and medical science, still largely condemned to empiricism, never fails to attempt a trial that offers some new hope." In her mind, the neglected science of Röntgen could produce a measure of that hope for these men, for, indeed, at the start of the war, "an injured person was *never* examined by X-rays."[30]

"My first idea was to set up radiology units in hospitals, employing the equipment that was sitting unused in laboratories or else in the offices of doctors who had been mobilized," she recalled. That would be a disappointing pursuit. Few hastily constructed hospitals around Paris had the electrical power to fuel coils that generated cathode beams. Unlikely to happen, she realized. Then, Curie wondered, could X-rays be taken to the battlefield? The French military medical service, the Service de santé, certainly hoped so. They were among those who saw the full potential of X-rays in battlefield medicine. But for actual portability? There was no idea how to get the machines to the patients.[31]

Perhaps she had heard of the engineer Georges Massiot. In 1912 he designed what he called a *voiture laboratoire de radiologie* (radiology laboratory car), using a ten-horsepower Peugeot automobile. The interior was packed with a generator, cables, coil, and tables for examination. He finished his first model, designated No. 1, the following year. It was such a novelty that in August 1914 Massiot unveiled his car, courtesy of the la Croix-Rouge française (the French Red Cross), at the Lyon Exposition. Other exhibits followed. Marie Curie may have been present at a demonstration of Massiot's unit at the Val-de-Grâce military hospital in Paris, sponsored by radiologist Georges Haret.[32] Haret was convinced of the utility of mobile radiology in warfare. Like Curie, he knew that greatest utilization would be in the countryside, where the wounded were. Thus, the need for motorization, some version of the automobile to take the bulky equipment two hundred miles and beyond.[33] Massiot's vans seemed ideal. Haret found two, loaded them with cathode tubes, coils, and plates and, with fellow radiologist Paul Aubourg, headed for the front. In the first seven months of operation, Haret's team completed over two thousand radioscopies and several radiophotographs on more than 1,800 wounded. His workers found hundreds of hidden fragments and bullets. So popular was the technique that shortly they were doing on average ten examinations each day.[34] Yes, Curie surmised, this was the answer: pepper the front with trucks and vans and their radioactive payloads. The territory was vast and numbers of wounded immense.

A woman of such passionate persuasions could not long refrain from engaging in the most feverish work of providing her beloved France with the very epitome of technology—that of the marvelous Röntgen ray. Massiot had dared to send his flimsy camions laden with radiology gear far into the country and had captivated ordinary surgeons now able to guide their searching fingers to metal slivers and broken bones previously unseen. Here, then, was her new calling, a marriage of science—her science—and the versatile automobile, that most intriguing of conveyances.

She designed her own *voiture radiologique*—her radiologic automobile. Portability was key. Like Massiot's, it must be self-contained. Everything to charge, discharge, and display radiology plates must be stored inside. That meant a powerful source of electricity—the electrical generator would connect directly to the automobile engine—coil, the ion-based Crookes tube, photographic plates, tables for patients, and dark space for development. In all, over two hundred pounds of equipment. She wanted twenty cars built and equipped. Could it be done? Few government funds were available. Rich in enthusiasm, the Service de santé was poor in cash. Who would pay for it? Curie the Nobel laureate had flirted with the cozy society of Paris. To them she would petition.

She approached an acquaintance, the well-connected historian Ernest Lavisse, a colleague from the Sorbonne who was now director of the new philanthropic Patronage national des ilitar (National Patronage for the Wounded). Lavisse was taken by her zeal and put the full weight of the patronage behind her. In fact, he made Madame Curie its "director of radiology."[35] With Lavisse's support, Marie had her first auto, a camion loaded with all her radiology accoutrements. Another donor, architect Paul Ewald, gave his personal automobile for a second radiology van. It might have been his luxury touring car, the "limousine" she referred to in her memoirs.[36] There were other supporters. Old friend Antoine Béclère, now director of radiology at Val-de-Grâce, came to her aid. Impressed by the work of Haret and Aubourg, he saw in Marie and her sway a means of getting more mobile radiology units to the front.[37]

And the grande dames and mademoiselles de la société rose to the occasion. She approached la Croix-Rouge française, a union of three volunteer services, l'Union des femmes de France (the Union of Women of France), la Société de secours aux ilitar ilitaries (the Society to Aid the Military Wounded), and l'Association des dames françaises (the Association of French Ladies), all repositories of benevolence. In fact, the Femmes de France, formed during the Paris Commune of 1871 and dedicated to rescuing the suffering victims of France during times of disaster, donated and outfitted Marie's prototype van.[38] She became quite the talk of Paris, touring the boulevards as if a new Joan of Arc preparing for electrical jousting with the invisible torments of war.

With the support of Béclère, the generosity of Lavisse, and willing French society, almost 700,000 francs were donated. Marie was able to outfit eighteen more vans, trucks, and limousines, which she turned over to Béclère's Service de santé. According daughter Ève, Marie kept one of these cars for her personal use, a sturdy, flat-nosed Renault camion painted regulation grey punctuated with a vivid red cross. Strictly a passenger at first, Marie soon tired of the chauffeuring. She got her driver's license in 1916 and, from then on, drove herself, even into battle zones, Red Cross armband proudly displayed.[39] Packed almost to toppling, she and her comrades chugged their way on rutted roads, carting their radioactive cargo with the power of a dozen horses to meet at the intersection of medicine and physics, burning through flesh with Röntgen's fluorescing beams to flush out the hidden derangements of splintered bone or the occult culprits of horrifying infections.

At first, her *petites Curies* (little Curies), as they were now called, kept their travels to one hundred kilometers (seventy miles) from Paris. Based in the city, when the call came, teams stocked equipment, engines were cranked, cylinders sputtered alive, and the wobbly cars sped off at thirty miles an hour to their destination. On board were driver, technician (called a *manipulateur*), and doctor (and many times Marie herself). On arrival, usually at a forward surgical *ambulance*, table, coil, and tube were unloaded, dynamo and cable attached for electricity, and the wounded brought in. Marie's favorite tool was the radioscope (fluoroscope) that spewed constant beams and gave real-time images of bones, sparing the stretch needed for photographic development. She herself piloted the device, panning up and down, providing a moving picture of internal anatomy. Surgeons flocked to her side to watch.

Marie Curie had never shirked from manual labor, nor did she now. She pitched in with the rest, unloading equipment, shooting images, and sweating with surgeons under the most adverse of conditions. According to her daughter Ève, she had even turned a stubborn crank on the car motor, changed tires, and cleaned a spitting carburetor. Comfort was of little concern to her.[40] More importantly, Marie Curie felt it was never beneath her to weather pressures and dangers of the battlefield, the functioning of her X-rays under hardships, and the stresses imposed by surgical workloads. Men certainly had to do so. In a letter to her daughter Irène, she mentioned one such experience near the Flanders town of Poperinghe in early 1915:

> After various wanderings, we've arrived here, but we can't make an attempt at working until we've made some modifications at the hospital. They want to build a shelter for the car and a partition to create the radiology room in a big ward . . . We hear the guns grumbling almost constantly. It's not raining, a bit of frost. We were welcomed at the hospital with extreme cordiality . . .[41]

The furrowed and cratered countryside was not kind to automobile travel. Lodging and food were unpredictable. Each journey demanded advanced planning, and Curie personally supervised arrangements, even to the point of loading supplies on trains when necessary to ease her timetable. In the end, it all came down to the battered men she saw and for whom she toured. "Nothing was so moving," she remembered, "as to be with the wounded and to take care of them. We were drawn to them because of their suffering and because of the patience with which they bore it."[42]

Still, Marie Curie was an intruder into the man's world of military medicine. At first, army bureaucracy forbad her to roam freely near the front lines. It was not until November 1914 that permission (apparently from General Joffre himself) was finally granted. She had been frustrated by the delays. In a letter to ex-lover Paul Langevin (with whom she still communicated—in secret perhaps?), she had written:

The day I leave is not fixed yet, but it can't be far off. I have had a letter saying that the radiological car working in the Saint-Pol region has been damaged. This means that the whole northern area is without any radiological service! I am taking the necessary steps to hasten my departure and am resolved to put all my strength at the service of my adopted country since I cannot do anything for my unfortunate native country just now, bathed as it is in blood after more than a century of suffering. [43]

But bureaucratic problems did not stop there. While Béclère's Service de santé was in full support, resistance to her mobile units persisted. Was it concern for the fairer sex or more basic jealousy? In fact, Georges Haret, that champion of mobile radiology, and now, later in 1915, director of radiology services for the minister of war, stood obstinately in her way. No more travel to the front, he decreed by official order. Curie was not intimidated. Surgical chiefs in forward hospitals were clamoring for her units. Service de santé headquarters in Paris would not do without her. Curie and her friends applied pressure. [44] Haret relented.

Her *petites Curies* had become crucial to wound management. So useful were X-rays at the front that, later in the war, the military set up fixed radiology posts in surgical *ambulances*. As indispensable as sterilizers, operating tables, and instruments, surgeons insisted on them. For example, around the active Verdun sector, in 1916, each surgical station, and there were a great many, had Röntgen's cathode tubes, coils, and photographic plates. They became part of the assembly-line processing of casualties, often required before any surgery was done. The larger evacuation hospitals, the Hôpitaux d'Origine d'Étapes (HOEs), in Froidos, Petit Monthairon, Vadelaincourt, Chaumont-sur-Aire, Landrecourt, Revigny, and Bar-le-Duc bristled with X-ray teams. Mobile surgical squads, the *groupes complémentaire chirurgicales*, and the *auto-chirs* did not operate without them. [45]

But as these units multiplied so did the need for workers to staff them. Curie understood. None of her *petites Curies* could operate without the coveted *manipulateurs*. What few technicians she had knew the machinery—setups, operation, maintenance, even interpretation of radiographs. She knew firsthand their value. A good *manipulateur* could literally run the entire unit. Daughter Irène, seventeen at the time, had been one of them, personally trained by her mother. She apparently delighted in the role, spending her eighteenth birthday locating shell fragments in a wounded soldier's hand—alone. "I spent my birthday admirably . . . except that you weren't there," she wrote her mother.[46]

Béclère, too, had recognized the need. He set up a school at Val-de-Grâce for male technicians, but qualified candidates were few and far between. Many were less desirable, with little background in physics or medicine, some perhaps hoping to shirk the draft.[47] Ranks were thin, and the competent men he trained were clearly not enough. It was then that Béclère reached out to Marie Curie. Could she open a school for women technicians—females were called *manipulatrices*. Curie, in her boundless energy, set to the task and immediately began recruiting women. The new Hôpital-école Edith Cavell, which opened in October 1916, would serve as her academy.[48] She intended to take nursing recruits (for whom the hospital and school were originally designed) and train them instead in radiology. In fact, she even enlisted laywomen, all the way from chambermaids to debutants eager to participate in the war effort. Her instructions lasted eight weeks: intricate concepts of electricity, the workings of the Röntgen tubes, use of radioscopy, and development of radiographic imaging. Marie was fiercely insistent they learn her material, much of which bordered on the incomprehensible. She drilled them incessantly—anatomy and physiology and reading of X-rays—knowing, as women in a man's world, they would have to be sharp and competent. From its opening in 1917, she graduated 150 *manipulatrices*, all of whom were immediately assigned to the front.[49] She had undying faith in feminist determination and potential. Her rigorous curriculum and conviction saw to that:

> The experience seems very conclusive. There is no doubt that the profession of [female] manipulator [technician] in radiology is perfectly suited to women of average education, provided that they have the intelligence, the training, and

a certain capacity for dedication essential to relate to sick individuals.[50]

Doctors skilled in this new radiology were rare, too. Antoine Béclère knew, with X-rays now an indispensable part of medicine, that more specialists were needed. He had written a number of memos in 1915 to the Director of the Service de santé pleading for more training resources at Val-de-Grâce for which he received modest support. Three hundred specialists, versed in X-ray methods *and* medicine, departed for the front as soon as they graduated—still not nearly enough, but they were the vanguard of experts equipped to decipher Röntgen's elaborate shadows.

The Great War spawned a new field of medicine—radiology. Almost forgotten in hospital back rooms, more of a curiosity than instrument, X-rays suddenly achieved such notoriety in just a few years to earn a prominent place in the health sciences. To a great extent, it was an immersive learning environment propelling the field forward, as historians Charles Bourne and Rethy Chhem maintain. The challenge brought by thousands of casualties and their shattered bones was met squarely by availability of a new medium once it could be brought to the bedside. And what better catalyst than the visionary determination of Marie Curie, who, driven by patriotism and an innate but profound restiveness—despite her many achievements—persuaded, coerced, and embarrassed bureaucrats to bring this modality to where it was most needed: the battlefields of France. The accelerating successes of X-rays would readily spill over into civilian practice and give rise to imaging techniques that would figuratively open the human body for inspection. "The opportunities for learning granted by the wartime medicine environment are equally as valuable to the study of the history of civilian medicine as they are for military medicine," Bourne and Chhem were to write.[51]

Marie Curie, though, deserves much credit. She was unarguably a central figure. In an article published in *Le Figaro* on February 14, 1922, Professor Henri Reynès from Marseille, chief doctor at the Miribel military hospital at Verdun, finally brought to light the unique role of Madame Curie—unbeknownst to the public at large during the war:

what must also be remembered is the important part taken
by Mrs. Curie in the progress of surgery, in particular with
regard to the first applications of X-rays, due to her initiative,
in the treatment of war fractures and looking for projectiles.[52]

Curie, the enigmatic feminist, had been a volunteer, an advocate, a
scientist, an innovator, and an educator. Her firm belief above all was
that women possessed the intellectual and emotional capacity for scientific and technological work and deserved an equal and respectable place
in the medical professions. At war's end, though, Curie was worn out,
physically and emotionally. The ennui from spent energy possessed her.
She had visibly aged in those four years. Nevertheless, quickly gathering
momentum, she returned to her fascination with radium, her new institute, and renewed research into applications of radioactive agents.[53] But
she could not easily leave the war behind. Marie Curie had been deeply
troubled by what she had seen on the battlefields and the tremendous
waste of mankind's youth. No doubt because of this, she felt compelled,
with that same fierceness, to rail against dangerous politics so damaging
to peaceful coexistence. She embraced the newly formed International
Commission on Intellectual Cooperation of the League of Nations, on
which she served for twelve years. Her desire was that the League of
Nations would promote global collaboration and stave off militaristic
designs. As for science, she had hoped her radium and its mysterious
emanations would be of immense value in the treatment of mankind's
diseases. Some of the public even touted the powerful, yet invisible,
rays as a cure for cancer and Marie, indeed, as that modern-day Joan
of Arc. In fact, radium opened new vistas of treatment. It and like substances would play a central role in cancer therapy over the next century
and beyond. Madame Curie's name would always be synonymous with
radiotherapy and her *petites Curies* that carried radiology into the modern
age of medicine.

As for Wilhelm Röntgen, the consummate scientist, he cared little
for the ramifications of his invisible rays. After being awarded the Nobel
Prize in physics in 1901, Röntgen continued his modest research in
Würzburg. Yet, the war would strip him of his assistants and coworkers,

all conscripted into the military. Without help, his research during the war dwindled and for all intents and purposes ground to a halt—as it did over much of Germany. Teaching now was his sole academic effort. His singular support for the Kaiser was a scribbled signature on the manifesto *Der Aufruf "An die Kulturwelt!"* (*Appeal to the World of Culture*) along with ninety-two other confreres: "we, as representatives of German science and art, protest in front of the entire cultural world against the lies and slander with which our enemies seek to defile Germany in the difficult struggle for existence imposed on it."[54] Later, claiming he had not read it, the aged wizard expressed regret for signing. Rationing and the privations of a war-torn country imposed hardships on Röntgen and his wife. He was reported to have lost forty pounds during that time. In 1919, his beloved Bertha passed away, and Röntgen slipped into obscurity, his indulgences reading and listening to music. After the Nobel Prize, he had shunned all recognition of his discovery, turning down titles of nobility and other invitations to the limelight. Colorectal cancer finally took him in 1923, a modest, reclusive genius.[55]

SEVEN

The Remarkable Harvey Cushing and His Journeys through the Brain

"It is amazing what the human animal can endure."
—Harvey Cushing, 1936[1]

On a Sunday in Paris in April 1915 a handsome man, slight of build, with features of patrician bearing, perhaps reminiscent of thoroughbred pedigree, had seated himself on a corner divan at a sumptuous dinner party highlighting such distinguished attendees as French prime minister Raymond Poincaré and American ambassador to France William Sharp. All were impeccably dressed in formal eveningwear save this one gentleman fresh from work, it turned out, at the Ambulance Américaine in nearby Neuilly-sur-Seine. Although not unaccustomed to such fine company, the hastily dressed individual, feeling rather embarrassed, sneaked off to a remote corner and quietly lit a cigarette, drawing deeply as pleasant repose from the day's havoc. Another dinner guest joined him, and without pause said, "I understand your name is 'Cushing.'"[2] And his new acquaintance, with a disarming smile, responded in the affirmative. Indeed, it was the American Harvey Cushing of Boston, that fine aristocratic Harvard surgeon whose reputation in matters of the brain had adorned him with a proper veneration. It seemed his newfound acquaintance had roomed with Cushing's brother at Cornell. A surprise, Cushing realized, that such a family connection could be found in this small corner of a world caught in the conflagration of a European war of still so little interest to Americans.

By now Cushing, almost an international celebrity, had settled into an unusual pace of surgery, far different than his operating schedule had been at the Johns Hopkins Hospital of Baltimore. He volunteered to provide surgical care at the Ambulance Américaine in Neuilly-sur-Seine. The Great War had swamped Parisian hospitals, and sympathetic American doctors and nurses were eager to respond. There may have been an element of romanticism in the whole matter, but it had stirred a desire in Cushing. As often happens in war, any romanticism quickly fled when he witnessed the indiscriminate carnage brought to his hospital. Its victims would come in bunches, with little notice, and in various forms of disarray, caked in mud and grime, wounds from the trivial to the ruinous. He was particularly keen on those victims of wounds to the head. That had been a focus of his in civilian practice, and now there was ample opportunity to break through the gloom cloaking these tragic injuries. The outcomes from bullets and shrapnel that penetrated skin and bone of the skull and drove deep into the jellylike substance of brain wreaked havoc on the composure of ordinary surgeons. Far too few of these unlucky casualties ever left the hospital, victims of bleeding and infection and a destroyed mind.

The story of neurosurgery during World War I is the story of one man—Harvey Cushing. And it is the story of countless young men caught in the crossfire of World War I, peeking above the parapets or stumbling through barbed wire and suffering the sudden volley of bullets and shellfire that tore through their flimsy metal helmets and into tender scalps, splintered bone and those grayish convolutions of intelligence that lie below.

Harvey Cushing, from a rich legacy of medical professionals—his father and grandfather were physicians—seemed himself destined for a career not just in medicine but in surgery. The Cushings were New Englanders by heritage but migrated to Cleveland, Ohio, in the early 19th century, where they quickly became pillars of the community. Harvey Cushing's childhood was embossed by a fierce determination to excel, and there was no doubt his aptitude for the sciences was exceptional. But it would be a particular surgical brilliance that would ultimately define him—even obvious before graduation from medical school. At Harvard Medical School he was a perfectionist, his dissections of cadavers, a mandatory rite of passage for any legitimate student of medicine in 1892, were artistic masterpieces; delicate nerves, arteries, and veins laid bare with the finest of strokes. Cushing dumbfounded his fellow students. Such outstanding medical school performance and an equally stellar year as house officer at the Massachusetts General Hospital earned him a coveted position as William Halsted's assistant resident in surgery in 1896 at the Johns Hopkins Hospital in Baltimore, Maryland. Halsted, a taskmaster for excellence, had designed a training program in surgery that rivaled the finest of Europe's. It was grueling labor he demanded, his trainees literally living in the hospital for the duration. After four years of study, including a tour of the most prominent European surgical centers, Cushing had obtained unquestionable proficiency in general surgery. Halsted was so impressed that he invited the young Cushing to join the faculty, and he promptly accepted. Despite a growing curiosity about the brain and nervous system, Cushing felt strongly that the basis of any specialized form of surgery was a solid mastery of surgery in general. It was the anatomic and physiologic foundation essential for any subsequent sally into finer fields of study.[3] Nevertheless, brain and nerves drew him in. His work with the very painful condition of trigeminal neuralgia—severe, unrelenting facial pain—severing and removing the Gasserian ganglion, the seat of the affliction, produced astounding results, freeing his patients from this distressing and crippling state. Before long, he was drilling and sawing through the skull bone to gain access to that wonderful organ of the mind—the brain. In all his attention to detail—an assiduous, exacting performance learned, in part, from his chief, William Halsted—Cushing was able to accomplish what so many others had failed to do: operate on the brain, remove disease, and provide an alive, conscious patient at the end.

The brain. That exquisite and enigmatic network of neurons and glial cells and billions of electrochemical connections. From basic physiologic oversight of fundamental functions of life to the elaborate architecture of the cerebral cortex, this masterful and complex organ has given rise to consciousness and thought processes characteristic of human behavior. How the grey convolutions and specialized centers evolved remains a total obscurity, as does the precise mechanism of reasoning, thinking, and conceptualizing. Involved in all this perplexity is the imposition of what some have called a spiritual motor—the soul. Does a soul indeed reside, perceive, and flourish immortally by virtue of cerebral input, or is this just the imagination of those who loathe to accept the inevitability of death? Regardless of ideas of immortality, soul and mind are inexorably linked in equally obscure fashions defying explanation. To wander into this vast living computer (and spiritual repository) is to invite disruption of pathways that, if extensive enough, will alter the neural grid in ways that affect behavior, emotions, and even cognizance. Journeying deeper might jeopardize motor and sensory function or, at the extreme, regulation of heart, lungs, and blood vessels. Paralysis, coma, and death are almost certain consequences of poorly planned and clumsy expeditions. Understandably, from antiquity, healers have been reticent to venture in, fearful of the dire consequences to follow. Yet, in the 20th century, the age of surgical marvels, scientists and surgeons stood poised—armed with an array of knowledge and skills—to violate the most sacred of organs.

The Great War provided the stimulus.

Head injuries, particularly those suffered on the battlefield, were the worst wounds inflicted. It was the immediacy of death that was so striking. In the age of gunpowder most victims died at once, the lead tearing through their brains, pulverizing the core of being so poorly understood but the fulcrum of humanness. Such men dropped immediately, no longer of this world. Attempts to revive were futile. For those less afflicted, those brought gasping and gurgling to harried surgeons, disruption of scalp and fragmentation of skull from various weapons, particularly gunshot wounds, provoked the temptation to intercede, gnawing on bone fragments with Stone-Age tools to try to elevate them from torn, swelling brain below. From antiquity the most common intervention employed on the skull for such injuries was trephining, the use of an augur-type device to burrow holes through the cranium for the purpose of releasing pressure, evacuating blood clots (or pus), and elevating in-driven skull fractures. In fact, the promotion of suppuration—pus—was felt by the medievalists as a necessary component of healing—an outcome that, in the era before antisepsis, was almost guaranteed to happen. Such meddlings often had fatal outcomes from the injury itself or the infection introduced. It was an impossible situation for patient and healer, the treatment often as lethal as the injury.

Even by the mid-19th century, there had been little resolution. Scottish surgeon George MacLeod, serving with the British army in the Turkish city of Smyrna during the Crimean War of 1853–56 compiled sobering statistics on the outcomes of his British troops suffering head wounds. Of those with mild injuries—perhaps some bruised brain—very few were lost, less than 1 percent. But with gunshot fractures and skull fractures, over one third died, and with bullets into the brain virtually all succumbed. Trephination hardly made a difference. Almost all subjected to that ancient procedure died.[4] "The mortality which attends the operation of trephining needs little proof, as it is one of the best recognized surgical facts," the sanguine MacLeod contended.[5] Indications to use the procedure must be well thought-out he advised, adding the generous comment that "the operation has failed as often as it has succeeded." Understandably, his position was:

> that as the symptoms calling for the use of the trephine have been so variously interpreted by men of experience . . . that as the good which has occasionally followed is ascribable . . . to other concurrent circumstances . . . and finally, that as the operation *per se*, is not devoid of danger, we should never have

recourse to the trephine, unless the indications for its use are very decided.[6]

With these experiences to draw from, it is no surprise that the common surgeon had no enthusiasm for head injuries. Most elected to treat them by watchful waiting. No ambitious operating. Only with reluctance, and only if there were signs of brain swelling—fading consciousness, usually—or brain infection, would surgeons dare to violate the skull.

Yet, thanks to a few intrepid souls, some progress was made in the closing years of that century. Rigorous efforts at asepsis seemed to help, and the ability to localize lesions in the brain by the symptoms and signs they produced aided clinicians in determining exactly where to trephine. Much of this work was done on animals, which had, of course, provoked an outcry among anti-vivisectionists. Nevertheless, it allowed British physician Hughes Bennett and surgeon Rickman Godlee to successfully locate a paralyzing tumor of the frontal lobe in a twenty-five-year-old man in 1884. Bennett localized the site, and Godlee pulled off a carefully planned operation to remove a piece of skull, peer beneath, and remove a tumor without incident. Even though the patient died a month later from complications, this was a significant achievement in the field of neurosurgery. Someone had actually survived surgery on the brain itself. As the two later reported:

> The chief features of interest in this case were that, during life, the existence of a tumour in the brain was diagnosed, its situation localized, and its size and shape approximated, entirely by the signs and symptoms exhibited.[7]

Cases like this stirred enthusiasm. Surgeons took a renewed interest in lesions of the brain. But, with poor skills and poorer understanding, their results were dismal. It mostly became a cognitive exercise for the non-operating neurology physician. According to the young Harvey Cushing, speaking before the Academy of Medicine in Cleveland in 1904, so often the neurologist identified a cerebral tumor, then:

An operator is called in; he has little knowledge of maladies of this nature and less interest in them, but is willing to undertake the exploration . . . and he proceeds to trephine. The dura is opened hesitantly; the cortex is exposed, and too often no tumor is found. The operator's interest ceases with the exploration, and for the patient the common sequel is a hernia, a fungus cerebri [brain infection], meningitis, and death.[8]

Cushing already knew that operating on the brain would need to be a patient, meticulous enterprise. Like no other organ, it tolerated so poorly any careless moves. These operations were not for the busy general surgeon who had only passing interest in cerebral matters. The two major problems were "bleeding and bulging"—hemorrhage from delicate cerebral vessels and swelling from tissue trauma.[9] Handling of brain substance, the consistency of gelatin and so central to the skills of surgeons such as Cushing, must be delicate, deliberate, and pains-taking; constant hemostasis producing a bloodless operating field in essence. Just as vital was adherence to absolute sterility. There must be no opportunity to contaminate the site with bacteria. Any residual hematoma (blood collection in the operative area) would provide ideal nourishment for microbes, and the consequences were too often fatal.

The more erudite of surgeons took up the standard. The Scotsman William Macewen demanded strict observance of two fundamental prin-ciples: immunity from inflammation—meaning strict asepsis—and local-ization of cerebral lesions through physical examination. He had been a house surgeon under Joseph Lister and was well versed in the nuances of antisepsis. As testimony, by following such mandates, Macewen claimed that of twenty-one "cerebral cases exclusive of fractures of the skull and other immediate effects of injury," there had been but three deaths and eighteen recoveries under his care.[10]

On the continent, the Prussian surgeon Ernst von Bergmann, like Macewen, a fanatic for strict asepsis, stressed the importance of sterility on head wounds. In agreement with his colleagues, Bergmann knew that penetrating head trauma was a setup for bleeding and infection. In particular, missiles and in-driven bone fragments frequently tore into the delicate, vascular meninges, the membranous covering of the brain, and lacerated brain tissue itself. Such events were likely to cause further bleeding. Conditions were perfect for infections to follow. Sometimes even the bacilli of gas gangrene would take root, injected far into brain substance by a bullet or bone fragment. The inevitable outcome in such cases, of course, was an ugly, tormented death. As dismal as the outcomes might be, such injuries forced the surgeon to operate. Bergmann was no reckless surgeon, though. Without violation of brain and its coverings, he urged fellow surgeons to refrain, for fear of planting infection in the vulnerable tissues beneath:

> knowledge of localities and routes by which we must proceed [into the cranial cavity] would not have justified us in opening . . . if the barrier against incision down to the cranial bones . . . had not been removed. This barrier was the occurrence of purulent meningitis . . .[11]

Bergmann had become a student of the brain and its response to trauma. He began to understand the consequences of brain injury. Aside from the destructive forces of the weapon itself, further damage could spread to affect vital areas some distance away and even disturb blood and oxygen supply. It all seemed a delicate balance that was so easily upset. The consequences could be surprisingly disagreeable:

> The primary cerebral lesions can be so significant that death follows quickly, be it through direct destruction of vital brain provinces or through impairment of blood movement in the brain, which sometimes disrupts, reduces and abolishes the nutrition of the most sensitive organ.[12]

He understood that brain injury often invited brain swelling, and that swelling might be responsible for disordering blood flow and nutrition. Once deprived of blood and oxygen, brain cells quickly died, and soon life was impossible. Bergmann was aware that trephination and rough handling of brain tissue only aggravated the situation.[13] Yet trephination could be lifesaving if it relieved pressure and restored oxygen delivery to crucial brain cells. Such decisions to operate must be made thoughtfully and carefully, and carried out with the utmost gentleness, he professed. Rough handling invited bleeding, always a constant threat. Once begun, control of bleeding from fragile arteries and veins was nigh impossible. Patients could literally exsanguinate. The force of his conviction gradually influenced surgical practice, and most soon realized that signs and symptoms of pressure on the brain demanded trephination in hopes of salvaging a dying patient. Few, though, were as gifted as Bergmann in the finesse of skillful operating.

The Swiss surgical wizard, Theodor Kocher, a clipped, humorless man known for his focused, scrupulous surgical techniques, certainly agreed. He was much aware of the disastrous effects of rising pressure on the brain within a rigid bony cranium, unable to expand. Pressure from brain swelling could close off nutrient arteries, and oxygen flow to cells would cease. He called it the anemia of "cerebral commotion"—the consequences of sudden forceful disturbances imposed on delicate neural networks. Anemia—the deprivation of life-sustaining blood—was lethal to nerve cells. "The increase in pressure causes displacement of fluids, cerebrospinal fluid, and blood," he had written.[14] Rising pressure was the cause. Kocher was even more ambitious in his treatment. He had gone beyond the simple drilling of holes in the skull. Craniectomy (or some called it craniotomy) was necessary, Kocher felt. He would remove large portions of the skull to allow the suffocating brain to literally breathe—swell forth but still receive crucial blood and oxygen. At the same time, he was careful not to intentionally disturb the dura mater. Violate it and be prepared for lethal infection unless strict asepsis is observed, he noted. Such radical surgery was not for the half-hearted or indecisive. His liberating technique "must be restricted to very specific cases" where there is certainty of underlying trauma that gives rise to compression. The thoughtless practice of "exploratory craniotomy . . . must be abandoned. The price at which you get the satisfaction of being able to carry out a thorough inspection of the brain surface is too high."[15]

Bergmann and Kocher were top surgeons of the era. Their quiet competence and foresight promoted a confidence in surgical care and instilled trust in their followers. Slowly, more of their colleagues boldly explored wounds of the head; more braved journeys deep into the brain. By the second decade of the 20th century, abstention from interference—the so-called expectant approach—had lost popularity. More likely now was the tendency to operate, and to operate early. Outcomes were encouraging; the Balkan Wars of 1912–13 proved that. A few military surgeons amassed considerable experience. After caring for thousands of casualties in the Balkans, both at the front and in rear-area hospitals. The Greek surgeon Pol Coryllos, for one, was inclined to totally abandon a watch-and-wait approach. "I am of the opinion that it is necessary to intervene in almost all cases of head wounds by gunshot and to intervene as soon as possible after the trauma."[16]

Onset of war in August 1914 gave surgeons ample exposure to all types of wounds, and wounds of the head were no exception. Those who decided on an aggressive approach—immediate exploration, cleansing, control of bleeding, and wound closure—once again seemed to reap a degree of success. One notable example was that of the Austrian surgeon Robert Bárány. Trapped and surrounded by Russian forces in the Przemyśl fortress in 1914, Bárány was forced to treat a number of soldiers with penetrating injuries to the brain. He immediately operated on thirteen of these, purging and closing all the wounds, including the scalp, at once. Out of necessity, because he was surrounded, Bárány kept these men with him, so he could see the results of his surgery. Of the group of thirteen, four died on the day of operation, each suffered catastrophic cerebral trauma. However, nine recovered and did not develop the dreaded meningeal or brain infections that so many surgeons feared. It appeared that, in fact, early operation on the brain following wounding had saved many.[17]

By 1915 British surgeons, too, made progress with head wounds. In the prewar years, the London surgeon Percy Sargent was a man devoted to disorders of the brain and spinal cord. He had been the celebrated Victor Horsley's assistant and displayed remarkable dexterity in his operations. His mentor, the gifted Horsley, was considered one of the true pioneers in neurological surgery at the close of the century. Sargent was enamored with his teacher and developed a fascination with the nervous system. Horsley, in turn, fed his young pupil the pearls of his trade, turning the eager doctor into a marvel of surgical expertise. With the winds of war, Sargent turned his full attention to neurologic surgery. By that time, he was an absolute wizard. Those who witnessed his skill could not help but be impressed:

> [Sargent exhibited] quick decision and rapid, skillful execu-
> tion [making] him the ideal neurosurgeon at the front, where
> there was often neither time nor facility for slow, meticulous
> operating and where twenty—not one—operations on the
> brain might have to be performed in a day.[18]

Yet, in Sargent's opinion, brain surgery had no business on the front lines. There was not the time or skill for such delicate and deliberate operating. Rough handling and hurried procedures were bound to stir up bleeding, extend damage, and foster later infections. Still, surgeons knew the urgency of operating on head trauma. There was little doubt quick intervention could save lives. The only alternative was rapid evacuation, a luxury seldom available in trench warfare. Sargent saw the consequences. By the time casualties reached surgical care, too many head wounds festered with infection or swelled with edema; the only recourse then was to widely decompress and debride. Rarely could operations be avoided, yet Sargent cautioned that "it must not be supposed that we are recommending extensive operations in all cases."[19]

His contemporaries agreed. At the Paris Inter-Allied Surgery Conference held in May 1917, doctors grappled with the dilemmas surrounding brain injuries. Once again, evidence pointed to early operation, but only at rear-area hospitals where skilled surgeons practiced and the patients could convalesce. Move them too soon and risk the dangers of hemorrhage. Such places like Bar-le-Duc, near Verdun, or Compiègne, or even Paris were proper sites. The muddy tents of British or French field hospitals were not. But battlefields would not permit these constraints. On the western front in all its filth and stagnation, such measures limited survival. Wounded men, oozing gray matter and teetering on unconsciousness, dawdled on stretchers while enemy fire poured in or litter teams were rounded up. Too little, too late produced fatality rates exceeding 50 percent. Outcomes like those of Bárány could not be duplicated. It was all pessimistic, deadly business.

◆

Harvey Cushing had worked with Kocher. He visited the master in Berne, Germany, in 1901 at the suggestion of his boss, William Halsted. By then Cushing was mystified by the brain. So few understood it. Even as an undergraduate at Yale, he had dissected a dog's brain and, at Harvard, had taken voluminous notes on the motor areas of the brain as they were known at the time. After his fourth year of medical school, while still at Harvard, Cushing had assisted surgeon John Elliot in two operations for brain tumors. Brave efforts indeed, Cushing acknowledged, but both patients died shortly after surgery. It was not until 1899, after completion of his surgical training, that Cushing attacked the debilitating disorder of trigeminal neuralgia. He spent countless hours perfecting his operation to remove the source of the ailment, the facial trigeminal (Gasserian) ganglion. But his sabbatical in Europe and studies with Theodor Kocher really piqued his interest. Cushing stood behind Kocher at the operating table and watched his movements. The maestro was like a concert pianist, instruments extensions of his fingers as if the flesh spoke to him. Now gentle. Now firm. Now quick. Now deliberate. The tissue parted for him almost by instinct. He was master of what lay beneath. This was Cushing's epiphany. In turn, Kocher was immediately taken with Cushing and offered him a research laboratory to study the effects of high intracranial pressure. It was a wise decision. According to Kocher's physiologist, Leon Asher, "Everyone in our laboratory was deeply impressed when Dr. Cushing appeared . . . From the very first he had all the eminent qualities and the great personality together with the wonderful charm."[20] A key factor in success with brain surgery, Cushing now knew, was control of rising intracranial pressure, and Kocher's laboratory afforded him opportunities to measure and correlate pressures inside the skull with critical functions of blood pressure and respirations, a landmark effect that would soon be called the Cushing-Kocher response.

A basic reaction of living tissue to trauma is swelling—officially called inflammatory edema. No different for the brain. However, firmly encased in a rigid, bony skull, trauma to the brain presented special difficulties. Jarring, bruising, or ballistic penetration to an organ the consistency of stout Jell-O produced an outpouring of blood-borne fluid that swelled the pliable interstices and even the brain cells themselves. In its bony confines, brain, unlike muscle or liver or intestines, cannot expand and, adhering to the physiologic interrelationship of pressure, flow, and resistance, intracranial pressure climbs.[21] The end result is compression of arteries and capillaries that could effectively shut off delivery of blood and life-sustaining oxygen. Brain cells then begin to die, and, before long, brain function ceases, perhaps irretrievably so. Bergmann had suspected it. Kocher understood it. And now Cushing embraced it as well. One compensatory mechanism, Cushing found, initiated somewhere deep in brain substance, was a signal to increase blood pressure in attempts to overcome the strangling pressure of tissue swelling. This was a major component of the Cushing-Kocher response.

Fascinating material for the young surgeon. In the course of all this, Cushing became a prodigious writer. After returning to America, in 1906 and 1907, he spent much of his free time working on a book chapter for William Keen's new five-volume opus *Surgery: Its Principles and Practice.*[22] It was to be like a bible for surgeons. Cushing's contribution was on surgery of the head. Initially limited to eighty pages, so detailed was he that it turned into eight hundred. Only with some resistance did he pare it down to a more modest 160 pages.[23] There was no doubt Cushing had a breadth of knowledge about neurologic surgery that few possessed. Even his mentor, the great Halsted, was suitably impressed:

> Dear Cushing, You little know how much I have hoped for a copy of your "Surgery of the Head" . . . I subscribe for Keen's surgery and had read much of your article with a great deal of interest & even eagerness, in that publication.[24]

And even prior to the war, he had worked out a system for dealing with head trauma, a not infrequent occurrence in civilian urban life. In typical Cushing fashion, his treatment would be thorough and method-ical. Simple skull fractures needed little surgical care, unless there were signs of high intracranial pressure. Then something had to be done to decompress the brain. More serious injuries that actually penetrated the bone, such as stab or gunshot wounds, deserved special attention. "Owing to septic complications a punctured cranial wound has long been accredited with especial danger . . . If the case presents itself early it is wise . . . to enlarge the wound . . . A button of bone which includes the puncture should then be removed with a large trephine."[25] Cushing went on to say that, if the dura mater—that tough outer membrane wrapping the brain—had been torn or punctured, it must be opened and the underlying brain exposed, examined, cleaned, and drained if necessary. If not done, infection was likely. He had already stressed the importance of a properly prepared operative field—head shaving, thorough asepsis, planned incisions, and control of bleeding. This was critical in any brain surgery.[26]

Needless to say, the onset of the World War in 1914 grabbed Cush-ing's attention. He had dabbled in affairs military and volunteered for service in the Spanish-American War, hoping for duty aboard one of the hospital ships off Cuba. Rejection. He was not needed near the front. Instead, he was relegated to the unglamorous role of handling cases shipped back to Baltimore. Hardly had his surgical talents been appreciated. Now at Harvard and chief of surgery at the new Peter Bent Brigham Hospital, Cushing got wind of his friend George Crile's efforts to send university doctors and nurses to the American hospital in Neuilly-sur-Seine, the Ambulance Américaine. "My dear George," Cushing wrote Crile, "I think it safe to say that Harvard University . . . can prepare to send a contingent to take hold [at the Ambulance Américaine] after yours has taken its turn."[27] Crile took him at his word, and after a flurry of details back and forth from Harvard to Neuilly, Cushing and his team were on board the SS *Canopic* March 18, 1915, headed for France.

On April 1, his Harvard group arrived, bedraggled from the long voyage in nasty weather. Work at Neuilly began soon, but few were the thrilling neurosurgery cases that had challenged him in Baltimore and Boston—at least for a time. "The actual surgery itself, it would seem, is not very difficult," he wrote from the hospital. Mostly, his time was consumed by exploring wounds of the arms and legs, removing damaged tissue and embedded foreign objects of war.[28] He had toured the battlefields—both French and British—visited Alexis Carrel's Hôpital temporaire no. 21 at Compiègne, and heard tales of the vicious German gas attack at Ypres that April ("the smoke was suffocating and smelled to some like ether and sulphur"[29]). And, on occasion, he was able to roam again within the cranial vault, picking out bone fragments and shrapnel from deep in the brain. To no one's surprise Cushing was an artist with his brain surgery, as if each move, no matter how small, flowed with a well-rehearsed proficiency. He had learned from Kocher. He had become his protégé. Few had seen anything like it.

He was back in Boston by the end of May and would not return to France for a full two years. During that time, he performed an extraordinary number of operations for brain tumors. In fact, it seems that, since 1902 and including both experiences in Baltimore and Boston, Cushing may have done almost eight hundred cases, all of which required that radical technique of skull removal called a craniotomy, permitting a wide view of the underlying brain and its pathology. Then he would remove large chunks of tissue with such elegance that blood hardly spilled. His exploits had made him something of a surgical star.[30]

But Cushing, the perfectionist, was bothered by what he had seen in France and the way war wounds of the head were handled. "There is no unanimity of opinion as to what should be the routine treatment of cranial wounds at first line hospitals," Cushing wrote after his return, in part based on his experience at the Ambulance Américaine. He seemed eager to compile his findings and share with surgical colleagues. Some surgeons in France, he had observed, preferred to treat immediately with trephination; others hurried to send the unfortunate victim farther to the rear. Of course, he saw only the ones who had been operated on beforehand. On more than one occasion Cushing felt it imperative to operate again—and again if need be—and extract more bone and shell and bullet fragments driven into brain but not retrieved at the outset. Haphazard surgery, he felt. He knew full well, like his British and French colleagues, that almost half of those with operations in frontline hospitals would succumb—

most from infections of the brain or meninges. And the farther back a victim had to travel for treatment, "the more gloomy becomes the prognosis." At the core was the fact that many military surgeons simply had no familiarity with head wounds and lacked the skills to manage them. Accordingly, there was a tendency to package the patient and send him on. This caused inevitable delays, improper treatment, and, very likely, poorer outcomes. These were complex injuries, Cushing felt, and proper treatment simply could not wait. Optimum outcome warranted a plethora of resources and skills not routinely found in 1915—whether at the field hospitals or base hospitals like the Ambulance Américaine. Surgery on the brain was so different than other aspects of general surgery.[31]

With all the fanfare of the United States' entry into the war, Cushing returned to Europe in May 1917, now officially a member of the AEF, the American Expeditionary Force, with the rank of major, commanding a full contingent of hospital personnel from the Harvard hospitals. His unit was named Base Hospital No. 5. On May 30, Cushing's Harvard team landed on the shores of France and, on a foggy and chilly night were transported to their hospital site, a run-down tent encampment of a former British general hospital just south of Boulogne. But his reputation had preceded him, and before long he had been summoned to tour forward hospitals in and around the neighboring Ypres salient. He drew in the likes of Sir Anthony Bowlby, consulting surgeon to the British forces, and Sir Douglas Haig, commander of the British Expeditionary Force in France.

As medical strategist for the British army, Bowlby's crowning achievement was taking lackluster clearing hospitals and expanding them into full-fledged forward surgical stations for the care of the dangerously wounded. These new casualty clearing stations, as they were called, seemed the ideal place to address head injuries. Operate on them early, the Allies agreed. Bowlby was in total harmony. Quick surgery could be lifesaving if done right. And his clearing hospitals were large enough to convalesce these patients until it was safe to move them.[32] He simply needed expertise in operative management, and Cushing the miracle worker was the ideal candidate. Casualty Clearing Station No. 46, then stationed near Proven, Flanders, would serve as the prototype. By late

July, 1917 Cushing was on his way to Proven. He was delighted. "We couldn't possibly be in a better place—simple, of course, but the whole equipment is far better than at . . . Camiers," he wrote.[33] His new hospital would be able to handle upward of 1,200 patients. The physicians would be needed. Another bloody offensive was being planned in Flanders.

Haig had orchestrated a third great offensive in the Ypres area, hoping to finally break through the German defenses and speed to the coast. His targets were German submarine bases in Belgium, a credible threat to transatlantic shipping. As so often happened in these great offensives, trench defenses—no matter how much they were pounded—were formidable obstacles. Germans were not about to be beaten, and held up well to British artillery and gas. The rain and flat floodplains of Flanders turned into a quagmire for troops and tanks alike, and Haig and his tactics stalled. The whole affair wallowed into a bloody, distasteful slaughter known as the Battle of Passchendaele. Tens of thousands of British troops were to be lost in a folly of attacks and counterattacks that would literally accomplish nothing.[34] It all began on Wednesday, August 1, and in a steady downpour. According to British prime minister David Lloyd George, "The Campaign of the Mud," as he described it, "will always rank as the most gigantic, tenacious, grim, futile and bloody fight ever waged in the history of war." It was a deplorable decision that he laid squarely at the feet of his commander in chief, Douglas Haig.[35]

Casualties streamed in quickly. Standing in mud and slosh and wearing a pair of rubber boots, Cushing operated from 8:30 A.M. to the next 2 A.M., his only nourishment generous portions of tea as a stimulant. The procession of head wounds seemed unending. Shrapnel pierced British Mark I helmets—not-so-lovingly referred to as the dishpan hat—and skull and brains beneath and demanded exacting extraction. Some men had lain in muck and rain, neglected for days, their wounds swarming with maggots. They were so covered in filth that it was almost impossible to tell where their injuries were. There was even one case of gas gangrene of the brain. "It's awful business," he recounted, "probably the worst possible training in surgery for a young man, and ruinous for the carefully acquired technique of an oldster," especially one with the extraordinary preciseness of Cushing.[36] The retrieval of metallic material from brain matter was an exacting and time-consuming affair, sometimes taking several hours to complete, all with the same attempt at sterility and hemostasis he insisted for his elective operations. In his thinking, there could be no compromise. Those who trained under him understood. One remembered: "His insight and skill in an emergency captivated me. Few words were spoken; much was accomplished."[37] Yet tolerance for imperfection was thin—poor outcomes and deaths of his patients plunged him into deep brooding, holding himself accountable above all.

The rain teemed incessantly, turning the ground into such a swamp that battlefield mud threatened to suck the wounded to their deaths. Of course, Cushing cared less about the elements and even less so about the British habit of heeding their mealtimes. He may have been slow in the operating room but he also wasted no time in such idle chitchat. All nonsense, Cushing felt. The operating table furnished his satiety, his glory. He would drive his American team to complete at least eight neurosurgical cases a day. These were desperately ill men with horrible wounds. Some had bullets and shell fragments well into their heads, near those vital centers in the stem of the brain. Death was millimeters away. Driven by urgencies, he operated for hours, food and drink frivolous luxuries he abandoned.

Harvey Cushing was no fan of slash-and-dash surgery, not by a long shot. He had seen the great Horsley do it while in England and had been appalled (Cushing was reported to have thought Horsley operated "like a wild man" and that "refinements of neurological surgery could not be learned from Horsley"[38]). His mentors Halsted and Kocher were nothing of the type either. Halsted had railed at such behavior. Kocher would have stood aghast. So, in Cushing's mind surgical bravado was the nemesis of brain operations. It was hack surgery, and he would have none of it. There would be criticism indeed leveled at him by both British and American commanders for not speeding along, especially in times of heavy casualties when patients were lined up waiting, but Cushing would not budge on this, preferring to do away with mealtimes and tea breaks in order to get the work done. The patient was better left untouched, he felt, rather than subjected to a hasty and ill-planned procedure (some head cases apparently died waiting for a place in his operating room, but it is very likely they would have died regardless). [39]

His method was deliberate: thorough shaving and cleansing of the scalp, removal of all bone around wounds of the skull, and gentle excavation of blood and damaged brain. For brain tissue, he used a special device—soft rubber tubing attached to a suction. This avoided use of his fingers. Of particular concern, though, was debris penetrating far into brain substance. This had always been a dangerous challenge for surgeons. If left behind it was sure to foster infection. If explored and removed there was a good chance that the prying fingers of the surgeon would damage more brain or start bleeding. Cushing would then wash with the wonderful hypochlorite solution of Alexis Carrel and Henry Dakin.

And then, for those metal pieces beyond reach, there was the magnet. It was called a "nail," but actually it was a thin wire inserted into brain and guided next to the metal. The wire was attached to an electromagnet and magically the entire apparatus was withdrawn, hopefully with metal adhered to the end.

It was not Cushing's invention, this magnetized probe, but it fascinated him. Who first thought of it? Electromagnetism had been a wonder of the fin de siècle. With its weird attractive and repulsive properties, some even thought it could exert mysterious effects on human health and disease—particularly the nervous system. As a result, electromagnetism too often bordered on quackery. Yet this use was different. Probably a French invention, marrying the invisible magnetic forces with surgery, extraction of magnetized "foreign bodies" (such as bullets or shell fragments) seemed a legitimate pursuit. Prior to the war, the Lyonnais ophthalmologist Etienne Rollet demonstrated the feasibility of removal of small shards of metal from inside the eye with his electromagnet. After war began, he marveled his contemporaries with electromagnetism by pulling pieces of German shell casings and metal-jacketed bullets from muscle and subcutaneous tissue as distant as 5–12 cm from the skin. [40] But it was the radiographer Etienne Henrard who combined the new X-rays of Röntgen with electromagnets. Henrard could now localize metallic fragments using three-dimensional coordinates—a process known as stereotactics—allowing surgeon Carl Janssen to push deep into brain substance with his magnetized probe and snatch these objects. It was all quite marvelous.[41] Patients hardly flinched, so little discomfort was involved. Yet, despite their successes Henrard and Janssen tempered their enthusiasm by not inviting disaster. Stay shallow, they cautioned:

> We were of the opinion that for the most part, only extract projectiles located shallowly and to leave those, which are more than 5 to 6 cm distant and do not cause real accidents. And yet, later, these "same small" projectiles can cause late fatal events [mostly abscess and brain infections].[42]

Cushing had first seen an exhibition at the Ambulance Américaine in 1915. One of the doctors there, a radiographer named Chaveau, introduced him to it. His first attempt was frustrating but eventually he pulled the shrapnel out, hanging on the end of the magnetized probe. Some might think it a display worthy of carnival sideshows: the tricks of invisible magnetism. But it was modern technology and much preferable to surgeons' stubby fingers rooting around in the depths of the brain.

Not that the procedure was flawless. It was tedious work docking a large electromagnet to the slender "nail." In those first cases of his, it often took several attempts to steer to the target. Yet Cushing remained calm, poised, unruffled, his patient demeanor so well suited to the fine motor movements needed in brain surgery:

> Let's try just once more! So I slipped the brutal thing again down the track, 3½ inches to the base of the brain, and again Cutler [his assistant] gingerly swung the big magnet down and made contact . . . and there it was, the little fragment of rough steel hanging on to its tip![43]

With the volume of head trauma now being seen, the technology had wide appeal. Belgian surgeon Antoine Depage sunk his magnetized wire into the brains of six patients at his seaside hospital at La Panne. Four survived free, now, of their cerebral rubbish. By 1917, electro-magnetism had become common practice for removing metallic fragments from the brain and elsewhere. Charles Willems's influential text *Manuel de chirurgie de guerre* emphasized that "immediate extraction of intra-cranial projectiles made a major advance by employment of a strong electromagnet introduced into the brain track to contact the projectile."[44] Like Depage, Cushing was now a disciple. In his work at Casualty Clearing Station No. 46 he boasted that he had used the magnet successfully eleven times in cases "in which the missiles would otherwise have been inaccessible."[45]

Haig would not relinquish his stubborn tactics, so the carnage in Flanders extended through October: thirteen separate attacks, by Cushing's count. He marveled at the stupidity of it all. Thwarted British assault after assault. The preparations became sickeningly familiar. Infantry brigades loaded with heavy packs struggled in the middle of the night just to reach their jumping-off point, usually in cold, relentless rain. Approaches to the front sometimes took hours. Then, once in frontline trenches, tired and soaked, commanders with those dreaded shrill whistles immediately piped them over the top. Into no-man's-land Tommies stumbled, toward objectives largely unseen. Exhausted, lost, they waded through muck the consistency of porridge up to their hips and into the teeth of enemy machine guns and artillery. "The conditions must be appalling," Cushing wrote in October. "An officer . . . says that a messenger he had sent back lost the tape [directional tape] and his sense of direction, wandered twenty feet away, and was found the next morning in a quagmire nearly up to his neck." He was alive when found but died shortly afterward.[46] The butchery from enemy fire was inhuman. Survivors slunk into shell holes filled with water. Those who could not keep their heads above the surface soon drowned. Others waited more hours before evacuation—if they lived that long. And then some were brought back to Casualty Clearing Station No. 46, their fractured heads full of metal and dirt.

Each attack brought a new crop of wounded in various stages of dying. On one particular Sunday morning, Cushing faced eight fresh head cases, all with pulped brain tissue full of splintered bone, bullet shards, and artillery slivers. Most were still awake and talking and eager to tell their tales. Some had been hit days before but lay in the mud until help arrived. Others arrived unconscious, their skulls broken, gray matter in total disarray, blood spilled throughout. For those, death was fast approaching, and Cushing in all his majesty could sometimes do so little.

Through it all, he was an inveterate record keeper. In the midst of his workload, he tracked all the head cases referred not only to his hospital but two others in the Ypres sector. Before his arrival, results had been discouraging. A full third of patients died before any surgery could be done. Of those who actually made it through operations, half lived and half died. Cushing changed all that. At Clearing Station No. 46 over a three-month period, he cut the death rate in half, down to less than 30 percent, and these were men with gored, bruised brains. Key to his success was that unaltered, compulsive routine: the shaving, the cleansing of skin, the careful debridement—scrupulous and detailed—followed by washing with the solution of Carrel and Dakin. It must be done the same way every time—and it must be done precisely—if survival was to improve. His case files contained every nuance of the patient and his wounds, how he planned his surgery, and particulars of the operation itself. These he would pore over in what leisure time he had, reflect, critique, and adjust for the next. There must be no errors. Precision was the target, and he aimed to nail it.

But there was also a personal side. With his patients, he faithfully recorded each soldier's name, rank, and unit—even their home addresses. He was enraptured by them, their suffering, the nobleness of their patriotism. With some he stayed in communication even years later—and they, in turn, adored him. His wife, Kate, kept one such letter:

> Dear Mrs. Cushing . . . In 1917—at Mendingham (No. 46 C.C.S.) I was a patient of the professor's—and had it not been for his skill and attention, I don't suppose I should be here to write this. . . . Twenty-two years have passed since he saved my life and now I have a son . . . [47]

One so affected by his patients could not help but be affected by the war. He had heard the stories of brutality and butchery on the battlefield and of the randomness of fortunes. He saw men who shook and trembled in trying to recall how they actually survived when so many of their comrades did not. His visits to the battlefields were sobering soliloquies, as he later wrote. Scenes worthy of hell: endless mud, tree stumps, and shell holes—a landscape stripped of beauty. On one visit to the front he saw:

> a waste unbelievably littered with debris of every kind, dead horses, derelict tanks, fallen and crumpled aeroplanes, cordite cans, shells, mortars, fish-tail bombs, broken and abandoned limbers, barbed wire, old trenches, water-filled craters . . .[48]

There was such a sameness to it; all so featureless that one could hardly tell in what direction lay friendly or enemy lines. There seemed only one constancy—the ever-present vestiges of humanity: half-submerged corpses in various stages of decay; an isolated foot or leg; a random fly-covered head; and the nauseating stench. It was a macabre graveyard of the unburied dead.

Cushing wrote and wrote, even more than his earlier days. He never seemed to tire of writing. Flanders looked to pull forth his most introspective nature. It was almost as if he were assembling his personal framework of neurologic surgery and his personal interpretation of war. In April 1918, he detailed his vast neurosurgery experience in France in *The British Journal of Surgery*. Never known for brevity, his report consumed 127 pages and involved 120 of his war cases in immaculate detail. He composed, in part, to dispel the pessimistic notion of brain surgery so many of his colleagues held. Cushing's conclusions? "The bad repute of cranio-cerebral operations from the standpoint of infection is, without question, largely due to delay—delay in transit, which may be unavoidable, unnecessary delay after admission, which often is avoidable," he said—shame on surgeons who tarried, he implied. Most cases had not arrived until well after twenty-four hours of injury so that all contaminated wounds had become infected—particularly those that pierced the brain—even before reaching his hospital. And as he had time and again, Cushing stressed his methodology of quick operation and meticulous, patient, and aseptic rituals. "There is every reason to believe," he wrote, "that by earlier operations, and by further improvements in technique along the lines of painstaking aseptic surgery, the accepted high mortality of cases . . . can be very largely cut down."[49]

Cushing rejoined his Harvard Base Hospital No. 5 in November, the unit having been moved to the port city of Boulogne. He and four of his friends settled in a leased beachfront villa for a more civilized existence than the desolation—and danger—of Proven.[50] It was a welcomed break. Much of the fighting on the western front was seasonal, and now it was winter. The next June, in 1918, he was ordered to pack up and head for AEF headquarters at Neufchâteau as senior consultant in neurological surgery. Pershing's American army was there in force and already embroiled in their own clashes. From action on the Marne, casualties had poured into American field hospitals in numbers that soon overwhelmed bed capacity. It was a picture that hearkened back to the early days of the war, when French and British wounded languished for days in the field, waiting to be evacuated. When they finally arrived many American boys already carried the swollen, smelly, discolored limbs of gas gangrene. Cushing pitched in and tried to bring order to chaos. No longer the neurosurgical specialist, he was the generalist, treating injuries of chest, abdomen, and extremities. His pace was frenetic, sometimes getting only a couple hours of sleep, once falling asleep on an operating table and tumbling off. He was one among many who did so and was quick to praise the young men who worked with him under tremendous strain. One surgeon later remembered:

> Dr. Cushing gave me but a kind word and in such a way that
> it did constitute one moment of glory in the dreadful months
> I spent operating upon the nontransportable wounded of the
> Second Dvision [AEF] during the campaign of 1918.[51]

In his role as senior consultant, Cushing now helped plan the Saint-Mihiel offensive in the late summer of 1918, and after that the Argonne offensive in the fall. When not actually operating he could be found visiting, surveying, calculating, and recalculating the numbers of hospitals to support Pershing's large-scale offensives. Yet, he could not help but push for neurosurgery centers that had seemed to work so well for the British, where head wounds could be better treated. He had even persuaded Colonel Alexander Stark, First Army surgeon, to position Mobile Hospital No. 6 for "head cases" at the village of Deuxnouds, southeast of the Argonne. Further pestering got him three more forward neurosurgical teams, at Souilly, Fleury, and Villers-Daucourt, forming a semicircle around the Argonne battlefields.[52] When Pershing's troops pushed into the Argonne, Mobile Hospital No. 6 proved to be a success. Over eight hundred head cases were routed there in less than three weeks. Cushing had taken great care to educate specialized surgical teams on the proper care of head wounds, hammering into them his standardized practices. Mortality must be kept low, he reiterated, and would be if they followed his tenets.[53]

A madman he had become; his pace unstoppable. Colleagues were amazed at his tirelessness, constantly on the move, visiting and checking on the field hospitals servicing American troops. Friend George Crile had been taken by "his incessant activity for improvement of the handling of brain cases."[54] But soon Cushing himself had become a victim. A peculiar ailment causing weakness of his legs had struck, confining him to bed for much of the time. For him the war would be over, not able for weeks to muster the stamina necessary for his time-consuming brain work. And for all, the war ended on November 11, 1918. Yet, Cushing the perceptive was in no mood to revel:

> There will be much celebrating, I presume, and drawing of corks—but perhaps not so much after all. That would have happened after the football game—a large dinner and the theatre—wine and song. This contest has been too appalling for that kind of thing, and there's a lot yet for everyone to do . . .[55]

He slowly recovered from his strange illness; some thought it might have been Guillain-Barrè syndrome or even a touch of that looming influenza virus.[56] In England by December, Cushing left for America on February 5, 1919. His steamship arrived in Hoboken, New Jersey, two weeks later, where he was met by Kate. And what of those days and nights hunched over men whose shattered bones and brains consumed his attention? What was he to make of it all? The war itself was immoral and distasteful, of course. There was some gratification that, for his part, neurological surgery had contributed far more to the conflict than even he had imagined it would. It was a time and place where he had merged the anatomy, physiology, and precision critical to surgery of the brain to accomplish what was heretofore unachievable—a reasonable chance of survival. He had injected a new paradigm that could be transposed onto civilian surgery and firmly anchored neurosurgery as a specialty all its own. Like-minded surgeons could now train, congregate, share ideas and skills, and provide for the waiting public a specialization that would raise standards of care.

Cushing's work during the Great War propelled neurosurgery to the forefront as a new surgical specialty. It had already been recognized by the Army Medical Corps at war's end as such. But the impact extended far beyond war trauma. Cushing was quick to point out that familiarity with head trauma did not necessarily translate to competence in "pathologic surgery"—the surgery of brain tumors, for example—in the civilian setting. Nevertheless, his methodical approach to head wounds—and his crusades to disseminate knowledge in this area—was a catalyst in forming the techniques needed to make neurological surgery a specialty of its own. It was in 1919, the war still a fresh memory, when Cushing had just presented a memorable paper on brain tumor statistics in his own inimitable fashion before the American College of Surgeons in New York, that the eminent William Mayo rose to declare, "Gentlemen, we have this day witnessed the birth of a new specialty—neurological surgery." And so it was decided. The Society of Neurological Surgeons, that first congregation of Cushing's followers, was born and the inaugural meeting held the following year.[57]

He had inspired a new generation of surgeons dedicated to surgery of the brain, spinal cord, and nerves, fueled especially by his exploits during the war. His case reports, his work ethic, his relentless desire to excel, and his dedication drew pupils in, eager to see him operate, to listen, and to absorb his knowledge. He alone became their icon. One later said of him after his death in 1940:

> His methods of treating head wounds at the front had proven revolutionary and many lives were thereby saved. I think he took deep satisfaction in visiting his various "teams" who were carrying out his operative technique.[58]

Harvey Cushing was the consummate surgeon-scientist—and the consummate educator. He relished the chance to disseminate newfound knowledge. Despite an admittedly large ego, there was no hint of self-aggrandizement. His discoveries belonged to the profession. It was his duty to teach, instruct, and, by example, instill. His hope: to relieve human suffering. Like other physicians of the Great War, Cushing's care of his patients was inexorably linked to an understanding of the basic principles of medicine. As a modern scientist, his practices were based on hypotheses, thoughtful experimentation, and assessment of the evidence. By scientific methodology lives were salvaged and enriched—he above others had shown that. But despite the specialized nature of his work, it was all still tied to total healing, both of mind and body. As characterized by physician-essayist Curtis Hart, Cushing "was both puritan and a patriot bound and determined to succeed and at the same time serve the common good."[59] Cushing himself was quick to point out: "I pray that neurologic surgery may never get so far from the home of general Medicine." Holistic care was paramount in his thinking. Cushing felt inseparable the human constitution and the human spirit. For Harvey Cushing, scientist, healer, and humanitarian were one and the same.[60]

EIGHT

Shattered Faces

"You have no right to ask men to endure such suffering."
—Surgeon and artist Henry Tonks, on the facially disfigured

Lance Corporal Ward Muir, a thirty-seven-year-old soldier-orderly at the Third London General Hospital, enjoyed his work and was even relieved he had not been picked for duty in France. He had tried twice to enlist, feeling that wearing khakis was his patriotic duty, but age was against him. Finally, on the third attempt he was accepted. But not for combat. He would be assigned to the Royal Army Medical Corps as a hospital orderly. As for orderlies, they were "honest souls capable of trotting about on errands from dawn till dusk and of being useful in countless ways." Generally, it was pleasant work; he even considered the staff—doctors, nurses, and orderlies—a "jolly" family of sorts. Mostly, his trusts were convalescing patients, the consequences of their wounding settling into a mundane ritual of dressings changes, bathing, meals, and socializing— almost a tranquility after the carnage of the battlefield. But there was one ward where happiness had fled, where it was hard to look a man in the face—or what was left of it—hard to meet him eye to eye. This was the ward that housed destroyed faces:

Hideous is the only word for these smashed faces: the socket
with some twisted moist slit, with a lash or two adhering

feebly, which is all that is traceable of the forfeited eye; the skewed mouth which sometimes—in spite of brilliant dentistry contrivances—results from the loss of a segment of jaw; and, worse, far worse, the incredibly brutalizing effects which are the consequence of wounds in the nose, and which reach a climax of mournful grotesquerie when the nose is missing altogether.[1]

Doctor Robert Tait McKenzie saw it, too. A Canadian citizen, he had departed Philadelphia at the outset of the war for England to serve in the same Royal Army Medical Corps—"to work for the welfare of the human race," as he saw it.[2] His abiding interest in physical training and fitness led him to develop specific rehabilitation programs for disabled soldiers for many of the convalescent hospitals around England. In this area his programs were legendary; he was truly one of the architects of modern physical therapy and rehabilitation. Of all these handicapped men, though, it seemed most disheartening to see the disfigured:

> Among the most distressing cases met with in military surgery are those in which the face has been so destroyed as to defy the best efforts of the plastic surgeons. The jagged fragment of a bursting shell will shear off a nose, an ear, or a part of a jaw, leaving the victim a permanent object of repulsion to others, and grievous burden to himself . . . After plastic surgery has done its best . . . there remains nothing but a living gargoyle.[3]

It was a peculiarity of trench warfare. Deep in their subterranean jigsaw slits, men were well protected from the neck down. Even bursting ordnance above, unless a direct hit, was survivable. But it was the forgetfulness, or maybe curiosity—or maybe even Mother Nature—that made foolish kids rise up above the parapets—just a peek or quick dash. One did get tired of the confines of earthworks, and at times one did feel an urgent nature's call. Maybe a quick glance at wide-open landscape might ease their claustrophobia. Or maybe a hurried trot to relieve oneself. Sure enough, across no-man's-land a sharpshooter, waiting patiently, would squeeze off a round and, in a blink of an eye, the jacketed bullet would smack into another teenager and either blow his brains out or, just as cruel, crease his face in ways that defied explanation. And then there was artillery. The murderous assaults of Verdun and the Somme and dozens of other nameless battlefields were intermingled with torrential bombardments, flinging metal fragments at blinding speeds into the faces of stooped, advancing infantry. At closer range there would be canister rounds, much like giant shotguns, spewing balls the size of walnuts. There some would lay, caught full-face in the barrage, bleeding and gurgling but quite awake: jaw, eye, nose shot away. Those chunks of metal were brutal: slicing off entire faces, leaving fully conscious horrible messes. Yes, *mess* was the only way to describe it, features the consistency of raw meat.

That was only the beginning. Alive, yes, but the start of a lifelong tragedy. Indeed, some might later think "would that I had died." In his essay "Handicap d'Apparence," David Le Breton made the following observation:

> The hierarchy of dread and rejection seems to put in the front line the man with the disfigured face . . . The man who "no longer has human features" . . . In our western societies the principle of identity is embodied essentially through the face. None of the skills to work, love, educate, live, prevents [the disfigured] from practicing because of his condition. Yet, he is sidelined by a subtle demarcation from which arises a symbolic tone all the more virulent since it is unrecognized.[4]

And the disgust, the pity began on the battlefield. Repugnance of such wounds was immediately apparent. Stretcher-bearers, seeing the clotted craters that gaped, a gurgling, moaning form beneath, would often leave the poor soldier for dead, and move on to more agreeable injuries. Many of these victims, sometimes blinded, barely conscious, could not get enough air pass their ravaged throats and suffocated unattended. Even those lucky enough to be carried by litter to the aid station, flat on their back of course, would choke on their own gore, unable to turn or sit and clear their airway. No one had the slightest notion or inclination to sweep away the gurgling cavities. At the advanced surgical stations, surgeons avoided such problems. Ordinary doctors, even those trained in surgery, had no idea how to care for them. Instead, facial wounds were wrapped with reams of gauze to hide the misery and marked for transport to other places: maxillofacial centers miles away. There was one in Amiens on the Somme battlefield and in Bar-le-Duc behind Verdun. It was here that specialists first examined the smashed and torn. Wounds were cleaned, shell pieces and bullets along with loose bone chips and teeth removed, and soft tissue (skin, muscle) loosely approximated. Surgeons attempted to close over yawning holes, but there was no reconstruction. Faces still looked horrid. Men still looked inhuman. Very often, swallowing was impossible, so feeding tubes were snaked down gullets or passed directly into stomachs. It was a pitiful sight, even to trained professionals. After the battle of Champagne in 1915, James Judd, volunteering at the Ambulance Américaine in Neuilly-sur-Seine, stumbled on such a case:

> Another boy was shot through the face sideways, the piece of shell tearing away a large part of the lower jaw and half his tongue. A fringe of lower lip hung down almost to his chest. He cannot speak, so writes notes asking for something to drink and whether he will ever be able to speak again. He is wonderfully brave and patient and after having been fed a few times he took his tube [feeding tube], funnel and pitcher of milk and insisted on feeding himself.[5]

Most such patients were kept no longer than a week before transfer back to skilled surgical teams. Doctors at most military hospitals had no means or time to deal with them.

Their reluctance was understood. Even from a professional perspective, these were impossibly complex injuries. The skin and bones of the face—the maxilla and mandible, nasal bones, eye sockets—could be cleaved, shattered, burnt, crushed, and gouged to the degree that human features were horribly altered or unrecognizable. At first glance, the victim often looked a grotesque monster. The human countenance was gone. Such mutilation could easily evoke revulsion, pity, disgust, and avoidance. And what of the spirit within? Also a victim; the defaced soldier stripped of dignity, hardly a man, hardly human. In no other conflict past or future were such numbers of marred men thrown back into society. Historian François Long estimated that from 11 to 14 percent of French wounded sustained trauma to the face, maybe as high as 15,000 such injuries.[6]

Weeks, sometimes months later, one could find them in those specialized hospital wards, the wounds now emitting a foul odor and the poor victims drooling saliva into bags under their chins. Long rows of the mangled, the monstrous, the misfits; caverns of the wretched. Yet, in a way, it was a small comfort to be at last in a place of fellow sufferers. Author Sophie Delaporte remembered one patient who later wrote:

"We could have despaired of everything if at our arrival in the hospitals, in our first contacts with the other wounded of the face, we had not had the reassuring impression that the very nature of our injury would bring us closer to each other in a completely exceptional way."[7]

◆

Before the Great War, before the times of carnage and catastrophic destruction, few surgeons cared much about the face. There were those, of course, who, from time to time, carved away giant tumors so noticeable that cosmetics demanded it. Yet to reconstruct was another matter. Elaborate methods to shift, insert, and arrange bone and skin were time-consuming and fraught with complications, many due to infections. For surgeons it was not popular business. Results were obvious, often discouraging, and not good for marketing.[8]

Hippolyte Morestin was the exception. Morestin projected a character of aloofness and competence; a man who at once stood out among others. He was of medium height, his face punctuated by a swirling mustache and goatee, yet his confidence—one might say quiet swagger—inflated an average build and set him apart. A solitary, private man, he shared little of his professional talents unless by pure example while operating, at which time he spoke freely, almost pretentious in his demeanor. There was an unpredictability to his temperament, sometimes placid, other times railing at any slightest imperfection in his team's performance. Of exceptional aptitude, he had left his native Caribbean island of Antilles to study medicine in Paris. Completing formal education, he began working at Hôpital Saint-Louis. Surgeons of the time, with availability of general anesthesia and asepsis, vigorously expanded the breadth of surgery to rid patients of cancerous lesions: wide swaths of surrounding skin, muscle, and bone taken with the tumor itself. Pathologists had warned of microscopic cancer cells lurking beyond the malignancy. Surgery was often a patient's only hope, to sweep out margins of normal appearing tissue as well. Craters left behind were secondary concerns, the price one paid for cure. Cancers of the head, face, and neck were particularly odious. Few surgeons had the gall to take them on. Facial distortions left from radical operations there were not easy to remedy. Patients recoiled at the sight of their mutilations and hid from the public. These pathetic creatures Morestin welcomed. He was a surgical artist, his canvas the face, his palette the genius that comes with innate talent to conceptualize. Morestin envisioned movement of flesh here, bone there, to restore natural flow of skin, the ridges, prominences, and valleys of humanness. To this end Morestin was a master of richly perfused skin flaps, those vascularized pieces of flesh he would advance, swing, and install into the cracks and crevasses holed out by cancer surgeons. He was gifted in the tactile: that sense of texture, of feel, of suppleness that allowed such fine techniques. It was patient, time-consuming work, sometimes three, four, or more operations were necessary before his desired result was achieved. On occasion, Morestin even gathered fatty tissue and rib bones to help in his facial contouring. By the first decade of the 20th century, his reputation was worldwide. Some would write:

> His experience in this malignant tumor surgery was exceptionally extensive; everything he has written on this subject will always be read with the greatest benefit by surgeons: it is a lasting and solid part of his surgical work. [9]

It was in the fall of that fateful year, 1914, that Hippolyte Morestin was summoned to the Val-de-Grâce military hospital as casualties streamed in with facial wounds. No one had seen anything like it. Hordes of gouged features, flesh and bones hanging like tattered fabric, snot and spit slavering from cavernous hollows. Few had any treatment, their injuries now festering mercilessly. Contractures, inflammation, and more deformity were the result, nature anxious to somehow remedy the insults. But Morestin looked upon these victims as one might jigsaw puzzles—not with pity but purpose. In his detached fashion, he was methodical as always. First came function. Workings of the jaw were crucial. Apposition of upper jaw (maxilla) and lower jaw (mandible)—along with rows of teeth—was needed for the simple act of eating and talking. Smashing bullets or shells often fractured and shattered mandible and maxilla; teeth were likely gone as well. Men could not chew, and slobbered and spit in garbled speech.[10]

These patients deserved special care, Morestin knew. Perhaps he had heard of the famous Düsseldorf Lazarett für Kieferverletzte (Düsseldorf Hospital for Jaw Injuries), set up at the start of the war. The talented contemporary, Professor Christian Bruhn, a dentist by trade, had already amassed a vast experience in industrial maxillofacial injuries and had anticipated that any future war would produce horrific wounds much more destructive than in prior conflicts. Eventually he procured a private hospital, which became his "Jaw Hospital," that afforded him almost seven hundred beds for his patients. Working with a team of surgeons, including the famous August Lindemann, his clinic produced a wealth of experience in the reconstruction of the jaw, much of the work involving bone grafting and prostheses to maintain proper dentition during the healing phases (for which Professor Lindemann was to become well-known). Frequently his patients wore external appliances much like modern-day orthodontics, which kept bone fragments together. Functional rehabilitation was the aim. To that end, he employed dietitians and physiotherapy specialists. Bruhn felt they were essential to successful convalescence of his reconstructions. He even set up workshops for his patients to resume their former skills and immersed them in writing, artwork, and concerts. His became one of the first multidisciplinary clinics in the world to specialize in facial trauma. Bruhn wrote reams about his work. They were famously published in volumes of *Die Gegenwärtigen Behandlung-swege der Kieferschussverletzungen* (*The Current Treatment Options for Jaw Gunshot Injuries*). [11]

So, these two pioneers, Bruhn and Morestin, alerted the profession to new techniques for sculpting the damaged face. Their focus first on functionality, the simple tasks of eating and talking, was paramount. Later, restoration of a suitable cosmetic appearance was the mission. Morestin had a name for his restorative efforts—techniques gleaned from the pioneering work of Charles Nélaton and Louis Ombrédanne, published in 1907—"autoplasty," (the name given by Nélaton and Ombrédanne). It involved the paring and lifting of skin to advance, swing, and fill gaps in anatomy. It was a tedious process, "a game of patience," he wrote. Cartilage, taken from ribs, was often needed to reconstruct forehead, eye sockets, cheekbones, and jaw. [12]

These procedures, though, were long and demanding. Bruhn and Morestin spent hours in the operating rooms on countless deformed patients. [13] For Morestin, his finished labors were a marvel around Paris. The lay press considered him a miracle worker for injuries that affected "the most human place of man": the face. [14] When Morestin spoke, as he did before l'Académie de médecine on March 13, 1917, the press was there, taking in before and after pictures. "I have rarely seen a more moving spectacle than that of these split, jagged, crushed, hollowed out, shapeless faces with thick ragged edges, infiltrated, bruised, literally monstrous," one journalist wrote. And then, on the "after" displays, after Morestin had shown the fruits of his talents, the same journalist continued: "but on the pages that follow each other in the album, here is gradually the order and the symmetry and the former beauty reborn by the wonderful art of the master surgeon." [15]

It was claimed that his unrelenting work, the endless hours of operating, his pedantic nature, and his deep empathies for these men contributed to an early, premature death soon after the war ended (or was he another victim of the great influenza pandemic of 1918?). He was gone by 1919. Paul Lecène and Henri Mondor, two well-known French surgeons, gave Morestin the highest of compliments with their praise that:

[Morestin] displayed unremitting activity and zeal during the five years of the war, and hundreds of the wounded were able to benefit from his exceptional skill; but the considerable fatigue he imposed on himself during this period certainly contributed to his premature death.

France, indeed, forfeited an icon with his death. Lecène and Mondor, unquestionable admirers, went on to say, "what a loss French surgery suffered when this elite surgeon died prematurely."[16]

While Morestin's techniques and strategies were impeccable, they may have been lacking what Bruhn so wisely had put into place: the holistic rehabilitation of these tortured creatures. Morestin's patients frequently entered a world hostile to their disfigurement, despite the miraculous wonders of surgery. Little prepared, they withered in a society that often shunned them as inhabitants of darker natures and the monstrous hunchbacks of war. And what of more personal matters, the intimacies of man and woman, the interplay of family and friends? In his memoir, *The Happy Hospital*, lowly orderly Ward Muir may have said it best:

Suppose he is married, or engaged to be married . . . Could any woman come near this gargoyle without repugnance? His children . . . Why, a child would run screaming from such a sight . . . To be fled from by children! That must be a heavy cross for some souls to bear.[17]

After all, the face is a portal to the soul. Whether glee, worry, or indifference, the multitude of features—the fine muscles that guide expression, slant and swivel of lips, eyes seemingly lit as if by incandescence—add credibility to the spoken word and convey warmth or cold as a condition to friendship or enmity. That which we highlight as most human, that which greets us at once upon meeting, then, is an animation brought about by that most complex of contortions to reflect an innermost regard—good or bad—most pleasing to portray and most difficult to conceal. Conversely, distortion of countenance in a ghastly manner descends into dominions of the monstrous and even demonic. Customary renderings of evil quickly alter visible appearances to be repulsive, hideous, and otherworldly. Such, then, was the anguish of these men whose sensitive natures now barricaded within vile distortions so as to project appalling and lurid images immediately fearsome. They were, at first glance, how they appeared: freakish effigies from satanic worlds.

This was not of their doing. These men shunned a world that they feared shunned them. Shrapnel had robbed them of dignity and tore at their hearts, mutilated by war as well. How could those most tender of emotions find their way to the surface, through the ravaged contours of war's remembrance? Love, that most basic of desires, might now be trapped forever below.

"Quel dommage," the French would say, "such a pity." There was nowhere to hide the ravages of facial trauma. Amputees were viewed as heroes; their artificial limbs a mark of bravery and endurance. Internal injuries were neatly tucked away beneath large abdominal scars. Not so those whose wounds were borne without concealment. "A man who did not look like a man, to himself and others, would not be able to live as one," historian Beth Haiken wrote. [18] David Le Breton added: "in our western societies the principle of identity is embodied essentially through the face."[19] Physiatrist Robert Tait McKenzie feared that such victims might become "a permanent object of repulsion to others, and grievous burden to himself. It is not to be wondered at that such men become victims of despondency, of melancholia, leading, in some cases, even to suicide."[20]

Morestin's patients banded together, forming their own support group. They called themselves *gueules cassées*—broken faces. Their journal *La Greffe Générale (The General Registry)* was a publication written by the patients themselves from 1917–18, a mixture of satire, pride, and practicality. These broken faces became a fraternity, united in their shared suffering and anxiety. True understanding, they knew, came only from those so affected. And, after the war, their fellowship matured into official groups, such as the Association générale des mutilés de la guerre (General Association of the War-Mutilated) and Union des mutilés et réformés (Union of the Disabled and Reformed), offering avenues of mutual support after *La Greffe Générale* ceased publication.[21] But probably the most influential would be L'Union des blessés de la face et la têt (Union of Wounded of the Face and Head), formed in July 1921, whose president, Colonel Yves Picot, was one of them, a *gueule cassée*. In January 1917 like a flash, an artillery shell exploded in front of him, shards puncturing his left eye and tearing off his nose. At Val-de-Grâce he underwent a series of painful reconstructions, there meeting other *baveux* (droolers) and sensing the need for some recognition of their bravery. He would crusade for social and political acknowledgement of all disabled but particularly his fellow *gueule cassées*. As for Morestin, despite their social stigmata, his "broken faces" adored him, calling him a miracle-worker, a *souverain contre les mutilations facials* (sovereign of facial mutilations). [22]

It was to this magnificent surgeon that a young British otolaryngologist by the name of Harold Gillies came. Gillies, a native of New Zealand, migrated to England for his training. He had shown remarkable potential and been hired as an understudy of the eminent King's own surgeon Milsom Rees. It was a sought-after practice on Harley Street, London, both lucrative and prestigious. But then war came and Gillies, feeling the patriotic tug, volunteered for service with the Red Cross. Preceding his trip to Morestin, early 1915 found Gillies at a Belgian field hospital near Boulogne. There he met the controversial and colorful dentist Charles Valadier.

Auguste Charles Valadier was a showman. A Parisian by birth, he had been educated in both medicine (or so he claimed) and "Dental Surgery" (verified, at length, from documents at the Philadelphia Dental College) in the United States. Valadier returned to Paris in 1910 after giving up a rather cushy New York City practice (the reasons remained obscure). With some effort, Valadier finally received a certificate of *chirurgien dentiste* from the University of Paris. The enterprising dentist promptly opened up a ritzy Place Vendôme office and began catering to the affluent of Paris. War caught him in a patriotic spirit as well, and, for reasons not entirely clear, he joined the *British* Red Cross, arriving at his duty station at Boulogne in a chauffeur-driven Rolls-Royce. [23] By hook and crook—but also, no doubt, by some degree of skill—the resourceful Valadier managed to convince British General Headquarters of the need for a face-and-jaw center (he had allegedly ceremoniously filled a good many of their teeth with gold), even though a few miles away another such unit had already been organized by the Harvard surgeon Varaztad Kazanjian.[24] Not to be outdone, Valadier commanded quite a production. Smooth of tongue and full of confidence, he coerced numbers of beds from the nearby Eighty-Third General Hospital and set up his face-and-jaw center in the small town of Wimereux. Fifty beds were now ready for facial trauma. He advertised his expertise widely, skills of facial reconstruction for which, should one ask, he seemed exceptionally suited.

Gillies and Valadier must have met there. For one thing, Gillies was drawn to facial surgery. He had devoured innovations on jaw injuries by Charles Nélaton and Louis Ombrédanne, including their remarkable transfers of flesh, and wanted firsthand experience. No better mentor than Valadier, it seemed, a man of exquisite taste and reputation. Let the show begin, Gillies must have thought, in his first encounter with the flashy Parisian. His biographer, Robert Ivy, gave this account:

> In Boulogne there was a great fat man with sandy hair and a florid face who had equipped his Rolls-Royce with dental chair, drills, and the necessary heavy metals. The name of this man, whose high brown riding boots carried a polish equal to the glitter of his spurs, was Charles Valadier.

He tagged along with Valadier to tour the jaw center, the progress of which, according to Gillies, "must go to the remarkable linguistic talents of the smooth and genial Sir Charles Valadier."[25] How exceptional was Valadier's unit is open to some question. Surely, there was no shortage of pomp and circumstance but perhaps less so of marvelous reconstructions. A fellow dentist, Ferdinand Brigham, who knew Valadier well, claimed that few patients were admitted to his special wards. Most, Brigham said, Valadier passed on to England. Moreover, Brigham went on, he had seen little innovation. For the most part, surgery mimicked that done at the Val-de-Grâce. Much smoke and mirrors, it seemed. Staid and sober Victor Horsley thought so when he visited in 1915, calling the whole business "fatuous."[26] However, the more diplomatic Brigham pointed out that Valadier authored a number of scientific articles on his facial surgery, highlighting his magnificent palatal and mandibular splints to hold bones and teeth in alignment during healing. And Valadier welcomed the help of general surgeons to cover soft-tissue defects and bony repairs. But make no mistake, they would never grab his glory. Valadier insisted he was the central figure, and, speaking to his dental readership, wrote, "you should be congratulated by general surgeons [for work done] far beyond your desires or expectations, receiving scientific recognition more than you deserve."[27]

Showmanship aside, Gillies was intrigued. He saw vast possibilities in this surgery to rebuild shattered faces. There was more to learn; who better to learn from than the famous Morestin of Paris. Perhaps Valadier had tipped him to the name—Morestin's reputation by now was almost legendary. So that is how it happened on a June day in 1915. Gillies paid his first visit to Morestin's clinic. The egotistical surgeon was warm and inviting on that occasion, and even asked young Gillies to watch his masterful attack on a facial cancer. Gillies was captivated:

> In the space of a single moment he could reveal the gentleness
> of a kitten and the savagery of a tiger. He received me kindly,
> and I stood spellbound as he removed half of a face distorted
> with a horrible cancer and then deftly turned a neck flap to
> restore not only the cheek but the side of the nose and lip, in
> one shot . . . at that time it was the most thrilling thing I had
> ever seen. I fell in love with the work on the spot.[28]

His second visit was not so welcoming. Morestin, now for some reason in a distinctly sour mood, barely recognized Gillies and grudgingly admitted him to his surgery. Little did Gillies care; he knew well his future passion, surgery of the face.[29] As for the grumpy Morestin, Gillies shrugged it all off. "Morestin was very unkind to me in the way of not letting me see his war surgery, but he was a very jealous and secretive person."[30]

Back to England for Gillies. The idea of a specialty clinic—like Morestin had—with surgeons and dentists skilled in the subtleties of facial reconstruction absorbed him. Gillies tapped his Harley Street contacts and soon had the ear of Sir Anthony Bowlby and Sir George Makins, both consulting surgeons to Alfred Keogh himself, director general of Army Medical Services. Keogh heard them out and was intrigued. He had already considered specialty units such as this in reorganizing the beleaguered medical services. Keogh instructed Arbuthnot Lane, director of the Army Surgical Services and commander at the Cambridge Military Hospital in Aldershot, outside London, to bring aboard the youthful Gillies (he was now but thirty-four) "for special duty in connection with Plastic Surgery."[31] Cambridge Hospital was a sprawling complex dominated by a lone clock tower, but surrounded by placid, bucolic landscapes. It had become a primary destination for Britain's innumerable war casualties. Lane himself sympathized with the wrecked faces that passed through. "The man who loses an arm, a leg, or is injured in the body, can go back to the bosom of his family, but the man whose face is distorted, no matter how much his family may love and cherish him, suffers most," he had said.[32] Lane would be the perfect boss and Cambridge the perfect location for the start of Gillies's healing crusade.

Promoted to captain now, Gillies argued that facial wounds should be segregated even on the battlefield. Clean them up, set them aside, and tag them. Then, swathed in white bandages, they could be funneled back to his unit in England. He even personally financed printing of casualty labels—distinctive enough to be recognized at a distance. At first, frontline surgeons balked. They were too busy to comply. It was just more paperwork. The Somme offensive in July 1916 changed all that. It would be the most murderous attack in British history. On the opening day alone, July 1, there were over fifty-seven thousand casualties, more than nineteen thousand of whom had been killed.[33] Numbers of arriving casualties went from enormous to incomprehensible, surgeons from busy to beleaguered. Now they were only too happy to cull out the facial wounds, tag them, and send them on—paperwork or no. In a ten-day period, two thousand sorted for Aldershot. Easy enough, perhaps, but new problems arose. Delays became logistical—and legendary. Once again, railways and motor transports were overwhelmed. Throngs of men idled on stretchers at train stations or in coach cars on railroad sidings, waiting their turn. Most suffered silently; many could neither eat nor drink. A miserable few begged to die. And not infrequently, some, mouths and throats full of clot and mush, their voices stifled, quietly expired in solitude.

But when they did come, Gillies's two hundred beds filled in a hurry. For so many casualties there were not nearly enough, nor was there space enough for his surgery. Even scarcer was room for rest and rehabilitation. Gillies went to Keogh for more. He had heard about Bruhn's hospital in Düsseldorf and wanted something like it: plenty of space to house, treat, and convalesce his cases who needed such intensive management. Setting down before and after pictures in front of him, Gillies convinced Keogh. It was all quite impressive. With his talents, facial features took on an almost normal form. Crevasses and cracks disappeared. Noses, eyes, and chins reappeared. It was a lengthy process, though. In the interim, men languished, sporting various tubes, flaps, and bizarre plates and prostheses. They still felt disagreeable to the passing glance and refused to be seen by family or friends.

Keogh had an idea. It turned out that a stretch of land in Kent had become available. On it sat Frognal House in the town of Sidcup just southeast of London. Frognal House was a stately redbrick Jacobean mansion. Centuries old, it was purchased in 1752 by a Thomas Townshend. His ownership passed down to descendants until the last proprietor, great-great-nephew Robert Marsham-Townshend, died in 1914. It was Robert's son Hugh Sydney Marsham-Townshend who sold the house and the 1,700 acres of grounds to the British Red Cross and Order of Saint John in 1916. Keogh would make it Gillies's hospital. Construction of building complexes Gillies needed for his work began in February 1917 and was completed by July.

The entire compound took on the appearance of a vast military encampment. The Frognal House itself was used for officers' messes downstairs and nurses' quarters upstairs. In back, hospital wards were located in huts arranged like a horseshoe, connected by duckboards as a circular walkway. Inside the horseshoe more huts were built to house operating rooms and offices. Extending right down the middle of the horseshoe was a long building filled with X-ray, therapeutic electricity, massage, photography, and specialized nose, throat, and dental clinics. There were even wards segregating Canadian, Australian, and New

Zealander patients—each with their own surgical teams. Altogether Gilles now had space for 320 patients. Doors opened on August 18, 1917, the facility now named Queen's Hospital, Sidcup. Gillies even took over parts of the town, commandeering houses as residencies for convalescing patients or for occupational or vocational training. Even 320 beds, though, would not be enough. By war's end, the main hospital expanded to 560 beds, and the entire enterprise could house nearly 1,000 patients.[34]

Gillies excelled at his work. Like Bruhn and Morestin, he became a surgical sculptor. Hideous faces morphed into human contours as if he had taken clay in his hands, fluted and massaged until anatomy corrected. Yet, for Gillies, it was painstakingly methodical. He would first study his maimed subjects. Missing and destroyed anatomy must be cataloged, skin assessed for blood supply and pliability, bone structure and dental architecture detailed. He looked and felt: injuries palpated, flesh kneaded. The new Röntgen rays were invaluable in plotting bone reconstruction. Gillies even used plaster casts to help design his surgery. Technology and artistry meshed in his hands in perfect combination. He was uncannily astute, his mind's eye foretelling each considered option.

With inventory taken, he began. First, further damage had to cease: scar tissue released, skin freshened and anchored. Then the skeleton itself—nature's scaffolding—must be repaired. "Disappointment is in store for him who would confine his repair to the surface tissues, heedless of Nature's lessons in architecture," Gillies cautioned. This is where the unflappable sculptor dominated. Haste had no place for the perfectionist, the one who must nip, tweak, and pull back to judge. Then make the finest of adjustments and judge again, as if the trims and scoring cut too much or too deep. "There is no royal road to the fashioning of the facial scaffold by artificial means: the surgeon must tread the hard and narrow way of pure surgery," he proclaimed. Artificial material, like "metallic plates and filigrees, celluloid plates, and injections of liquid celluloid, solid pieces of wax, and injections of molten wax" is anathema when bone from the patient himself can be used, he wrote. Such diddling in the absurd caused atrocious results. Gillies preferred rib grafts: bone and cartilage that could be split, bent, and angled—the patient's own biologic material—to frame a jaw, giving function and form. He was like a blacksmith, as if he were forging, drawing, and molding bone to form those flowing angles and curves characteristic of the living veneer.[35]

Function was paramount, just as Morestin had insisted. Chewing and phonation demanded an upper and lower jaw that coapted and anchored teeth, skills that demanded expert dental help. Correct apposition of teeth made all the difference in biting and grinding food. His dentists were superb in that regard. Gillies would then wallpaper the inside of the mouth with skin-like membranes to discourage scarring and preserve gumlines for healthy dentation. If not done properly it would be, Gillies had found, "a supreme cause of plastic failure."[36] So, here he was at his finest, piecing together fragments that remained, filling in with bone and cartilage, giving prominence to the upper lip, the angle of the jaw, the point of the chin. He bestowed consonance on his ravaged subjects.

Then the softness must be found: the gentle contours, the rounded nose, the grace of lips, the fullness of cheeks. Flesh of the face must be used, yes, but sometimes there was not nearly enough to cover. Gillies worked the pliability, the elasticity of skin to rotate, stretch, advance, and cover gaps left by hot shrapnel or smashing bullets. This was the autoplasty of Nélaton and Ombrédanne and popularized by Morestin, the peculiar property of dermis and epidermis to yield and conform. But there was need for more. For Gillies it was the art of tissue transfer, forming tubes of vascularized skin—even muscle—to arch from shoulder, neck, or forehead. His flesh transplants were particularly useful in reaching areas in need of thicker covering, such as nose and prominence of the chin or those subtle hollows that gave the face animation. The new pedicle would grow to its attachment with fresh blood vessels, and, after some time, was cut away to become as a native member of the face. This was a talent that went far beyond measurements and suturing. It required an innate sense of tension, flexibility, and mobility and a projection of how such bulbous tissue would eventually temper to become like normal features. Key was the tenuous blood supply. Failure to keep the grafting alive from its source could spell disaster for reconstruction.[37] "The plastic surgeon must early acquire an instinct for forecasting the viability of the flaps he uses," he wrote.[38] But even Gillies was not immune to failure and loss. One soldier, burned horribly about the face, underwent pedicle flaps generous enough to cover his whole countenance. The tenuous blood supply dwindled, however, and the flaps turned gangrenous. "The patient gradually sank and died twenty-four hours after the operation."[39]

His operations were sometimes hours long. Under such conditions, sufficient anesthesia was critical—not too much and not too little. Chloroform and ether were the choices, but Gillies used the new endotracheal tube because it allowed him free access to the face. The old open-drop method had obvious disadvantages in these patients, the cloth mask an insurmountable obstacle, often covering much of what needed repair. Never before had communication between surgeon and anesthetist been so critical. "In this class of surgery there should be more than usual cooperation between the surgeon and the anesthetist, both in regard to watchfulness over the patient's condition and in manipulations involving the airway," he wrote.[40] Now placed a short distance away, no longer could anesthetists have immediate access to the pupils or feel of the skin to judge the effect of their vapors. Pulse at an extended wrist was all. The rest was up to the surgeon.

Gillies was careful to chronicle the passages of his subjects—they numbered well over two thousand—from pitiable distortions to faithful restorations. The injuries, as seen in his 1920 textbook, *Plastic Surgery of the Face*, were horrid, his ability to reconstruct defects of the maxilla, jaw, and nose nothing short of astounding. The steps he carefully laid out in sequence; the final results displayed full-on without apology, his camera unflattering but honest. Yet, the black-and-white before and after images were nothing short of phenomenal. One could not help but admit that his work excelled.[41]

Gillies, though, was first and foremost a scientist. Each case provided lessons of immense value to him and his colleagues. But the stark clinical display of results could not reflect the emotional toll suffered by his patients. Expression of the soul within the caged, damaged faces would fall to serendipity.

Mild-mannered surgeon Henry Tonks had become disenchanted with his Red Cross service in France. A man of many talents, Tonks had completed his surgical training in London, serving as a house surgeon under the great Sir Frederick Treves. As it turned out, during his apprenticeship with Treves, Tonks had taken up a side interest in painting. Studying at the Westminster School of Art, he developed a certain proficiency and was even granted a faculty position at the Slade School of Fine Art in 1892. For a time, it seemed, he was happy to leave medicine for the world of hues and shades and tints and tones. Focusing on pastels and watercolors, he was heavily influenced by impressionist painters of the era. With time, he matured his artistic talents and linked up with avant-garde artists and writers like novelist Lady Cynthia Asquith and portrait master John Singer Sargent. Tonks managed to hold some exhibits of his work over the next several years, even traveling to Europe with his new companion Sargent.

Like so many others, the war caught him in a patriotic fervor, and January 1915 saw him in France, not as a surgeon but as an orderly at the Hôpital Temporaire d'Arc-en-Barrois, a British Red Cross hospital behind the lines near the Argonne Forest. There was a flood of casualties from the Champagne offensive of 1915. It was all so dreadful for the impressionable Tonks. "The wounds are horrible," he wrote to art collector Geoffrey Blackwell, "you have no right to ask men to endure such suffering."[42] At the same time, he felt compelled to display the gruesome suffering that he watched, and turned once again to the emotional outlet of painting. Having seen enough, he was back in England after a few months, organizing a British field hospital for Italy. His duty there was distinctly disheartening, mostly dealing with housekeeping chores such as dirty linen and kitchenware.

Feeling of little use as a doctor, Tonks somehow managed to get himself reassigned to the Cambridge Military Hospital at Aldershot as an orderly. It was there that his path crossed with Gillies's. In fact, Gillies, aware of the artistic talents of the new orderly, sought him out to sketch the course of his patients. Tonks assented, happy to immerse himself in his artwork: "I am doing a number of heads of wounded soldiers who had had their faces knocked about. A very good surgeon called Gillies who is also nearly a champion golf player is undertaking what is known as the plastic surgery necessary. It is a chamber of horrors."[43] But Tonks understood well the skill of his collaborator. They were the perfect team, both aware of the need for anatomic precision in planning reconstructive surgery. Hours were spent by Tonks in the operating theater with Gillies and others, carefully sketching the steps needed and displaying sequential drawings as part of the case record. But it would be the later pastels of these same men that would captivate Gillies and the world of art. Gillies fully knew that stark black-and-white photography often failed to represent the true nature of the wound. Tonks's portraits, with the strokes of impressionism, brought out a color dimension and a more profound view of troubled inner dealings in these men. They were no longer the mechanistic exposés on photographic plates. Their images now spoke of animation and sentiment, evocative of so much more empathy.

Meanwhile, Gillies continued his work: restoring functionality and humanness to victims of war. Rearranging the face in such pleasing manners would be a hallmark of the new plastic surgery. The ancient Greeks called the process κόσμησις (cosmesis: an adorning). Cosmesis in a strict sense was an ordering of the body. It was cosmesis that Gillies and his teams pursued: producing human features that provided acceptance and expression. This was a novel dimension to reconstructive surgery. Generations afterward would be the beneficiaries of Gillies's work, the foundations of what would be known as aesthetic surgery. From another Greek word, αἴσθησις (sensation, feeling), aesthetics would be the presentation of features through which individuals could indeed feel, sense, and perceive. Gillies's biographer Reginald Pound called this craft a "strange new art."[44] Indeed, it would be more embellishment than assembly.

Gillies insisted on even more. He wanted to provide the holistic care offered by the likes of Bruhn in his German clinic and that seemed lacking in Morestin's Paris clinic. Holistic, again from Greek, meaning "the whole." Gillies believed in total rehabilitation; not just functional and cosmetic but psychological, social, and vocational. "No effort should be spared to give these men a fresh interest and a new start in life, lest many drift to the towns on their discharge from the Services, only to become mere objects of pity and recipients of charity," he wrote.[45]

From a purely medical standpoint what was absolutely critical to recovery? Nutrition. The protein and calories required to unite, weld, and configure rearranged tissue were substantial and involved a concerted effort to maintain. Such cases as that of Reginald Evans were typical:

He [Reginald Evans] was in fact very thin because his injuries prevented him from eating properly and what he euphemistically referred to as "the food problem" was a permanent condition. He was far from alone in this as many medical case notes from Sidcup conclude with the comment that the patient must be restricted to "a mince diet."[46]

For many men whose mouths and jaws were destroyed, who were without teeth, this task fell to blue-frocked nurses, their flowing white caps and aprons reminiscent of medieval nuns. Indeed, they were often called "sister," and their bedside attention bordered on religious conviction. It was they who piecemeal fed their subjects, bite by bite, each spoonful a painful passage for those freshly sewn lips and gums. Each stage of repair—and for many there were a number—was a separate challenge, a separate demand for more calories. Men would spend weeks in recuperation shrouded in bandages, some blind or blinded by their dressings, not a few unable to take any food, to chew and swallow. Total stays of up to two years were not uncommon. Nurse Catherine Black offered one perspective during her time at Aldershot:

The problem of feeding was acute, for very few of the patients in that ward could take even a particle of anything solid, and yet their strength had to be kept up at all costs. So we had to ring the changes as best we could in two-hourly feeds . . . tomato soup made with milk, Benger's food, iced coffee, egg flip. Often we would use as many as three hundred eggs a day in that ward alone.[47]

In between meals, other nursing duties, of course, prevailed. Dressing changes were intricate and usually painful rituals. Some wounds needed daily irrigations. Bathing was essential, a task few patients could complete unassisted. Even walking from the toilet to bed could be a challenge. Yet it was that undefinable touch of femininity that played loudest on those sometimes boisterous, sometimes forlorn hospital wards. Men—many teenage boys, really—who worried their masculinity had been stripped keenly needed acceptance by the pretty, starched girls who attended them. Smiles, soothing strokes, and sympathy gave them hope that wives and girlfriends just might feel similarly. American volunteer nurse Elizabeth Walker Black was asked by one French soldier:

> Tell me, Mademoiselle . . . do you think she will care for me when I return, a poor *mutilé* [mutilated one] with a changed face? She always told me how handsome I was, so much more so than all the other men. Maybe she will marry Jean after all, when she sees what they have done to my face . . .[48]

Fresh breezes and sunshine were meant to uplift spirits as well. Men were encouraged to "take the air" around Sidcup. There was plenty of time for it. Gillies was in no hurry to move from one operation to another; healing must be complete before tackling the next stage. It was not unusual to see men alone or in pairs strolling about the town. But the reality of their plight followed them even then. Blue painted benches were scattered along the footpaths. These were reserved for the facially disfigured and alerted towns-people to beware: monstrous appearances might await those folks who sat there. Yet, the sight and smell of nature were crucial. It was restorative, as the lushness, the aroma of greenery, the sounds of life often are. Even in the bleakest of weather, it was a far cry from the death and decomposition of no-man's-land. And there was more. Patients were given opportunities to train in various skills that might benefit them in civilian life after discharge. According to excerpts from the *Rotherham Advertiser* of January 1917:

> Extensive gardens and a farm of 100 acres are attached to the house, where they . . . will be instructed in outdoor occupa-tions . . . In addition, workshops will be provided for practical instruction in estate carpentry and other handicrafts, and work in connection with electricity, agricultural machinery, and motor traction.[49]

At the very least, it was distraction from painful operations and bandage changes. Some of their work was of such notoriety as to attract the attention of the queen herself, as the London *Times* reported in December 1917:

> The Queen, Princess Mary, and Princess Helena paid a visit on Sunday to Chelsea House . . . and inspected there an exhibition of children's toys and beadwork and woodwork articles made by the soldier patients of the Queen's Hospital, Frognal, Sidcup.

The report went on to relate that the crafts were made by men who had suffered facial disfigurement. In extreme cases, where some of the patients experienced depression even to the point of suicide, the article read, the work "had brought a powerful counteracting interest."[50] There was no more sound endorsement of the value of these simple projects in adding substance to their healing.

Gillies's work at Sidcup lasted long after the Armistice of 1918. Traumatized faces filled the wards, workshops, and walkways for months and even years afterward. In 1920 Harold Gillies published his textbook *Plastic Surgery of the Face*. It was almost entirely based on his war experience, yet he took lessons learned and applied them to civilian practice. He was all but certain that such techniques would be immensely beneficial in peacetime as well as war. Birth defects, trauma, and cancer all fell under the purview of the facial plastic surgeon, he foresaw:

> It is not sufficiently recognised [sic] how readily the skill developed in this branch of war surgery is directly applicable to the relief of disfigurements met with in civil life. Ugly scars resulting from burns and accidents, deformities of the nose and lips, hare lip and cleft palate, abnormal protrusion or ill development of the mandible, moles, port-wine stains, all abound, and are not only the constant source of the greatest distress and anguish, but materially lower the market value of the individual. There is also a vast field in the obliteration of marks of operative interference, such as removal of malignant growths.[51]

Through the efforts of Morestin, Bruhn, Gillies, and others, World War I proved the catalyst for plastic and reconstructive surgery.[52] In France, Hippolyte Morestin never saw the fruits of his labor. His grand operations and startling results, though, were not lost on his pupils and admirers. The miracles of Val-de-Grâce spread quickly throughout Paris to enthrall the finer set of Parisian society. Eventually, they even captured the passion of surgeons for whom resculpting of the human frame was the pinnacle of surgical refinement. One student of Morestin's, Raymond Passot, opened a practice of reconstructive surgery in Paris after the war and, with his partner François Dubois, became the darling of Parisian circles with their wonders of aesthetic surgery. Yet Passot was always aware of his roots. In his textbook of 1933, he could not fail to acknowledge the broken faces whose terrible destruction had given birth to his new specialty:

> To you my glorious comrades, the *Gueules cassées* ["broken faces"], who by addressing me with your medal of recognition, brought me one of the most moving days of my life, I dedicate this book. By working with all their hearts on your poor faces, plastic surgeons have acquired the skill which enables them, now, to face other problems of which I will try, here, to show the social importance.[53]

And for the maimed men who benefited from their savior Morestin, no such organized system of rehabilitation and societal reentry had been furnished to them at Val-de-Grâce. It was to be provided by their own initiative, L'Union des blessés de la face et de la têt, which provided a range of support for these patients once they had been discharged from the hospital.[54] It helped restore the deeper scars of their injuries, those of the heart, and taught dignity, worth, and their honorable place in post-war France. Their motto? Sourire quand même (Smiling just the same).

Still, above it all, The Queen's Hospital at Sidcup would be considered by many as the cradle of modern maxillofacial surgery. For the professional, Gillies's cases were a superb depiction of the careful planning and staging of facial reconstruction and continued to serve as a workbook for future plastic surgeons. For the war-disfigured, it was a testament to the redemptive capabilities of modern surgery to resurrect those vital qualities of expression, emotion, and acceptance.

Of all those whose fortunes were tied to the disfiguring brutality of the war, one has to finally turn to Harold Gillies as the Father of Facial Surgery. His holistic efforts to rehabilitate mutilated men lent an element of compassion essential to their complete healing. Yet, to dissect further, it was his technical proficiency that brought facial reconstruction out of the back rooms of surgery and into the modern age of aesthetics. As his supporter and admirer Arbuthnot Lane said in his introduction to Gillies's textbook:

> It was largely due to him [Harold Gillies] that such rapid progress was effected in this special and difficult form of surgery, of which little or nothing was known before the war. Methods were employed and scrapped with great rapidity as improvements were devised. [55]

But with a visionary like Harold Gillies one cannot separate the technical—the tangible—from the intangible. It was awareness of the inexorable connection of structure and spirit that gave his work life. The destitute figures who entered his clinic had wounds far deeper than the apparitions that haunted their dreams. It was Gillies who reached in to soften, massage, and rearrange those distortions as well.

Prior to World War I, few combat-related mutilations of the face occurred. Covered only by flimsy cloth caps, most head injuries were immediately fatal. Now the steel helmets of Allies and Central Powers provided some protection of the brain but very little of the face. Withering wounds could occur sparing cranium but annihilating countenance. The psychological impact of disfigurement for these wounded soldiers was profound. Little did they care to exhibit the scars of their service. For them, only to appear "normal" and unnoticed was the desire.

Historian and sociologist Jay Winter has likened the Great War to an indelible cultural awakening. "The images, languages, and practices which appeared during and in the aftermath of the Great War shaped the ways in which future conflicts were imagined and remembered," he wrote.[56] Indeed, the *gueules cassés*, the men with broken faces, were a perfect illustration. But more to the point, these walking reminders of the carnage had benefited from the likes of Christian Bruhn, Hippolyte Morestin, and Harold Gillies. Scholar Marjorie Gehrhardt cogently observed that "*gueules cassés* evoked, on the one hand, the brutality and destruction that human beings were capable of, and the technological and scientific prowess they could achieve, on the other."[57] Plastic surgery catapulted into mainstream medicine, fostering connections with dental surgery and prosthetics and aiding in the development of anesthesia and antiseptic methods that, in turn, facilitated recovery. From the dehumanizing effects of facial disfigurement and the haphazard treatment of them on the battlefield, specialty care as developed in Düsseldorf, Paris, and Sidcup systematically introduced processes to restore humanity, dignity, and anonymity, which these men craved. These became the very pillars of the new art of reconstructive surgery.

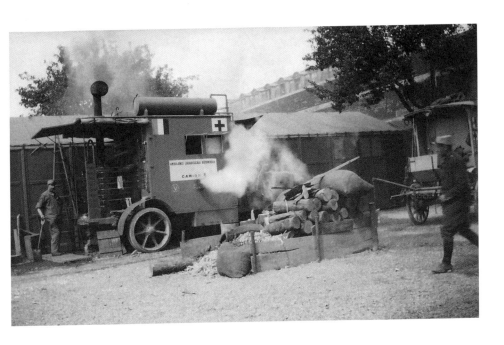

ABOVE: Gosset-Marcille Ambulance Chirurgical Automobile (auto-chir) 21 (Archives Dr. E. Chassaing). BELOW: French surgical hospital near Sainte-Menehould, Verdun sector, 1916 (Musée de Service de santé).

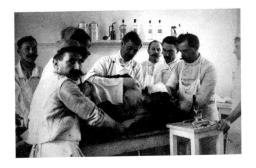

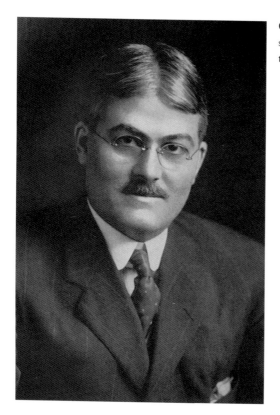

George Washington Crile (1864–1943) student of hemorrhagic shock and blood transfusions (public domain).

A French-Canadian field nurse administering a blood transfusion for a Moroccan gunner at Auxiliary Hospital No. 3 at Troyes, France (personal collection Michel Litalien).

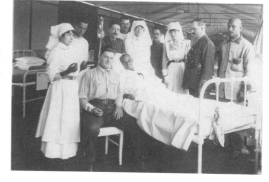

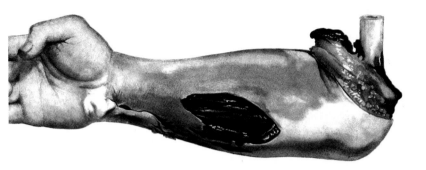

ABOVE: Amputated arm displaying the horrid features of gas gangrene (from British Medicine in the War, 1914–1918, the British Medical Association). BELOW: Alexis Carrel (1873–1944) innovative physician who, together with chemist Henry Dakin, developed an antiseptic regimen to prevent gas gangrene (Library of Congress).

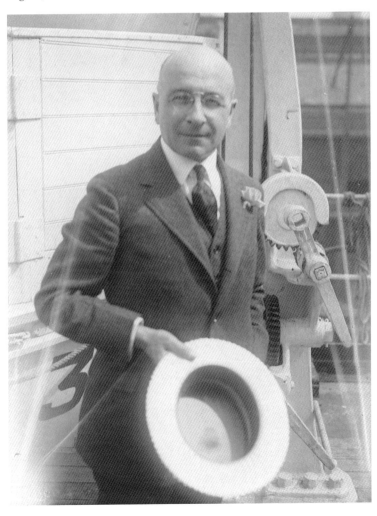

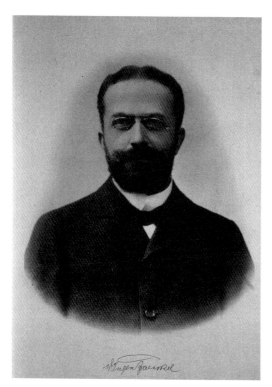

Eugen Fraenkel (1853–1925) German pathologist and bacteriologist who identified the bacterium responsible for gas gangrene (public domain).

The dead following the first gas attack, 1915 (British Library/ Science Photo Library).

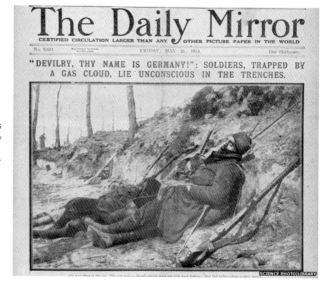

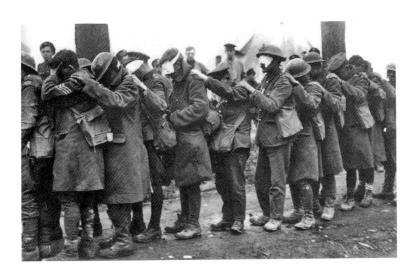

ABOVE: British troops blinded by gas (probably mustard) near Estaires, France, 1918 (Imperial War Museum). BELOW LEFT: Wilhelm Conrad Röntgen (1845–1923) discoverer of electromagnetic radiation (public domain). BELOW RIGHT: Maria Skłodowska Curie (1867–1934) Nobel laureate and champion of field radiology services during the war (public domain).

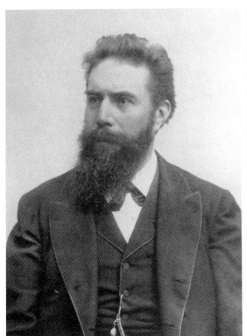

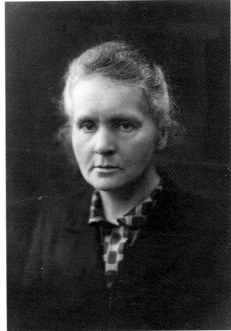

The eminent Harvey Cushing
(1869–1939) Father of Neurosurgery
(public domain).

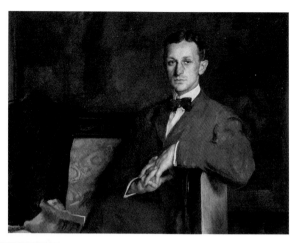

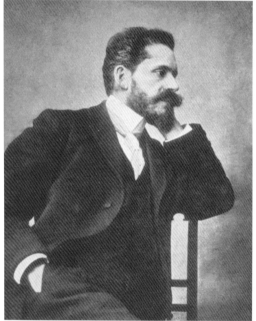

Hippolyte Morestin (1869–1918) French
innovator and reconstructive surgeon
(National Library of Medicine).

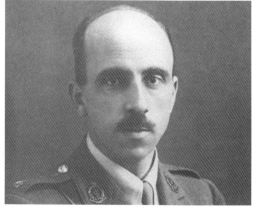

RIGHT: Harold Gillies (1882–1960)
New Zealand pioneer facial surgeon and
humanist (Queen Mary's Hospital Archive).

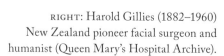

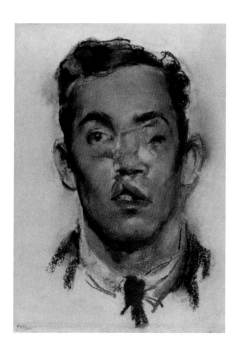 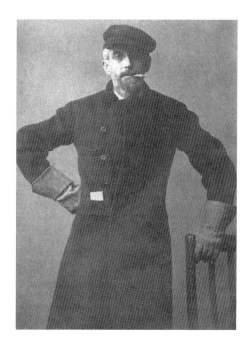

ABOVE LEFT: Henry Tonks' color portrait of facial disfigurement seen during the war (Royal College of Surgeons). ABOVE RIGHT: Hugh Owen Thomas (1834–1891) creator of the Thomas splint that revolutionized orthopedic care during the war (public domain). BELOW: The "Thomas splint" of Owen Thomas (National Archives, UK).

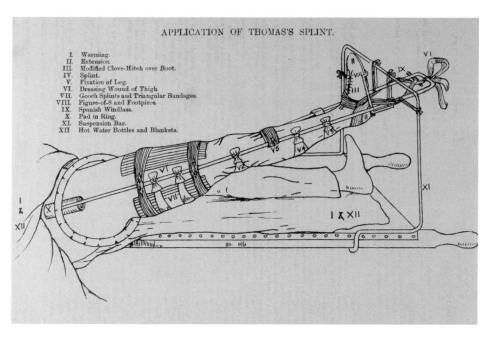

APPLICATION OF THOMAS'S SPLINT.

I. Warming.
II. Extension.
III. Modified Clove-Hitch over Boot.
IV. Splint.
V. Fixation of Leg.
VI. Dressing Wound of Thigh.
VII. Gooch Splints and Triangular Bandages.
VIII. Figure-of-8 and Footpiece.
IX. Spanish Windlass.
X. Pad in Ring.
XI. Suspension Bar.
XII Hot Water Bottles and Blankets.

William Halse Rivers Rivers (1864–1922) physician and psychologist dedicated to the rehabilitation of war's invisible wounds (National Portrait Gallery London).

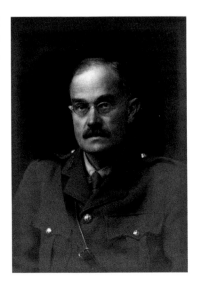

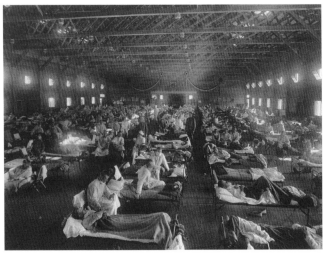

Converted warehouse, Camp Funston, Kansas, where the first influenza cases were housed in 1918 (public domain).

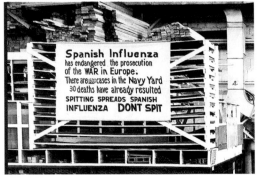

Sign appearing in Philadelphia Navy Yard warning of influenza contagion (Library of Congress).

NINE

Owen Thomas, His Splint, and Nephew Robert

"simplex, sigillum veri" ("simplicity, the sign of truth")
—Herman Boerhaave (1668–1738)

If there was one humble device—so simple as to be crude—that revolutionized fracture management during World War I most, it would have to be the flimsy-appearing orthopedic splint invented by Hugh Owen Thomas, with its remarkable benefit for men suffering war fractures of the leg.

Hugh Owen Thomas, known as Owen Thomas, came from a long line of Welsh bonesetters. These gifted men of the Thomas family had practiced their skills for generations on the island of Anglesey (where Owen was born).[1] The Thomas clan, it was said, was blessed with a dominating character, severe disposition, and commendable dignity.[2] On the whole, Welsh bonesetters were known locally as *meddygon esgyrin* (bone doctors) and were quite popular among the common laborers of Wales, who suffered with some frequency physical injuries from manual and industrial work. In 19th-century Britain, bonesetters were the manipulators of fractures, sprains, and joint disorders. Many had side interests in blacksmithing or farming. Some were even industrial hands themselves. Their origins stemmed from the nuns and monks of the British Isles of the 16th century, and they were likely spin-offs of the medieval barber-surgeons, available and affordable healers to the vast peasant workforce. Most were self-taught, or learned from one generation to the next in apprenticeships. For example, in more modern times, after the eldest Evan Thomas died in 1814 a tablet was erected to his "extraordinary gift of nature" acquired "without the aid of education or any other advantage."[3] But in their best light, these pragmatic healers were adept at applying a variety of techniques to counter pain, stiffness, and inflammation. For example, the use of bed rest and confinement of an extremity with compressive splints, commonly made with plaster of Paris, was a familiar prescription. Of course, there was a dark side. Not all were so admired. In some cases, bonesetters were viewed as quacks and charlatans who did much more harm than good.[4] The Apothecaries Act of 1815 would help change that. The decree mandated that all practitioners, even surgeons, be compelled to receive formal training in anatomy and chemistry in addition to at least a six-month apprenticeship. It was the beginning of the incorporation of surgeons into the erudite medical community. Thus would the end arrive for familial bonesetters.

As for Owen Thomas, his great-grandfather washed up on the shore of Anglesey after a shipwreck (he may actually have been of Spanish origin). He was found and adopted by a local couple (the Thomases) and given the name Evan.

As he matured, Evan seemed to have a talent for healing physical injuries, skills learned working with livestock on his family's farm. He married a local Anglesey girl and fathered four sons, one of whom, Richard Evans,[5] seemed even more gifted. Another healer. They had become a family of bonesetters, and their skills earned a good reputation and a good living.

Richard sired seven children, including three sons. All were bonesetters. One, another Evan Thomas, intended to travel to America but, upon reaching nearby Liverpool, found he hadn't enough money for the fare. Evan settled in Liverpool and began treating industrial injuries with such acclaim that he developed his own practice as a bonesetter. It was on a visit to Anglesey, though, that Evan's wife quite unexpectedly delivered Owen.

The island of Anglesey sits just off the northwest coast of Wales, separated by a slim sliver of channel called the Menai Strait. The island is over 270 square miles of sublime Celtic countryside inhabited by fiercely proud Welsh people steeped in their ancient language (Ynys Môn is the Welsh name for the place) and always suspicious of their not-too-distant English brethren. In the 1800s much of the island, which incorporates the small detached appendage of Holy Island and other smaller islets off shore, was used for animal husbandry—cattle and sheep. They were hardy people who tended the land, thrifty and industrious, as was the Welsh custom. Some have described them as of "modest character and aversion to ostentation." Despite the restorative atmosphere of the country, city life had begun to take on a more hectic pace with the intrusion of industries, a much-needed swing toward modernization, as some Welsh felt. Anglesey—and all of Wales—was, in the eyes of entrepreneurs, a blank canvas ready for the plucking. Yet, contemporary collusions would create an uncomfortable juxtaposition of nature and modernity—the tranquility of agrarian existence pitted against the invariable poverty of urban life.[6]

Owen was raised in Rhoscolyn, on Anglesey's Holy Island. He was a frail, nervous child, a worry to his mother, with whom Owen formed a strong attachment. She fostered an interest in books, an idle hobby fit for solitude and intellectual comfort. And Owen devoured them with a ravenous scholarly hunger. Returning to the Welsh mainland at age thirteen, he immediately bonded with his uncle, Owen Roberts of Saint Asaph, not too far from Liverpool. Roberts was a respected physician and a kind man who steered the young Owen toward a career in medicine. Roberts was a pillar of his community, a man of "Christian bearing, sterling friendship, and uncompromising honesty of character," as his obituary in the *British Medical Journal* depicted him.[7] In fact, Owen spent a good many hours at his uncle's side watching the practice of medicine. It seemed the career for him, following in his family's footsteps. But Owen's father, the traditional bonesetter, knew the business was changing. He admired Owen's passion but demanded his son receive a formal education in the medical arts.

Thus, at age twenty, Owen was off to medical school in Edinburgh. While his schooling was of excellent caliber, surgical decisions seemed quick, such as amputation for tuberculosis, a condition treated more conservatively by his father. There was less patience, he thought, for ailments of bone and joint. Surgeons were aggressive, eager to swipe with knife and saw, less tolerant of nature's slow pace. Nevertheless, he graduated in due order and was admitted to the Royal College of Surgeons in 1857.[8] From Edinburgh Owen traveled to London and Paris, as was the custom of the day, and finally settled in Liverpool to practice with his father. It was then that the time-honored methods of his father and the newfound teachings of modern surgery clashed. Certainly, Owen admired his father. "I watched for many years the extensive practice of an untrained gentleman [referring to his father], and, to do him justice, record here that he never failed to secure a perfect restoration of [radius and tibia] fractures," he said later in life.[9] It may have been that father and son were too much alike in temperament and character.

In any event, differences could not be resolved. Evan retired to Anglesey, and Owen moved his medical clinic to Nelson Street, close to the Liverpool docks, in 1866. In those days, Liverpool was a gritty, port city, bordering as it did the right bank of the River Mersey as it opened to the Irish Sea. The shore was lined by seven miles of docks extending from Hornby to Herculaneum that were a major center of overseas British commerce. Solid masonry warehouses fronted the water, so imposing as to appear impregnable to even ships of war. Most often, immense stores of animal, vegetable, and mineral freight—corn, wheat, lard, cotton, tobacco, and all sorts of manufactured goods—from every corner of the globe were displayed, filling huge sheds and awaiting transport inland. Dockworkers were indispensable in the whole process of unloading, cataloging, and shipping imported items. They were of two persuasions: "lumpers," who emptied payloads from the ships' holds, and "porters," who received cargo on the docks to weigh, mark, stow, and load off onto transports. Each job was grueling physical labor and carried its own risks to life and limb. Their recreation, when time permitted—indulgence, some might say—was found in the bawdy taverns not far from the waterfront, where liquor flowed and drunkenness reigned.

The town itself was a migrant's paradise (a large number of Irish and Welsh immigrated in the 1800s) but was, in reality, a grim arrangement of working-class neighborhoods and hapless throngs of meandering plain folk in search of market or liquor. *Squalid Liverpool* was a phrase used to describe certain districts of the city in 1883, within a stone's throw of the Mersey, areas of offices and warehouses containing nearly half the population of the city. Behind them were tightly packed, tiny, dilapidated houses and dank alleys, plagued by "the blankest, most appalling poverty, cut off from every grace and comfort of life," residents living their frugal existence without leaving the neighborhoods. These areas were called by some "fever dens," as distempers raged among the unsanitary conditions. They were locations graced with poverty, abuse, and rampant illness. Residents were of necessity a thrifty lot, who, rummaging for bargains in terms of medical care, were much more likely to frequent the odd healer than traditional (and expensive) licensed practitioners.[10]

Those same tough longshoremen were particularly prone to trauma. They bullied crates and spools and bales all day on the pier, then bullied pints of ale at the pubs, and finally, in fits of drunken rage, they bullied one another. What could a man do who barely scraped enough together for food and family? He fought. He fought the pallets shifting toward the docks and he fought the bloke next to him at the bar. He fought everything. He fought his fate. Broken bones, bruises, and blood were the price; then they came to Owen, and he would fix them to fight again.

Owen Thomas was immensely popular. There was never an occasion of refusal. Each man, monied or not, was his client. He understood them just as his father had. He understood their poverty, their frustrations, their physicality. He understood the anger they vented on the swinging cargo, the liquor, and sometimes their wives. And he had a remedy: rest, a prescription he may have learned from his father. For orthopedic problems, it was ideal. Work on the docks was almost a seven-days-a-week mandate with little time off. That kind of labor irritated inflamed muscles, tendons, and joints. Counterproductive, he knew. Inflammation would never subside, sprains never repair. Rest must be "enforced, uninterrupted, and prolonged," he said.[11] "The defective part must have the greatest amount of relaxation from the performance of its usual function during the abnormal state," he explained.[12] Complete immobilization was the only path to healing. Some contemporaries might agree, but the common method of slathering limbs in rigid plaster of Paris seemed barbaric. Encasement like this, Owen thought, applied more pressure to injuries, restricted blood flow, and retarded recovery. Immobilize, yes, but liberate the tissue, encourage circulation. Here was his solution: a new type of splint, simple in design and effective in binding:

> The upper crescent is formed of an iron ring 3/8 of an inch in thickness . . . the ring is nearly ovoid in shape and is covered with boiler felt and basil leather; from its upper and lower portions two iron rods pass down to the lower end of the machine. . . . Across the two bars is stretched an apron of basil leather to support the limb. [13]

So how did it work? He lodged the padded upper crescent against the bony ischial tuberosity in the groin and the ridge of pelvic bone on the side. This anchored the splint against the pelvis. Then the struts of the splint would extend below the foot and be secured by cloth supports under the leg. The foot was then wrapped so that traction could be applied, drawing the foot down against the bottom frame and extending the entire limb. In this configuration, the leg remained immobilized at rest and even during ambulation, which was still possible, if somewhat awkwardly. It was perfect for knee problems.

Owen found in short order, though, that his splint came in handy for managing fractures of the thighbone as well, a devastating injury for dockworkers. Some of these, compound fractures (open fractures) where the bone ends have broken through the skin, led to amputation. Fear of gangrenous infections was real, and amputation the expedient solution. Yet, Joseph Lister had revolutionized such conditions with his antiseptics, so that amputation could be avoided. Owen saw that his splint, when applied to straighten the fracture ends and put them in alignment, was an unexpected antidote that best promoted healing of fracture ends without shortening of the leg. Once in place, nature could do the rest:

> In cases of compound fractures, it is my custom to place the limb in an apparatus which retains it immovably fixed

[speaking, of course, of his splint], so that there is no occasion to disturb its immobility for the purpose of changing bandages or dressings, until it has recovered. [14]

Of course, some surgery was necessary. Bone ends poking through skin needed to be set back inside. Then he would clean the wound, remove blood clots and loose bone fragments, place bandages, and apply his splint. He cautioned, though, against too much meddling. Even as Owen Thomas was a scientist, he was also a minimalist. Let the body heal by its own mystical design, he believed. "The crying evil of our art in these times [1883] is the fact that much of our surgery is too mechanical, our medical practice too chemical, and there is a hankering to interfere, which thwarts the inherent tendency to recovery," he wrote. The physician should do nothing more, and nothing less. As for his ingenious splint, he offered: "men admired my splints as if I were a blacksmith, but the principles on which they were framed they never could see."[15] Rest went hand in hand with healing.

It was to the modest little house at No. 11 Nelson Street, Liverpool, that a young Robert Jones, nephew to Owen Thomas, came with his mother, Elizabeth, on holiday visits. For young Robert, the meetings with Thomas seemed magnetic. Thomas, though thin and pale, was a forceful figure, inquisitive, inspiring; his vitality much larger than the frame that contained it. Robert immediately latched on. And Robert, very much the intellectual and scholar—and quite influenced by his uncle—did not hesitate in deciding on a career in medicine. He attended the Liverpool School of Medicine. There was no question that Robert would be a surgeon. Years of informal apprenticeship with his uncle on Nelson Street, watching the splint-makers, and accompanying Thomas on rounds had instilled an unquenchable thirst for surgery and a profound interest in orthopedic problems. He unfailingly passed his examinations by the Royal College of Surgeons. Shortly after graduation, Robert Jones joined his uncle as a professional assistant. He was but twenty-two years of age. While both were keen on the surgical arts, the large share of their practices concerned ailments of bones and joints. Learning from his uncle would land him in good stead. "A man who understands my principles will do better with a bandage and a broomstick than another can do with an instrument-maker's arsenal," his uncle claimed.[16]

Indeed, Jones absorbed a great deal working with Owen, but, as his confidence built, he longed for his own practice. While he had been granted a number of honorary positions in hospitals around Liverpool, a major opportunity surfaced in 1888 with an appointment as consulting surgeon to the Manchester Ship Canal. Jones leaped at the chance. The construction project, with all its machinery, would generate countless orthopedic crises needing attention.

As for Owen Thomas, the delicate little man with boundless energy and keen intelligence never left No. 11 Nelson Street. He remained doctor to the poor, the crippled, the warehouse workers, and the stevedores of Liverpool. While his reputation spread far and wide and his splint became a staple of orthopedic care, he never lost sight of those much more in need of his attention. He died of pneumonia on January 6, 1891. It seemed he had taken a chill while visiting a patient, perhaps even a victim of the influenza epidemic of the day. He was but fifty-six. Thousands thronged to his funeral, and hundreds of dockhands formed an honor guard. "It was impossible for anyone to know him intimately without being moved to admiration by the purity and unselfishness of his life," his obituary read.[17]

Robert Jones had an unwavering loyalty to his uncle. He soon moved back to the house on Nelson Street and began caring for Thomas's widow, Elizabeth, and did so until her death shortly before the onset of World War I. Jones also took on the formidable practice of his uncle and all the dockworkers who flocked for care. Discarding the mantle of "bonesetter," Jones, with his academic background, intended to modernize orthopedic care. In fact, he was one of the first to purchase Röntgen's marvelous machine just months after its first report. He and fellow physician Thurstan Holland along with physicist Oliver Lodge used it to find a bullet in a young boy's wrist—almost certainly the first radiograph performed in England.[18] By 1909, Jones was considered "one of the greatest of living surgeons."[19] His contributions to skeletal surgery had been astounding. His reputation spread internationally.

By that time, fractures of the femur, even those open fractures so lethal just a generation past, were now survivable—without amputation—thanks to Lister's antiseptic remedy and lengthy traction—sometimes eight weeks or more at bed rest. In the new 20th-century Britain, seldom did civilians die of such injures; in one large collection of cases, only a few percent failed to recover.[20] The key was immobilization. Fracture ends needed stillness in order to form callus that will eventually unite bone ends. A few surgeons even tried fixing the fractures together by plates and screws, a method now termed "internal fixation." Jones's practice was no different. He was a superb technician. Unlike his colleagues, though, the focal point of his treatment was the splint of his uncle Owen Thomas. Jones had such confidence in the device that he once claimed: "the Thomas knee splint is incomparably simplest and best. I have often fixed a fractured thigh in this splint and sent the patient home in a cab."[21] Jones, the general surgeon by training, had now become the new specialist in muscular and skeletal conditions. He embodied the modern-day version of his ancestors' bonesetter practices. Liverpool, all of Britain, and even America embraced him as the architect of orthopedic care.

Like many British physicians, Jones welcomed military service—a sense of duty, not obligation. He held a position in the Territorial Force—a reserve organization for the regular army. That would all change with onset of war in 1914. He was promptly placed on active duty and, at fifty-seven years of age, made a surgeon in the Royal Army Medical Corps. Because of his unique specialty and impressive reputation, Jones soon became director of military orthopedics with a rank of major (he would eventually rise to the rank of major general).

Doctors, of course, faced dreadful conditions on the western front in those early days of 1914 and 1915. Enormous numbers of injured swamped frontline surgeons and precluded any type of meaningful care. Devastating injuries of the head and trunk killed many almost at once. Of those surviving, most suffered wounds of the limbs. These ranged from the trivial to the terrible. Surgeons encountered men carried or crawling back brandishing horribly mangled arms and legs filled with mud, blood, and the ravages of warfare. Their patients were little more than bewildered boys who now left childhood behind and wished for nothing more than a cigarette and the safety of starched sheets. Some were in traumatic shock. Hemorrhage, pain, and pulped muscle wreaked havoc on their systems, pale, clammy, apathetic appearances the telltale signs.[22] Fractures in particular caused ferocious pain. Patients were warmed, hot tea and morphine given, bandages applied and, with broken bones, a cumbersome splint called the Liston splint was fixed. Named after a famously brutal Scottish surgeon, Robert Liston, the device was strapped to the outside of the fractured leg all the way up to the rib cage. A bulky binding of bandages hopefully secured the whole affair in rigid immobilization.[23] While suitable for civilian practice, the apparatus fared poorly in the trenches. Ushering wounded through the narrow zigzag slits was particularly unnerving. Victims were contorted, lifted, dropped, and jostled in such a manner that the splint hardly worked. Manhandling like this grated bone ends together, nerve endings on edge, firing exquisite agony at each movement. And, just as serious, grating ripped into muscle and blood vessels. More bleeding. Worsening shock. The death rate for thigh fractures was staggering. British surgeon William Macpherson painted a gloomy picture in his medical history of the war: "gunshot wounds causing fractures of the femur were among the most fatal injuries met with in the war." Almost two in ten died outright, and nearly one half never left the continent alive.[24] Prewar methods—including Liston's splint—had failed hopelessly.

Berkeley Moynihan was a man of distinction. His father had been a military man and earned the Victoria Cross for courageous action in the Crimean War. Sadly, he died at an early age, leaving Berkeley, two sisters, and their widowed mother to subsist on a meager government pension. Such deprivation imbued the boy with a true ethic of industriousness and ingenuity. In fact, Berkeley entertained some thought of the navy himself before entering medical school in Leeds, England. After graduation he focused on surgery, and, from there, his career was meteoric, ascending the ranks of academic surgery and showing that peculiar knack great men seem to have for wisdom and authority.

It was in that capacity as preeminent surgeon and scholar that landed him in France in 1914 as a special consultant to Alfred Keogh. Moynihan had no doubt that his dear Britain was on a moral crusade to rid

Europe of malicious militarism. He was reported to have said at one point: "[t]his is a moral war. It is a holy war if ever there was one. It is deep down a war between conflicting and discordant and unconformable moral systems."[25] But this holy war had not provided the best for Britain's finest young men. Conditions in France were appalling. Field medical services floundered and wounds festered. Moynihan called back to Keogh and told him in no uncertain terms: "[for one thing] [t]he treatment of compound fractures is deplorable; the country will soon be flooded by men doomed to deformity and crippling. If something is not done about it a scandal will break over your head. This is a war of orthopaedic surgery. You must appoint a director of military orthopaedic surgery."[26]

Robert Jones heard the same stories and planned his own battle-field tour. Like Moynihan, he correctly supposed that the war would generate mobs of casualties with smashed limbs. "Deplorable," he echoed Moynihan's comments to another of Keogh's consultants, Major General Sir George Makins.[27] Who in their right mind could ignore the rows of men with swollen, smelly, deformed legs, he wondered. Robust callus and proper union of bone ends was a dim wish under the circumstances. More likely, crutches, canes, and wheelchairs would be their fate. Men were hardly getting any treatment at the field hospitals. Instead, they were splinted, wrapped up, and hurried off to crowded, seedy evacuation trains, ripe for neglect and spreading infection. Even at base hospitals in Paris or Boulogne their treatment was uncertain. Some had already suffered the consequences of long delays with spitting pus and bone spicules of osteomyelitis or fracture healing so poor that crippling disability was assured. Few would be fit for civilian life.

Liston's splint and the pervasive plaster of Paris were at the heart of the problem. As for both methods, skin breaks and muscle trauma from open compound fractures simply could not have the *débridement* and cleansing prescribed by the likes of Carrol and Dakin. By January 1915, disenchantment with the methods was clear. The prestigious *British Medical Journal* voiced their opinion in an editorial that month: "[s]everal cases of compound fractures of the femur were included in a large convoy of Belgian soldiers from Antwerp provided with the most rudimentary splints and all extremely septic. This proved a pitiful spectacle."[28] Jones hated the plaster cocoons (plaster of Paris). It was a "filthy method," he proclaimed. The disgusting plaster "mops up discharges like blotting paper, and becomes horribly offensive." Some doctors thought the rifle, wrapped to the broken limb, made a better splint. Why not his favorite Thomas splint instead? It seemed to him the perfect solution, particularly for hauling patients through the ankle-deep mud of trenches, into rickety ambulance vans, and along bumpy, uneven roads. All the while, with traction, the bone ends would move into alignment as muscles began to relax, free of constant irritation that caused them to spasm. "The general use of these . . . splints [Thomas splints] . . . would be an incalculable boon both to the surgeon and the patient," he wrote. And here was the critical part. With the leg still in traction, wrappings were porous enough that deep open wounds could be examined, washed out, and re-bandaged. It was all so sophomoric, yet Jones knew that many inexperienced surgeons caring for wounded had no clue. Due to their negligence and misinformation, femur fractures were becoming "the tragedy of the War," he felt. Unless surgeons were taught the convenience of his splint and how it provided easy access to dirty wounds and bone—all the while keeping traction and comfort—there was no doubt the tragedy would continue. [29]

Jones was not alone in his conviction. He had his followers, but, in the early days, there were precious few. One notable was Noel Godfrey Chavasse. Chavasse was a handsome lad and gifted athlete who attended Oxford and ran the 400-meter at the 1908 Olympics. His academics hardly suffered through all this as he earned top prize in his medical school's final examination. Chavasse first met Jones in 1909 while still in school. In 1913, he returned to Liverpool to become his house surgeon, a coveted position. Despite his aristocratic background (his father was bishop of Liverpool and founder of Saint Peter's College, Oxford)—or perhaps because of it—Chavasse was drawn to the military. He accepted a commission in the Royal Army Medical Corps, even while he was apprentice to Jones.

War soon found him in the trenches, attached to a Liverpool regiment. Chavasse thrived on action, feeling much more at home in rat-infested trenches than the "cushy" life of hospitals farther to the rear. "A Field Ambulance is no place for an active young chap. It should be only for older men with wives and families."[30] At Guillemont, France, in August 1916 he prowled no-man's-land searching for victims of a failed offensive that left many of his men dead and wounded. For that, he received his first Victoria Cross. For those brought back with terrible leg wounds, he used the Thomas splint favored by Jones. The results were almost immediate relief of pain. In fact, Chavasse had written to his mentor in June 1917 that "every aid post now has Thomas splints in stock. But I have been carrying one about on my medical cart for the last two years. I hope we shall be able to save more fractured thighs."[31] On August 4, 1917, around Passchendaele, Chavasse's short life came to an end. After once again refusing shelter and crawling through the cratered grime separating British and German trenches in search of comrades, Chavasse was finally in the relative safety of his aid post when an artillery shell landed squarely on it. Such is the randomness of war that even heroes are not immune. His injuries were extensive. He lived a few days, but at the last, his heroic stamina failed him. Young Chavasse died at a casualty clearing station at Brandhoek. He was but thirty-three. He was posthumously awarded a second Victoria Cross. When Jones heard the news, he was devastated. Chavasse's father wrote to him, "our most dear boy loved and honoured you . . . your life and work were one of the great formulative forces of his life." The loss of his former pupil and friend was one of the deepest blows of the war for Jones.[32]

And then there was Major Meurice Sinclair. Sinclair quickly grasped the utility of Thomas's splint and began using it while at No. 2 Casualty Clearing Station in 1914. Later, at a general hospital in Wimereux, he really saw the advantage. That simple splint of Owen Thomas permitted meticulous wound care—so critical to men transferred to him—and reduced mortality from femur fractures almost in half by 1918. Sinclair was nearly evangelical in his campaigning for its wider use. Jones admired his passion. "He [Sinclair] reminds me more of Hugh Owen Thomas than any surgeon I have met," Jones said, "in his scrupulous attention to and effort mastery of mechanical details, and his zealous struggle for the salvation of the limb."[33] Sinclair could not imagine treating a leg fracture without it.

In January 1916, Jones himself was asked to visit British hospitals in France. His reputation might encourage rank and file medical officers to use his splint. In a whirlwind of touring, Jones performed like an evangelical revivalist, giving lectures and demonstrations in Boulogne, Calais, Étaples, Abbeville, Le Tréport, Rouen, and Le Havre, as well as countless casualty clearing stations. It all had an impact, Jones's preaching and Sinclair's sermonizing. By late summer, they had enlisted other supporters. Surgeon McCrae Aitken, an obvious Jones disciple, delivered a scathing rebuttal of skeptics by pointing out the splint's versatility in relaxing the spasm of injured muscles and easing fractured ends into alignment. Aitken explained "the extraordinary way in which . . . fracture of the femur treated on a Thomas splint comes in due course to a state of complete muscular rest."[34] Then, once aligned, proper healing could begin. By November the following year, classes were required for medical officers in the proper application of the splint in first aid stations right at the front. "Splint Drills" were even devised to ingrain the steps required to immobilize fractures "about the knee joint or upper part of the leg." It was all so simple, doctors agreed, this splint could be slipped on and secured and patients warmed up and then shipped back to surgical hospitals. Signs of shock, so characteristic of broken thighs, seemed so much less.[35] Thomas's splints fast became part of the medical lexicon. In countless lean-tos, crumbled buildings, and dugouts, mud-soaked, rain-drenched, bone-tired doctors could be heard to say again and again, for their men with pulverized thighs "where's them Tommies [meaning Thomas splints, of course]?"[36]

Keogh understood, too, that treatment of leg fractures extended far beyond the battlefield. Neglect and inattention at any step of the way could cause untold disabilities and future problems in healing. Proper treatment started at the trenches and continued through convalescence. The danger of infections, poor union of bone fragments, and bone shortening—all factors in disordered management—loomed large for these men. Drawing on battlefield experience, Keogh understood that "few surgeons see their patients from the beginning to the end." But this was exactly what fracture patients needed. Orthopedic care was specialized and had such an impact on future disability and earning potential. He argued as much in Jones's 1917 textbook on military orthopedics.[37] Keogh's remedy was a fracture hospital, dedicated to those with skeletal trauma. His prototype was the Alder Hey Hospital on the outskirts of Liverpool. It had originally been designed as a workhouse for the poor, then, in 1914, a place for sick children. Then Keogh took over. Four hundred beds he set aside for war fractures. Who to head the effort? Without question, Jones was his man for this task. His appointment, though, ruffled not a few feathers among the more erudite of London surgeons, but Keogh was undeterred. Jones it was. Not surprisingly, Jones willingly accepted. The success of Alder Hey led to the development of other fracture hospitals throughout the country. Keogh would later say of Jones's accomplishments there: "the early days of orthopedic work in the War, when its importance had to be vindicated and established . . . to you and to you alone the successful result has been due."[38]

Early application of the Thomas splint and proper cleansing of the wounds brought about a remarkable improvement in survival from thigh fractures. By the end of 1915, the use of the Thomas splint was mandated at base hospitals and many field surgical hospitals. Doctors from dressing stations to casualty clearing stations familiarized themselves with it, practiced with it, and became proficient at applying the splint, even over battle uniforms. "No lesson has been more clearly taught by the experience of this war than the necessity for the efficient splinting of fractures at the earliest possible moment after injury," said Colonel Henry Gray in his 1919 textbook, *The Early Treatment of War Wounds*. Almost without exception the Thomas splint, he maintained, was the preferred method to provide "self-contained [leg] extension."[39] Its utility lay in ease of placement and that it could stay in place during transport and further wound care, all the while maintaining the traction needed to keep bone ends in alignment.

By 1918, the outlook for men suffering fractures of the femur had brightened. Official figures for that year alone showed that of over 4,500 femur fractures treated by conservative measures (meaning no amputation) in British armies, fewer than one in ten died, a dramatic reduction, considering that over half perished in the first year of the war. According to historian William Macpherson: "the chances in 1918 as compared with those in 1914 of survival with a useful limb of a man with a gunshot wound of the thigh with fracture of the femur constitute a striking tribute to the success of military surgery."[40] This simple device, thought up by the son of a rural bonesetter, alleviated so much pain and disability during the war and to the present day that it has to be one of the most notable achievements produced by the Great War.

TEN

Shell Shock

"More life may trickle out of men through thought
than through a gaping wound."
—Thomas Hardy [1]

The great English novelist and poet Thomas Hardy was no stranger to warfare. He was seventy-four when the Great War started, and he was of the generation that remembered and venerated the veterans of the Napoleonic Wars—those brave Brits who turned the tide at Waterloo—and the more recent Boer Wars. Yet, to Hardy war was an ambivalent incursion. On one hand, he loathed it as a consequence of social inequities: the reckless gambling of working-class lives by the ruling castes pursuing their imperialistic designs.[2] On the other, he seemed enamored with the spectacle of war, the patriotic themes, the soldierly enthusiasm, and the pomp of military parades. Still, in 1914, it did not take long for the disillusionment of battle to strike full force. Patriotic impulses had now given way to horror, suffering, and misery. It all led, in his mind, to a renunciation of the joie de vivre, now replaced by base natures, brutal and unmerciful. It was a folly of romantic soldiery thrown against the unromantic butchery of modern combat.[3] Such disgust he would feel that Hardy would join the ranks of war poets who vented their frustrations in verse at the ironies and miseries of this great conflict. This was a war not characterized by the chivalry of bygone eras but by the demonic inhumanity of men gone mad. This was a war that would bleed not only the red blood of its heroes, but the very sanity of its combatants.

Sanity indeed. Soon affected by the disheartening tortures of trench life, the human mind in its complex quirkiness made known a turmoil boiling within. Across the Channel, on the western front, in the waning months of 1914, strange cases of paraplegia appeared, affecting small numbers of British soldiers subjected time and again to withering shellfire. In the published medical report, their examinations had all the trappings of traumatic spinal cord contusion—as if actual blows had been delivered—even though no sign of external injury could be found. The men eventually recovered; yet, because there was no obvious wound, they were called "hysterical," their condition relegated to "neurasthenia."[4] Shortly after this report, another one surfaced. Authored by physician and psychologist Captain Charles Samuel Myers, it appeared in early 1915 describing three soldiers shaken by the force of high explosives. They were nearly blinded and, over the next days, voiced vague complaints of shivering, insomnia, and emotional volatility. Myers found that their visual fields—the scope of their vision—was altered, suggesting a true disturbance of their central nervous system. To varying degrees each soldier, more or less, slowly recovered. Myers, who had been sent to France with the Royal Army Medical Corps as consulting psychologist, was puzzled by his patients' peculiar malady, and considered that it was due to the concussive effect of shellfire. He called the syndrome "shell-shock." Yet, he was not convinced it was due to concussion of the blast and also supposed "the close relation of these cases to those of 'hysteria' appears fairly certain."[5] Back in London, William Aldren Turner, known as Aldren Turner, a distinguished neuropathologist at the National Hospital, Queen Square, was equally baffled. He considered that cases were either due to the violence of a shell explosion or, more telling, a reaction to physical strain, sleeplessness, or exhaustion. Some men, he gauged, were almost stuporous, dull, lethargic. Some had no recollection of their trauma—or any recent memory at all. Others were even deaf, mute, or blinded. They were like men suffering "surgical wounds of the head," but these men were nothing of the kind.[6]

Thus began one of the great psychological mysteries of all time: what happens at the extremes of stress to that most fragile, complex, and misunderstood of all natural workings—the human mind? Why did combat generate such bizarre behavior? Was it, in fact, the sudden, violent concussion of bursting shells, or something more subtle, more sinister? Such strange carryings on that would cause some to accuse the victims of malingering, of a weak and cowardly temperament. The image of soldierly bearing had been fractured. Gone were the colorful warriors of Waterloo or Sir George Colley's fated but proud legion in South Africa. No, far from it. These present sorts were men beset by the rigors of subterranean life, who day after day suffered the battering of artillery and the cutting efficiency of machine guns, of numbing cold, of drenching rain, and of vigilant insomnia. Who day after day faced the imminence of sudden annihilation by an enemy few had even laid eyes upon.

Neurasthenia was the label given. While the humoral theory of medicine had long since died out, the idea of temperaments had not. In the Victorian era, medical men recognized that each personality was affected by specific morbid afflictions. The nervous manifestations were no exception. Ebbs and flows of psychologic behavior had, more or less, to do with the nervous energy within—the nervous temperament. Sensibility to external stimuli provoked different reactions within the individual: excitability, irritability, and exhaustibility being prime examples. And all, to some degree, it was thought, were influenced by heredity. In other words, there was a genetic influence passed on through generations. Therefore, individual supplies of nervous energy were limited and varied, depending largely on hereditary capacity. For those exhibiting a diminution of their nervous energy, then—nervous exhaustion—physicians applied the term *neurasthenia*. Some people simply were prone to early depletion and more likely to suffer the ills of neurasthenia—profound anxiety, despair, fear, insomnia, fatigue, and listlessness among them. [7]

Because of the weird quality of symptoms, it had fallen into the catchall of the hysteric, or for men, the hypochondriacal. But, in fact, not, experts might propose. Aldren Turner wrote in his 1910 textbook that neurasthenia was "a condition generally associated with a lowered state of the general health . . . characterized by symptoms of mental and physical fatigue." Emotional jolts and physical injuries were likely to contribute. Yes, hysteria was linked to the female disposition—that excitatory behavior brought on by "all forms of emotional disturbance—shock, fright, worry, or grief."[8] Neurasthenia was different. Sufferers were often dull, depressed, listless. Liverpool pathologist Thomas Glynn considered it a "traumatic neurosis," a consequence of injury or fright. Those affected complained of physical problems—stuttering speech, hearing disorders, trouble walking or keeping balance. Glynn felt it was an ailment mostly found not in women but in men. He theorized it to be a "weakened nervous organization brought about by the abuse of tobacco and alcohol . . . and unhealthy or arduous occupations and unhygienic surroundings."[9] Such emasculating tendencies were in startling contrast to attitudes fostered in Victorian and Edwardian England, where men were expected to be exemplars of self-discipline and emotional discretion. Any expression of feelings was considered giving way to "womanish wailings." Such behavior was not only unmanly; it was also blameworthy.[10]

There was nothing about it to admire. Prior to the war neurasthenia was considered "the refuge of the destitute." Little changed with the onset of hostilities, despite the ugliness of combat. Army doctor Charles Wilson spent three years in the front lines with the Royal Fusiliers. He was distinctly hostile to the idea of war neurosis, rather considering it a character flaw or simply outright cowardice. While admitting that shell bursts could stun a man ("disheveled minds," he called it), others who cowered "were plainly unable to stand this test of men. They had about them the marks known to our calling of the incomplete man, the stamp of degeneracy." Streaks of compassion in this physician seemed to be sorely lacking. But sadly, he was not alone in his perception.[11]

The British had come across such soldiers in the campaigns in South Africa in 1899 and 1900. It was a rarity then. Surgeon Morgan Finucane reported nine cases of delayed recovery—listlessness, sleeplessness, and the like—after suffering gunshot wounds or nearby explosions. Each injury had indeed traumatized nerves; two were direct head wounds, one man was knocked senseless by a shell explosion. Slow recuperation was blamed on some undefined motor or sensory impairment considered "psychical" ("nerve shock" was yet another term used). Finucane thought actual concussive damage to the fragile brain less likely.[12] Aberrancies to military honor. Blemishes on unblemished character. Rare curiosities, in the most masculine of endeavors. Such matters were largely ignored.

But in 1914 the British were taken by surprise. No one expected it. Those strange curiosities began trickling in. Brave young Englishmen would fight as they had always fought, with pluck and vigor, of course. "I do not think psychologists will get many cases, although shock plays a great part. Such cases as I had improved rapidly with rest and good cheer and watching their brave companions. Lowered vitality plays a great part; rest and stimulants seem required," one doctor predicted.[13] Yet, by November, cases piled up. No longer was this just a curiosity. The numbers could not be ignored. One who sounded an alarm was Lord Knutsford, chairman of the London Hospital House Committee. He published a letter to the editor of the London *Daily Mail*:

> There are a certain number of our gallant soldiers for whom no proper provision is at present obtainable but is sorely needed. They are suffering from very severe mental and nervous shock due to exposure, excessive strain, and tension. They can be cured if only they receive proper attention . . . If not cured, these men will drift back to the world as wrecks, and miserable wrecks, for the rest of their lives.[14]

At first, physicians were urged to brand such blighted patients as neurasthenics out of kindness rather than their supposed inclination to think them insane or unworthy.[15] Oddities in temperament, even ethnic differences, they were told, might dispose to sudden prostration, queer pains, enfeebled legs, headaches, or insomnia. These were nervous systems in disorder and disarray. The prescription for recovery: rest, massage, hypnosis, not to mention more exotic means such as electrotherapy.[16]

In fact, German doctors had recognized the same symptoms in some of their troops. Falling heavily under the influence of the great Sigmund Freud, German academicians attributed this strange behavior to Freudian psychology—emergence of repressed psychic conflicts. The label of hysteria surfaced there, too; an implication that the entire picture was one of a flawed character, of cowardice. Hysteria equated with weakness—a blemished constitution—and little empathy flowed for these troubled young men.

There was one naysayer, though. Hermann Oppenheim stirred controversy with his theory of *traumatischen Neurosen*—traumatic neuroses. He insisted that psychological trauma—perhaps precipitated by physical injury—had an organic (i.e., physiologic) cause. He even suggested that there could be hemorrhaging into the brain disrupting nerve pathways and affecting secretion of important "trophic" substances by the nerve cells themselves. It was nothing new. He had seen it before:

> Vigorous young people from all walks of life, mostly peasant boys, who went into battle with the familiar enthusiasm of the last war [presumably the Franco-Prussian War of 1870], with courage and strength, hardiness and steadfastness . . . came back afflicted with war [traumatic] neuroses.[17]

Science backed him up. In 1915, Swiss researcher Franchino Rusca demonstrated the concussive effects of blasts in rabbits. In numbers of these animals, injury to the lining of the lungs, arteries, and intestines could be seen at autopsy even though there were no external signs. In many animals, these proved to be lethal injuries. He held that similar internal trauma occurred in humans subjected to high explosives. Some died instantly, sometimes without a mark on them, and in these, he suspected the same hemorrhagic lesions in the brain stem, areas controlling basic respiratory and cardiovascular function.[18]

Psychiatrists joined in. The German Robert Gaupp, a protégé of the famous Carl Wernicke and assistant to the great Emil Kraepelin of Munich, used the term *commotion cerebri* (cerebral commotion) and argued that such "traumatic brain damage" does occur as a result of violent explosions. But Gaupp felt there was more. It was this subclinical damage that "created a readiness for the occurrence of hysterical conditions," which he still felt were at the crux of most neurotic behavior.[19] Gaupp explained that in some zealous men, of impeccable character and fortitude, the nervous system could not reconcile with the dangers and horrors that war brought. In these men, an abrupt explosive event shatters the soul, as if "a sudden storm broke on the nerves," and that tenuous hold on inner strength flees. Control ceases. The exhausted soul attempts escape.[20]

It would be a universal phenomenon among the armies of the Great War. The informal French "trench newspapers" so popular among the troops expressed candid thoughts of the soldiers themselves, free from censored government publications. These periodicals described the horrid effect of massed artillery on beleaguered infantrymen:

> Soon the noise becomes hellish; several batteries thunder out together. Impossible to make out anything. Shells fall without interruption. He feels his head is bursting, that his sanity is wavering. This is torture and he can see no end to it. He is suddenly afraid of being buried alive . . . He imagines the terrible agony of death.[21]

These were not the back alleys of Liverpool or Whitechapel, where a man could fight a decent fight. These were cowering places meant for the timid, the whipped, the half man to await his slaughter. It was war unlike any other, where hoped-for bravado quickly fled and steely courage submitted to the simple matters of survival. Few men who had hunkered in shell-shattered trenches were immune:

> In the *mêlée* there are no handsome young leading men who mouth fine words and stick out their chests . . . as the shells rain down, there are only weak beings flattened on the ground by their instinct for self-preservation because the ability to utter fine phrases has never been needed as a prerequisite for dying.[22]

The contentious Parisian neurologist Jean-Martin Charcot had predicted this. His work in nervous system diseases would earn him the title of "Father of Neurology," his contributions legendary.[23] Not so taken by the concussive effects proposed by Oppenheim, Charcot nevertheless reasoned that extreme violence could stagger the mental machinery. He had written: "the nervous shock, or commotion, the emotion almost unavoidably inseparable from an often life-threatening accident, is sufficient to produce the neurosis in question." It was, he said, a form of traumatic hysteria, *le grand ébranlement psychique* (the great psychic shock). And fear was the most potent of emotions triggering the unbalancing. In his thinking—and this was critical—while traumatic hysteria resulted from a combination *diathèse* (some sort of constitutional predilection) and an agent provocateur, it was a legitimate medical ailment, irrespective of the moral judgments and character assassinations of skeptics. And what was his *diathèse*? Not the pampered life of the well-heeled, it seemed. Instead, the grit and grime and daily inequities of common laborers whose lives were barely in their control would erode fortitude and resilience. [24] In Charcot's time, "the hysterical men of the working class . . . who fill the hospital wards of Paris today are almost always somber, melancholic, depressed, and discouraged people." It was as if he were already gazing into the future at those same corridors later occupied by disturbed souls stumbling back from the trenches. [25]

Indeed, it would be so. Men flocked to hospitals suffering any number of aliments that, at first glance, were not caused by direct physical injury. Hysteria and emotional shock were labels attached to such disturbances: those men with peculiar paralyses, hallucinations, disordered emotions, a perceptual unwinding—sometimes totally adrift from reality. "Mental anaphylaxis" some called it; psychic poundings again and again coupled, perhaps, with physical exhaustion as well. "The subject becomes unable to bear the emotional shocks properly" and, in a term used so often, suffers a nervous breakdown. As for those loud, earth-shaking artillery blasts that literally stunned soldiers? Of course, they were unnerving for the moment. But to shake up a nervous system in such a bizarre fashion did not seem likely. [26]

Yet, in truth, no one had ever witnessed such firepower unleashed on troops. High explosive shells were filled with combustible material known as lyddite, melenite, emmensite, or trinitrotoluol, all of which have as a base the volatile picric acid (trinitrophenol, more commonly known as TNT). Projectiles weighing from a few pounds to nearly a ton and containing up to two hundred pounds of TNT arched indiscriminately toward opposing armies at speeds exceeding one thousand miles per hour. Explosive forces were enormous, calculated at almost 120,000 pounds (60 tons) per square inch. The kinetic energy released on impact was so stupendous that it would shatter the metal casing of the shell—and anything in the vicinity—to smithereens. For larger-caliber shells, anyone caught in the open up to one hundred yards away was simply obliterated.[27]

Sudden expansion of these explosive gases created powerful shock waves that could tear limbs from trees and disassemble brick houses. Troops were aware of it. The living had to clean up the messes. No longer were the dead men or boys or friends or soldiers. Mutilation and dismemberment were so complete that the unrecognizable mounds of flesh were simply referred to as "things."

For those not immediately blown to bits, a supersonic blast of pressurized air still passed through their bodies. Not infrequently, groups of men could be found dead, as if in a state of suspended animation, but without any physical injury, the suddenness of their concussive death attested by morbid poses of daily living: eating, smoking, sleeping. Others were flung feetfirst into the air or buried alive by a blast that collapsed their trench.[28] Such eruptions were quite capable of ripping fragile arteries and veins lining the intestine, liver, and lungs. It was almost certain that tiny vessels in the brain also shattered. Chief British medical officer Sir Anthony Bowlby testified that "the mere explosive force of the gases of a large shell exercises great powers of destruction . . . [and] is sufficient to kill." In the only case of such a casualty in his experience, at autopsy the brain contained numerous petechial hemorrhages.[29] Perhaps, too, that kind of battering about tore at delicate connections of infinitesimally small nerve fibers. Enough disruption and maybe thought processes themselves jumbled.

Soldiers were petrified of these bombardments, some lasting hours or even days. Artillery duels literally carpeted no-man's-land, transforming an already bleak panorama into the cratered surface of the moon. The cacophony of sound, rain of dirt and mud, trembling of earth, and screams of terrified men produced by detonations sent many soldiers into a maddening frenzy. Troops would rather endure anything but shelling. British Duchess Millicent Gower, that patriotic socialite, like many well-to-do British, had established an *ambulance* in Namur, Belgium, in the opening days of the war. She had witnessed the effects of the big German siege cannon on the human frame and the incessant shelling of the city. Barely escaping with her life, she returned to England, where she described her experiences to the press:

> The man who had lost his voice was beginning to whisper. All he could say was, "J'ai peur, j'ai peur" ["I'm afraid, I'm afraid"]. These words seem ordinary words from a child or a woman, but they were terrible coming perpetually from a strong man under such circumstances. One gathered from them an idea of the horrors he must have seen and heard. The wounded gave me terrible accounts of the new German siege guns. When the shell explodes it bursts everything to smithereens inside the forts. The men who are not killed and wounded become utterly demoralized and hysterical, even mad, in awful apprehension of the next shot.[30]

British infantry officer Siegfried Sassoon witnessed it firsthand: how bravado with comrades in their trench dungeons soon deteriorated into nightmares of solitary fear, as if so many times they had been taken to the abyss of madness and, before long, fell in:

> Shell-shock. How many a brief bombardment had its long-delayed after-effect in the minds of these survivors, many of whom had looked at their companions and laughed while inferno did its best to destroy them. Not then was their evil hour, but now; now, in the sweating suffocation of nightmare, in paralysis of limbs, in the stammering of dislocated speech.[31]

Or sometimes no speech at all. A few ghoulish creatures, almost catatonic, said nothing, as if words could not escape souls so choked by fear that mouth and tongue rebelled by stillness, protesting the waste of it all with silent terror.

Hysteria? Neurasthenia? What tiny disturbances of neurons and fibers in brains knocked about by the tonnage of TNT expended on them caused chaotic nerve impulses, both motor and sensory, both conscious and unconscious, no one could tell. Was this, in fact, a demonstration of that popular 19th-century concept of nervous energy depletion?[32]

Charles Myers, the author of that first report in 1915 describing shell shock, came to develop an abiding interest in these altered states. It all happened quite by serendipity. Myers was far removed from the battlefields of France in August 1914. In fact, he was on a climbing expedition in Switzerland, purely an invigorating holiday. He had been, at Cambridge, a physician specializing in experimental psychology, even traveling to the Torres Strait of Australia with men by the name William Rivers and William McDougall, die-hard anthropologists.[33] He was totally absorbed by all of it. But such was the impact of war that he scurried back to Cambridge, traveling through the near panic and chaos of embattled Paris. Once home, and now with Britain committed, he put aside his anthropology interests for more pressing matters: medical service for his country's soldiers. The problem was, at forty-one, Myers exceeded the maximum age for military commission, even for a physician. Connections with alumni of his Saint Bartholomew's Hospital solved the problem. He was put in contact with the Duchess of Westminster, Constance Lewis, and persuaded her to add him to the roster of people slated for a voluntary hospital in France. It seems that the lovely duchess, embittered by her loveless marriage to the duke, the immensely wealthy Hugh Grosvenor, snatched any distraction—patriotic all the better—to leave London.[34]

So, the duchess, Myers, and troop were off to Le Touquet, near Étaples in the Pas-de-Calais. Myers immediately busied himself with setting up a registrar for the wounded, cataloging their injuries and personal information as a novel inventory of medical matters. This caught the eye of the army's director general Sir Arthur Sloggett, who forthwith offered Myers a commission in the Royal Army Medical Corps. Not too long after that, Myers encountered those disturbing cases of disheveled behavior—brought on, he thought, by nearby artillery detonations—that he termed shell shock.

It must be, he reasoned at first, that neural pathways in the brain unhinged in some fashion with the wallop—the shock—of an exploding shell. Maybe those shock waves disrupted fine connections with the "lower, emotional regions." It was for this reason that he chose the term "shell shock." It was not long, though, before he realized that there were other contributing elements that had more to do with ill-defined human natures. Just maybe, these mind troubles occurred not because of any physical injury (as fellow psychologist Frederick Mott was trying to blame), but by the internal trauma of events and circumstances culminating in one sudden, giant event—like a shell burst—that seemingly tipped the scales and produced a decompensating psyche unable to adapt.

Myers's 1915 piece on shell shock in *The Lancet* caught the attention of Aldren Turner, now elevated to consultant in neurology for the War Office. Impressive, Turner thought, and chose Myers to head investigative work on so-called war neurosis cases in France. Turner suspected a number of these patients were actually malingerers and wanted Myers to ferret them out. It turned out Myers was an excellent choice. He approached the matter in an objective and methodical manner, interviewing and examining victims in exquisite detail. Indeed, a few were, in fact, malingerers. Most were not. Myers determined that many men—almost a third in his estimation—were simply exhausted by the rigors of trench life and the terrors of combat. A few days' rest and they were good to return to duty. Of the remainder, a sizeable group needed evacuation to England.

Turner agreed. It was a reasonable plan for keeping men near the front. A period of relaxation was often curative to calm the jitters of front-line service. And it conserved manpower, if not dignity. Myers worked out a plan of what he called "mental wards" in casualty clearing stations and base hospitals on the Continent, all designed to handle milder war neurosis casualties and return them to their units. He was just in time. The disastrous Somme offensive of the summer of 1916 generated huge numbers of shell-shocked soldiers, totally spent from the slaughter of those pointless assaults.

Gordon Holmes was a product of the renowned National Hospital, Queen Square, a famed neurological research institution (officially known at the time as the National Hospital for the Paralysed and Epileptic). He was a dashing figure, outgoing, even boisterous. Not unexpectedly, he and Charles Myers differed sharply in their approach to the treatment of shell shock. Holmes had become one of the dominant neurologists at National Hospital and, some said, the leading figure in British neurology in the early 20th century. More the unbending clinician, he had no tolerance for shell-shock victims. "He never liked those people," as one colleague put it. Another admitted, "Holmes had no time for neurotics and hysterics, and less . . . for psychoanalysis."[35] He was an anatomist, physiologist, and rationalist. What could not be examined, measured, and proven must be discarded. He had studied under the great Hughlings Jackson, premier neurologist of the Belle Epoque. The response of the spinal cord to trauma and the visual cortex of the brain were Holmes's interests, quite the leap from the mind games of Myers. It was no secret that hysterical behavior rankled him—and his colleagues at National Hospital. There was no patience for such frivolity. Attitudes like his permeated the place. In fact, psychiatry in general had little standing there. How Holmes, then, managed to wrangle the position of consulting psychologist to the army from Myers was anyone's guess. It might have been a trivial matter of bearing. Holmes was tall, athletic, outspoken; Myers the opposite: a bit chunky, thoughtful, reserved. In any event, Myers took it poorly. Resentful, he suspected it was a calculated move by Holmes to fatten his chances of a lucrative practice after the war.[36] Angry and frustrated, Myers returned to England and asked for a new assignment. In November 1917 he was posted to a recently opened psychiatric hospital in Maghull to assist Richard Rows in training young medical officers to treat shell shock cases.[37]

MAUDSLEY AND MOSS SIDE, MAGHULL

Gordon Holmes's hard-nosed approach notwithstanding, the British were unequaled in their study of shell shock. Britain's leading neurologists, psychiatrists, and psychologists rallied to the effort. The result was a system to care for these disturbed men centered around specialized institutions. The names Maudsley; Moss Side at Maghull; National Hospital, Queen Square; and Craiglockhart would come to signify hospitals designed to furnish enlightened treatment and foster research for this new breed of war victim—and, in fact, for the mentally afflicted in general. Besides the compassion of Charles Myers and the rigid science of Holmes, there was a litany of brilliant minds who searched logical explanations for the baffling behavior of so many addled men.

Frederick Mott had a long and distinguished career in the unraveling of mental illness. He had studied under the indomitable Henry Maudsley, the leading psychiatrist of his day. Maudsley was a firm believer in the organic nature of psychiatric disease, quoted in one of his lectures as saying, "Mental disorders are neither more nor less than nervous diseases in which mental symptoms predominate, and their entire separation from other nervous diseases has been a sad hindrance to progress."[38] And, for sure, the convictions of the teacher had infected the student. Mott became an anatomist and physiologist, fascinated with the neuron and its interdigitated relation with others in the nerve pathways of the brain. He was a firm believer that biochemical and anatomic alterations of neurons could affect the workings of the mind and even thought processes. He may have also been influenced by the Russian Constantin von Monakow in Zurich, who proposed a theory he called *diaschisis* in the 1890s. Diaschisis was the traumatic disruption of connections between functionally related parts of the brain. Whether edema or physical injury was the cause was not entirely clear, but symptoms were seen as altered mental states or even as extreme as flaccid or spastic paralysis. It was, more or less, a functional standstill among groups of neurons. All seemed reversible, though. With time, symptoms might abate and recovery be permitted.[39]

Mott, too, witnessed the flood of shell shock cases returning to England. He first focused on the effects of physical trauma. Like Myers, he realized that "the employment of high explosives combined with trench warfare [had] produced a new epoch in military medical science." The repetitive detonations so frequently described by victims of shell shock just might have so disrupted the minute workings of nerve cells in the brain and spinal cord—even on a microscopic level—that, combined with other fatiguing influences such as terror, loss of sleep, and physical weariness, could deplete what he called the "neuro-potential." This, in itself, might give rise to that purported neurasthenic behavior. He did not exclude a certain temperamental predisposition to all this. A more timid, retiring sort, albeit desirous of doing his duty, might have less ability to cope than one not as insightful—some might say, more callous. Mott even postulated that inhalation of carbon monoxide gases from explosions or bubbling of tiny amounts of nitrogen in the bloodstream caused by sudden atmospheric pressures generated by blasts might contribute to deranged workings of the brain. So, Mott's best guess was that shell shock followed concussive injuries superimposed on the inner exhaustion and futility of this new type of war. [40]

He had his critics. In rebuttal, British surgeon Captain Harold Wiltshire offered a study of 150 cases during a 12-month tour of duty in France. He claimed that in those suffering obvious external wounds from shellfire, he could not recall a single case of shell-shock symptoms—"the wounded are practically immune from shell shock." Mott's theory was hogwash, he proclaimed. Instead, Wiltshire attributed bizarre neurologic symptoms to an underlying exhaustion brought about by continual fear. Like others had maintained, some abrupt emotional event triggered psychic decompensation. Wiltshire may have underestimated the effects of repeated shelling. The official British committee of inquiry into shell shock, convened after the war, did not:

> No human being, however constituted, however free from inherent weakness, however highly trained to meet the stress and strain and the wear and tear of modern warfare, can resist the direct effect of the bursting of high-explosive shells. [41]

It was not, as Wiltshire claimed, the same "functional nervous affections of civil life." Nothing was civil about the brutality of trench warfare. Wiltshire might have been overly optimistic in his portrayal of wounded troops as "cheerful" (was it because they had a ticket out of the trenches in

an "honorable" manner?) and the observation that "our troops in France
are very well fed and free from epidemic diseases" ("moderate cold and
exposure tend to improve rather than diminish physical well-being").[42]
Life in the ground and under fire definitely did not improve a sense of
well-being—nor did bone-chilling cold or constant rain.

Mott was undeterred by such misrepresentations. In fact, it
was Mott who suggested to his mentor Maudsley, years before,
the construction of a specialized hospital to treat mental cases far
removed from the psychotic denizens of contemporary insane asylums. Mott's idea was a center dedicated to rehabilitate neurotic—not
psychotic—disorders. He argued that mental illness in its earliest forms
could be cured outside the prisonlike confines of sanitaria. Mott had
been heavily influenced by his visit to the clinic of pioneer psychiatrist Emil Kraepelin housed at Ludwig-Maximilians-Universität in
Munich, Germany. Kraeplin was also a believer in the biologic basis
of mental disorders. His clinic, a vast research palace, focused on cataloging case studies, conducting research, and classifying psychiatric
diseases, plodding through the spectrum of mental disorders. Mott
intended to mirror his efforts. It was an ambitious idea, but Mott made
his case, appealing to benevolent natures, as he wrote in the respected
journal *Archives of Neurology* in 1907:

> A fruitful field of study in psychiatry would be those early
> cases of uncertifiable mental affection termed neurasthenia,
> psychasthenia with obsessions, mild impulsive mania, melan-
> cholia, hysteria and hypochondria . . . such patients are often
> in the hopeful and curable stages, and these . . . could not fail
> to yield valuable results . . . [in] the causation, prevention, and
> cure of insanity.[43]

Maudsley was convinced. With Mott as the scientist and Maudsley
the rich benefactor, the hospital became reality. In overall design, Mott's
hospital, in fact, resembled Kraepelin's Munich clinic: short-stay wards
totaling 144 beds interdigitated with pathology laboratories, library,
dispensary, and administrative offices. The building was finished in

1915, located across the road from the Fourth London General Military Hospital (King's College Hospital). It was suitably named for its major sponsor, Henry Maudsley. However, before it could be used, the Maudsley was requisitioned by the War Office for use by any infirmed war veterans. It was not until 1916 that Mott finally convinced Alfred Keogh to admit shell shock victims there.[44]

The Maudsley project was all part of Aldren Turner's scheme. With his position as consultant in neurology, Turner had the ear of Alfred Keogh. While no fan of Mott's concussive theories, Turner was well aware that more and more shell-shocked troops needed specialized care, and hospital beds in France were badly needed for other casualties. For those cases not quickly improving, the next echelon would be England. Turner proposed mental "clearing hospitals" there. Mott's Maudsley Hospital was to be one of those. The most severe, psychotic patients would be sent on to the asylums of Napsbury and the like. To put these types at Maudsley—certified lunatics—would simply be too volatile and disruptive. Mott agreed. His Maudsley would be "particularly valuable for the treatment of the more serious cases of war psychoneuroses and psychoses."[45] Keogh signed off.

Mott knew full well that therapy for shell shock centered on a trusting bond between doctor and patient. He promoted an "atmosphere of cure," even invoking a spiritual infusion. "It is faith that saves or heals," he said. Meetings, counseling, physical activity, reeducation, and rest were critical components of the recovery. For those with corporal infirmities such as paralysis, stammering, even mutism, Mott permitted a slow, patient process of rehabilitation.[46] As for causation, he still believed in the concussive potential of shellfire. The knocking about in cannon-sodden trenches was irrefutable and correlation with infirmities substantial. Such trauma often produced little if any outward signs of violence.[47] There would be no place in his program for insinuations of cowardice or flawed character. These men had an organic illness.

However, the Maudsley Hospital was not meant to provide long-term care and rehabilitation. Turner intended deeply disturbed cases—those who could not easily shake their internal demons—to be cared for on mental campuses like the former Moss Side State Institution located in the town of Maghull, just outside Liverpool, National Hospital, Queen Square in London, and a place called Craiglockhart, in Scotland.

The Moss Side House, stateliest of the buildings on the grounds outside Maghull, was erected in the 1830s as one of the grand mansions built for a wealthy merchant named Thomas Harrison. His estate was otherwise featureless—an expanse of undeveloped pasture. Harrison's descendants sold the estate in the 1870s. A cluster of buildings soon arose, barracks really, in 1878 as a convalescent home for children from Liverpool workhouses. By 1910, it had become a convalescent home for boys only. Not for long. In 1911, Moss Side was to be turned into a colony for epileptics. However, the Mental Deficiency Act of 1913 changed even that plan. So called "idiot", "imbecile", and the "feeble-minded" youths could be institutionalized by parent, guardian, or authorities.[48] Moss Side was to be one destination for these unfortunates. But before the first patient could be admitted, the War Office took control. Moss Side Hospital was to become the destination for, in the words of Aldren Turner, "'borderline cases' [of war neuroses] which require more special supervision than could be given in hospitals."[49] After homeland "clearing hospitals" like Maudsley, Moss Side would be the next tier of care for shell shock victims.

The problem was that in the fall of 1914, as it was about to open, Moss Side had no medical staff. The two young physicians assigned had transferred to France, eager to serve with the British Expeditionary Force. An obscure neuropathologist by the name of Richard Rows, then at the nearby Lancaster County Lunatic Asylum, appeared, willing to take the job for a modest salary of £450 (£44,000 in present currency). Rows was fascinated by diseases of the brain and spinal cord. As a pathologist, he was fixated on the microscopic changes invoked by different stresses. But as a pathologist, he had little familiarity with intangible mental issues such as shell shock and war neuroses. No mind; the position captivated him. In his innate inquisitiveness, he would lend an air of science to these disturbing soldier-patient ailments. He turned to his colleague, the Australian Grafton Elliot Smith, chairman of anatomy at nearby Manchester University. Smith was a recognized expert in the framework of the brain to the extent that his wide-ranging knowledge of human neuroanatomy and anthropology made him a leading figure in neurology. In fact, he became a tremendous resource for Rows as the program at Moss Side matured. In turn, Smith recruited another prominent neurologist and fellow faculty member, Tom Hatherley Pear, a psychologist who lent fresh interpretations of the mind, different from dominant Freudian views. Smith also managed to entice neurologist and anthropologist William Rivers. They had met after Rivers's Torres Strait expedition, examining Rivers's anthropological specimens. Rows, Smith, Pear, and Rivers would form the core faculty at Moss Side. It would prove to be a stellar assembly.

Like at Maudsley, treatment was compassionate. While highly individualized, the essence was a thorough understanding of the emotional damage that terrors of war had wrought. "The patient must be approached *without prejudice*," they emphasized. Doctors at Moss Side must "ponder of the sufferer's mental wounds with as much . . . care and expenditure of time than would be given to physical injuries." Central were psychological analysis and then reeducation, meaning development of practical strategies for coping. These men, Pear and Smith maintained, had not lost their reason or their senses—or their minds. Far too often all those were sharpened, reliving again and again the gruesome tales of death and dismemberment that they had witnessed and for which they too often held themselves responsible. Of paramount importance was careful examination so as to arrive at a correct diagnosis. Only then could an appropriate treatment be developed. Therapeutic methods incorporated varying degrees of firmness and sympathy, occasional isolation (although this was usually considered ill-advised), hypnotic suggestion (only if combined with other techniques), and psychological analysis. Talk therapy was usually encouraged. It was a method of rationality and practicality. Confronting fears, allowing them to surface, analyzing, dissecting, and explaining was key. Such exposure to deep-seated terrors reduced the magnitude of inflated anxieties to more manageable forms.[50]

NATIONAL HOSPITAL, QUEEN SQUARE

More controversy surrounded the treatment at National Hospital, Queen Square, in central London.

The National Hospital for the Paralysed and Epileptic opened in 1859, funded by voluntary and philanthropic donations. At first only ten inpatient beds and outpatient clinics were available. Yet, at its founding, it was the only hospital in the United Kingdom that confined its efforts to diseases of the brain and spinal cord. It would shortly become the premier hospital for neurological diseases and attained an international reputation for its commitment to service, education, and research. National Hospital had become the "temple of British neurology" and its staff "a priesthood for the spread of the neurological faith of Britain."[51] But the hospital, despite its glowing reputation and charitable care, was never distant from financial ruin. The war itself may have been its saving grace, for the British government donated generously in the care of its wounded veterans.[52]

It was here that the unconventional but revered neurologist John Hughlings Jackson (he was known by his middle name, Hughlings) dissected the convulsive pathways of epilepsy. His explanations for these enigmatic disorders, based on a rigid foundation of anatomy, pathology, and physiology, would become the new "neurological method." But he was a rationalist. Disease must be seen and measured to be believed. Therefore, there could be no unconscious component to the human mind. There, too, was the neuropathologist Charles-Édouard Brown-Séquard, a master of pathology of the spinal cord. It was where the great Sir Victor Horsley had marveled his admirers with the complexities of brain surgery, heretofore forbidden territory, performing over 130 operations in a 13-year period before the turn of the century.[53]

The philosophy there was one of pragmatism and physicality. Hughlings Jackson had advanced the guiding principle of concomitance, whereby the brain and the mind are distinctly different and function in parallel rather than as an integrated unit. Diagnosis of neurologic disorders concerned the sensory and motor alterations detectable on examination (a sensorimotor machine in Jackson's eyes). Not so with mind disabilities. This had the effect of creating a cleft between scientific neurology and the vagaries of psychiatry. At the National Hospital, neurology clearly dominated, pushing aside more subtle issues of mental health. It would never be so obvious as with treatment of shell shock victims. Clinicians there had little time for such trivialities. It was not a lunatic asylum and the faculty were not alienists.[54]

Following Lord Knutsford's letter to the *Daily Mail* in November 1914, National Hospital opened its doors to the shell-shocked of France. At first, only one ward serviced these cases. After Turner formulated his plan and National Hospital was to figure heavily in it, three additional wards were prepared. From 1914 to 1919, over 1,200 soldiers with various neurologic or psychiatric conditions were treated—at Turner's insistence. Well over one third had no discoverable organic disease. For these, twelve different diagnoses were leveled, including shell shock, neurasthenia, traumatic neurosis, depression, and hysteria. Reflecting, perhaps, a disdainful bias, the academicians subtly shunned such cases. Day-to-day management largely fell to the house physician Lewis Yealland. Yealland, an energetic Canadian researcher, preferred the term *war neurosis* to *shell shock* or the other host of labels. With an ingrained sense of the empiricist, he felt most comfortable with men who had some obvious physical infirmity such as paralysis or loss of speech. He was far from convinced that the shock of explosion had much to do with the bizarre tremors, paralysis, deafness, and inability to speak some cases exhibited. He was even more puzzled by the aimless, depressed patients with headache, exhaustion, nightmares, and insomnia. Yealland was tempted to label them as hysteric ("nothing the matter with them") but, in his psychologist brain, understood that clearly something was amiss. For one thing, he believed these individuals were somehow defective: below average in intelligence or had "unstable" personal or family histories. Yet, combatting the "weakness of the will and intellect, hypersuggestibility and negativism," as he perceived hysterical behavior, was a challenging proposition. It was here that Yealland and his junior partner, the electrophysiologist Edgar Adrian, departed into the macabre. Yealland devised a three-pronged program: suggestion, reeducation, and discipline.[55] Central to recovery, they felt, was the use of electric current. It was a method called *faradism*, for those who did not quickly respond to other forms of therapy. Electrical charges could awaken paralyzed limbs, correct awkward movements, or stimulate the mute to talk. While usually of a mild nature—some tingling, often not unpleasant—Yealland did not hesitate to increase the strength for stubborn cases:

> The current can be made extremely painful if it is necessary to supply the disciplinary element which must be invoked if the patient is one of those who prefer not to recovery, and it can be made strong enough to break down the unconscious barriers to sensation in the most profound functional anaesthesia.[56]

Electricity was still something of a mysterious energy to laymen and, by power of suggestion, the patient felt its use could be curative, even if accompanied by excruciating discomfort. With relief of their symptoms, patients were reassured that their malady was gone (reeducation) and that they had recovered. Of course, Adrian and Yealland touted astounding successes. With a variety of ailments—deafness, mutism, aphonia, various types of paralysis, and gait disorders—the two claimed victory in 95 percent (Adrian would later admit that there was a high relapse rate).[57]

It was treatment in line with attitudes about mental disease at the National Hospital. Certainly, faradism to the point of pain seemed heartless, yet shell shock and war neuroses were medical mysteries. National Hospital, the home of rigid experimentalism, did not offer a kinder, gentler approach for these subjects. It was only a matter of time as understanding evolved that Yealland and his techniques would be demonized. Historian Elaine Showalter labeled him as "the worst of military psychiatrists."[58] He was even vilified in popular literature. Novelist Pat Barker portrayed the indifferent Yealland, in her World War I book *Regeneration*, busy applying electrodes to the back of a young private's throat and zapping him until the poor devil begins to talk—all contained, word for word—in Yealland's factual *Hysterical Disorders of Warfare*:

> It has been my experience with these cases to find two types of patients; those who want to recover, and those who do not want to recover . . . it makes no difference to me which group you belong to. You must recover your speech at once.[59]

Was Yealland truly a brute? Did he lack compassion? Was his treatment of these war veterans insensitive and demeaning? As barbaric as it might seem today, faradism was widely practiced therapy in the latter half of the 19th and early 20th centuries. Hysterical states, such as globus hystericus, seemed particularly responsive. Women were often the target, afflicted, as it was thought, by such perturbations of emotion thought to emanate from that most enigmatic of organs, the uterus. Neurologist Wilfred Harris attacked such women with electrodes to the back of the throat, presumably until they declared their cure. More to the point, the Scottish physician Samuel Sloan claimed success with faradism for "psychic neurasthenia," even using it on the brain (through the scalp, of course). As late as 1935 zapping still occurred. Edinburgh neurologist Ritchie Russell wrote: "strong faradism can be used very effectively as a suggestive measure in cases of flaccid paralysis, aphonia [mutism], and hysterical gait."[60] Treatment was controversial, to be sure, promptly abandoned by some of the great minds in psychiatric disease such as Sigmund Freud. Nevertheless, faradism was not torture and Yealland surely not a monster. It rather speaks to the perplexities of shell shock and other forms of war neuroses and the desperate attempts by legitimate practitioners to find curative therapy for these embattled, indeed internally tortured, individuals. If nerve pathways fall prey to short-circuited electrochemical provocations, then a jolt of electricity might help.[61]

CRAIGLOCKHART

The kinder and gentler approach of Moss Side, Maghull, was a fruitful experience but only for the enlisted man. Officers in need of further help would be shunted to Scotland and a location called Craiglockhart in a village named Slateford, just outside of Edinburgh. Must not one keep hushed the mental woes of Britain's elite officer caste?

High society of the fin de siècle hyped the power of water as providing healing and health. Hydrotherapy was the name and became the rage. Throughout Great Britain a number of spas promoting water cures opened to accommodate those eager for pampering. One such resort was the hydropathic spa near Edinburgh. The massive Italianate-baronial structure known as the Craiglockhart Hydropathic, built in 1877, housed the main attractions: Turkish baths and swimming pools where up to 120 guests could enjoy the soothing mineral waters and experience a rejuvenation of body and soul. It was but a twenty-minute taxi ride from the city, built into the side of Wester Craiglockhart Hill, four hundred feet above sea level. The house overlooked both the Forth Valley and the Pentland Hills. From their parlors and suites on the upper floors, lodgers had a commanding view of the expansive estate and, in the distance, the city of Edinburgh. Despite its imposing architecture and holiday venue, the hydropathic operation fell on hard times and was sold to James Bell in 1891, who revived the facility and placed it on firm financial footing.[62]

In 1916, however, because of the swelling numbers of British soldiers suffering from shell shock, the War Office requisitioned Craiglockhart as a hospital for Turner's cases. Officers only were hospitalized, those suffering from the peculiar neurotic afflictions of battle. These were men failing quick recovery in France or on arrival at Turner's clearing hospitals in England. They needed longer help. The imposing Craiglockhart, appropriately out of the public's eye, was thought to be the perfect place. A medical staff was quickly assembled, and the talented physician, psychologist, and anthropologist William Halse Rivers Rivers recruited to lead the effort ("Rivers" was, it seems, intended both as a given name and a surname).

William Rivers was born in the "hop" country of Kent in southeast England. He schooled in Brighton and the posh preparatory academy of Tonbridge (Kent). From here, Rivers had aspirations of qualifying for Cambridge, but a serious illness, probably typhoid fever, laid him low, missing qualifying exams, and effectively erasing that career track. He would choose medicine but in a distinctly attainable fashion, hoping to enter the Army Medical Corps. In 1886, Rivers graduated from the University of London and Saint Bartholomew's Hospital with his baccalaureate in medicine. From there the young Rivers traveled as a ship's surgeon to Japan and North America, and returned to England to earn his MD degree and fellowship in the Royal College of Physicians. After another year as house officer at Saint Bartholomew's and a year in private practice, Rivers landed a position as house physician at the National Hospital, where he, too, fell under the spell of Hughlings Jackson, physiologist Michael Foster, and Victor Horsley. His interest in the nervous system and the intricacies of human behavior deepened.

Rivers left the National Hospital after one year, but his career path had crystallized. A visit to Jena, Germany, and the lectures of Otto Binswanger and Hans Berger cemented that notion. Toward the end of his stay there, he wrote in his diary, "I have come to the conclusion that I should go in for insanity when I return to England."[63] The following year he went back to Germany and the clinics of Emil Kraepelin, now in Heidelberg, where he studied the effects of various substances like coffee, tea, alcohol, and drugs on mental activity. Recognized now as a rising star and with his connections at National Hospital, he was invited to move to Cambridge and the academia that had eluded him a decade before. It was there that he did much of his research on the senses, firmly convinced of the interplay of physiology and psychology. In particular, he focused on visual color and space perception and wrote the chapter on vision for the sixth edition of Michael Foster's *A Textbook of Physiology*, published in 1900.

During his time at Cambridge, Rivers headed the psychological section of the Cambridge anthropological expedition to the Torres Strait of Australia. The primitive nature of the Torres islanders fascinated him as a manifestation of unfettered psychology. During this trip, he laid the foundation for genealogical investigations as an invaluable tool for sociologic studies of remote cultures. In 1908, he was off to the Solomon Islands in the South Pacific, where, again, he employed novel methods of ethnological research to unravel genealogies and kinships among the Melanesia inhabitants. Such work engrossed him and brought him in closest touch with fundamental human interaction and behavior.

When war erupted in Europe, he was once again in the South Pacific. Returning soon to home, he accepted Elliot Smith's offer of a position in July 1915 as a civilian psychiatrist at Moss Side Hospital, Maghull. Here he met Richard Rows and Tom Pear. And here he found a settledness that perhaps had long eluded him. Colleague and friend Walter

Langdon-Brown saw a different Rivers during the war. "It was not really until the war that Rivers found himself and discovered his remarkable aptitude for the treating of psychoneuroses. I think it was because he had to heal himself before he could heal others."[64] Charles Myers, who worked with Rivers at Maghull, felt the same: "He became another and a far happier man. Diffidence gave place to confidence, reticence to outspokenness, a somewhat labored literary style to one remarkable for ease and charm."[65]

In 1916, Rivers was commissioned as a captain in the Royal Army Medical Corps, an aspiration he had fancied since adolescence. Yet, now it would put him in the compromising position of maintaining army standards of discipline and disability while honoring his true commitment to the mental health of patients. In October of that year, he was transferred to the mental hospital at Craiglockhart. He would stay there until the end of 1917. Leery of a dark, foreboding asylum, Rivers found the place surprisingly agreeable. Its inmates, though, were not so sure. Siegfried Sassoon, one of his more famous patients in 1917, described it as "a gloomy cavernous place." Sassoon recalled, "the War Office had wasted no money on interior decoration; consequently, the place had the melancholy atmosphere of a decayed hydro."[66] Rivers and his staff did what they could. The bedrooms had changed little since their hydro days. They were described by Rivers as small, but with the surge of patients they needed to accommodate two or three occupants. This was a distraction for some. Sassoon, the inveterate writer, commented that little could be accomplished while his partners were awake. There was, to be sure, scarce personal time, but darkness brought out the worst. "One lay awake and listened to feet paddling along passages which smelt of stale cigarette-smoke; for the nurse couldn't prevent insomnia-ridden officers from smoking half the night in their bedrooms . . . One became conscious that the place was full of men whose slumbers were morbid and terrifying," Sassoon went on to write.[67]

William Rivers turned out to be a leading figure in shell shock and war neuroses. His mannerisms, intelligence, and practicality earned him high respect and reputation as a healer in mental disorders. By midsummer 1917 he was the dominant personality at Craiglockhart;

almost two thirds of the patients were under his care. Before him sat men troubled by inward fears of many natures. Few, he believed, had truly suffered from impacts of explosive concussions. Instead, the deep-seated demons of repressed horror and guilt had worked damages of profound qualities. There were those lame, mute, blind, or deaf who looked for all intents hysterical. Others simply faded into states of lethargy and insomnia punctuated by nightmarish fits or restless agitation. For these, the neurosis-plagued, Rivers offered help, his underlying premise that there was a *"conflict between the instinct of self-preservation and certain social standards of thought and conduct, according to which fear and its expression are regarded as reprehensible."* [68]

And then there were those who had left reality behind, who now existed in delusions, rantings, and obsessions far beyond mental stability. These were the psychotics not long for Craiglockhart. They soon transferred to places of lunacy and bantered about their encasements in alternate realities.

In those times, Sigmund Freud still ruled the psychiatric roost. It was Freud's belief that "traumatic neuroses" existed in response to awful events that permeated the conscious and filtered into the subconscious. "Any experience which calls up distressing affects—such as those of fright, anxiety, shame, or physical pain—may operate as a trauma of this kind," Freud had declared. [69] Rivers agreed. Egregious fright, anxiety, guilt, or shame could wound the victim as surely as bullets and bombs. There was a close interplay of physiology and psychology, one impacting the other to the point, he now observed, of physical infirmity. War was so much different than any normal day-to-day experience that the sights, sounds, and smells were a new insult on the psyche. The military tried to prepare men for this, but it was an almost impossible task. For the common soldier of the Great War, often poorly educated and emotionally immature, the war created impotency and despondency. Stuck in muddy trenches, he faced a daily danger of sudden annihilation. Sometimes the only solution in his mind was a physical debility that removed him from danger. Anxiety and fear mounted until they literally erupted from the subconscious, as difficult to tamp down as spewing lava. "Controlling social factors have been weakened by exhaustion, illness, strain, or shock, so that the motives arising out of the instinct of self-preservation have gained in power," Rivers later wrote.[70] Even for the better-educated officers, coping skills were incomplete. They, too, anguished from fear, doubt, and duty until the stammering incongruity of it all washed over them.

Between October 1916 and March 1919 over 1,700 patients with shell shock were treated at Craiglockhart. Almost half returned to full duty.[71] The cornerstone of treatment was, once again, an abiding trust between doctor and patient. Beyond that, the key in many cases was to unlock the repressed memories of war. Those swirling recollections, embedded in brains by the sheer magnitude of fear and doubt, had to be freed as surely as the demons of possessed souls. Talking, probing, and interpreting—time and again—were the enduring methods needed for liberating inner tortures. At the same time, staff members offered solutions, education, and coping skills for men who surely would carry their vivid mental monsters into the future.[72]

◆

After the Armistice, after the fighting ceased, veterans hobbled back. In Germany, amidst the hordes of maimed, victims of shell shock received little empathy. Deutschland had been humbled, the economy was in shambles, a generation of young men had been wiped out, and blinded, amputated, disfigured sons, husbands, and brothers were everywhere. In Teutonic fashion, commiseration, then, for tattered minds was low priority. Mental anguishes—the queer aberrations of expression, gait, and reckoning—were viewed as hysterical and therefore of an "unmanly, pathological nature." These misfits possessed a feeble and reprehensible constitution, it was assumed; simple dregs who shirked battlefield duties, abandoned comrades, or malingered for pensions.[73] As for Oppenheim's concussive theories, German psychiatrists moved on, unconvinced. More likely, they opined, it was a muddled masculinity or underlying psychological weakness. Yes, Freud's traumatic neuroses and repressed memories still held sway, but superimposed on a flawed character. Despite the censure, pragmatism won out, however. Something had to be done with this mob. It seemed inescapable to historians Stefanie

Linden and Edgar Jones that German psychiatrists saw themselves as servants of the state and national cause. As such, their obligation was to restore functionality. Was there genuine concern for the well-being of their patients? That is not entirely clear.[74] Nevertheless, any treatment that would return sanity or productivity was justified. Hypnosis, locked wards, isolation, anesthetization, electricity, and even radiation were all tried. More probative efforts mirroring Moss Side and Craiglockhart were just not feasible; simply too many cases.

The British were more curious and, it seemed, more compassionate. Shell shock in all its forms needed interpretation and explanation. In 1920, at the request of Parliament, a committee of inquiry was set up to study the "different types of hysteria and traumatic neuroses commonly called 'shell-shock.'"[75] In forty-one meetings, committee members, doctors, military authorities, and civil servants interviewed fifty-nine "witnesses," including such figures as Gordon Holmes, William Rivers, and Richard Rows. The committee's report was issued two years later. They disparaged the term "shell shock." It was a poor label for the different manifestations of war neuroses. And, importantly, the committee found no link with cowardice. These victims exhibited no signs of timidity during battle. It was only afterward that the symptoms struck, as fears and terrors that could no longer be subdued surfaced. Some witnesses testified that it was no wonder such horrors devoured sanity. Trench warfare was in itself insane: the powerless hunched below ground as explosives rang out again and yet again, or until the shrill whistle of another suicidal charge, or the cunning sniper's bullet found its mark. It was, as Freud imagined, a condition born of fright. "The most appalling thing," one doctor said, "was the feeling of inaction, tied to the trenches." Of Mott's concussive theory? No proof, the committee felt. While no human being could withstand the repeated concussive effects of shelling, there was seldom evidence of organic injury of the nervous system. War neuroses were largely emotional states. "From the evidence presented to us, it appears that the purely emotional variety of shell-shock, which forms 80 percent of all the cases, is brought about by a great variety and combination of causes": mental exhaustion, loss of sleep, constant battle racket, poison gases, cold, and rain. And most disturbing for these addled veterans, war neuroses were not battle casualties. No compensation.[76]

In January 1919, Charles Myers contributed an article to *The Lancet* on his personal familiarities with shell shock victims. His experience had been indisputably substantial. "No medical officers have felt the strain of war more severely than those engaged in the treatment of functional nervous disorders," he began. Myers was now convinced that the commotion of shell blasts played a minor, albeit precipitating, role. Nevertheless, he did not rule out contributions of "internal secretions" or loss of some higher control yet ill-defined. Treatment remained uncertain. He finished that these disorders, mixed though they may be, had opened the field of neuropsychiatry to vast opportunities for investigation and research. "Up to now the field has been almost wholly neglected," he ended. "Far from being barren, it is rich with the possibilities of valuable results."[77]

It was a most puzzling of times. Modern warfare had ushered in a modern—and enigmatic—psychological strain. The Freudian idea of ill-contained repressed and disturbing mental images of emotional trauma would become a 20th century buzz phrase: post-traumatic stress disorder. Such troublesome phenomena were a curious blend of nature and nurture that still provoke incomplete comprehension. For one, history professor Tracey Loughran concluded that "there was no straightforward transition to a psychological understanding of the war neuroses: psychology, physiology, and biology were all inseparably blended in many theories."[78] Meanwhile, for the heroes themselves, martyrs of the trenches and all that was evil, in midnight hours grief swept over them as sudden as the clap of thunder, and, as if flooded in tears, they forevermore swam in seas of sorrow.

ELEVEN

Death Rides upon a Pale Horse: The Influenza Pandemic of 1918

*"And I saw, and behold, a pale horse, and its rider's name was
Death, and Hades followed him; and they were given power
over a fourth of the earth, to kill with sword and with famine
and with pestilence and by wild beasts of the earth."*
—Revelation 6:8 (Revised Standard Version Catholic Edition)

There was to be much killing in this first of the World Wars. Hundreds of thousands would never return home, buried now in the soft earth of France, Belgium, and Russia. Some deaths were inflicted from without and some from within. The advent of an epidemic—soon to be pandemic—from the tiniest of enemies, human viruses, would approach the devastation wrought by the mightiest of shells. Invasion of the interior of the human body was as subtle and painless as high explosives were blatant and pounding.

The illness known as influenza had been around for centuries. The origin of the name remains obscure but may have come from the 12th-century Italian *influenza di freddo*, meaning "influence of the cold," from a time when the environment was thought a major instigator of disease: those miasmas bubbling out of bad air or rotting soil.[1] The influenza contagion of 1918 had the most obscure of beginnings. It likely started in the most obscure of places—a remote county on the plains of Kansas not far from the towns of Garden City, Dodge City, and Liberal. How did it arise and what caused it? That remains a mystery. Blame fixed on the new hosts of bacteria, but none could be held accountable. It was not the Pfeiffer bacterium at all, named after the German bacteriologist Richard Pfeiffer, although many would claim that it was. The cause of this influenza was much tinier. It proved to be a novel avian-like virus, not likely to have infected humans before 1918.[2]

In the small farming community of Santa Fe, Kansas, in February and March 1918 reports in the local paper emerged that described sudden onsets of a respiratory illness. The local doctor was so concerned about the number of cases he reported them to national public health officials. In the April 5, 1918, *Public Health Reports*, eighteen cases of influenza—of a severe variety, the report said—were identified in Haskell County. There were three deaths.[3] If not for that, the entire matter would have been forgotten, as the local plague ebbed as quickly as it had surged. But from Santa Fe and other farms around Haskell County, young boys had been recruited for the army and were traveling back and forth to Camp Funston, a training camp near Fort Riley, some miles away in the middle of the state. In the morning of March 11, 1918, the first soldier at Funston became ill. "Patient Zero" by common lore was a company cook, Private Albert Gitchell from Haskell County, who reported to sick call with a sore throat, fever, and muscular pains. He was banished to the infirmary's contagious ward. The second case followed almost immediately. Corporal Lee Drake appeared with a fever of 103 degrees and identical symptoms. By lunchtime, over one hundred soldiers had reported sick, and by week's end there were over five hundred.[4] Over a three-week period ending March 29, eleven thousand cases had been treated at the base hospital.[5] And more disturbing, some of these young men worsened and died. Eighteen-year-old laundress Jessie Lee Brown was terrified by what she saw. Soldiers were dying so fast that bodies, she heard, were being kept in a warehouse. She wondered if she would be next.[6] Yet, no one quarantined. Solders trained, hopped troop trains, and sped throughout the country. Then, laden with incubating virus, got onto troopships to France.

Training camps were virus breeding grounds. The Army Medical Department would see weekly admission rates from influenza begin to rise by late summer 1918, and by September 22 climbed sharply in camps across the United States.[7] Without warning, men became sick in a fashion not typical of previous influenza illnesses. They suffered severe headaches, chills, pain in the back and legs, and fevers to 104 degrees. It was all overshadowed by a hacking cough and feeling of breathlessness. In army posts across America, from mid-September to November 1, over three hundred thousand cases of influenza were reported: one in five soldiers sickened.[8]

Camp Devens (later Fort Devens), Massachusetts, a seven-square-mile cantonment just outside Boston, earned the distinction of the first hot spot in the United States. The sentinel case of influenza occurred on September 8. The influx of recruits had seriously overcrowded the post, with almost ten thousand men housed there. Barracks were filled wall-to-wall with young men breathing, eating, and sleeping close to one another. Just one week after the first case, men flooded the camp hospital: 1,200 admitted in just one day. Within a month, Devens had recorded eleven thousand cases and over seven hundred deaths. On one day alone ninety patients died.[9] Further movement of troops into the fort was curtailed. Experts arrived to unravel the perplexing plague. Bacteriologist Victor Vaughan from the University of Michigan visited the camp that fall and was struck by "the utter helplessness of man in attempts to control the spread of this disease." It depressed him beyond words.[10] It was almost certain that other camps around the country would shortly be affected, and, indeed, they were. At Camp Dodge near Des Moines, Iowa, over ten thousand men were stricken and nearly two thousand died.[11] Almost ten thousand cases were admitted to the hospital at Camp Meade, Maryland, in little over a month. Wards spilled over with three times the normal census.[12] At Camp Lee, Virginia, whole buildings were set aside as "battalion hospitals." Eighty were eventually reserved. Regardless of the exact cause, the sickness was clearly a contagion and terribly communicable. Doctors hoped that what is now called "social distancing" might help. Every attempt was made to provide one hundred square feet of space for patients but, with the vast numbers, that was doubtful.[13] Just as at Camp Devens, consultants were summoned to provide some guidance for prevention and treatment. The surgeon general sent Rufus Cole and William Welch of the Rockefeller Institute and Victor Vaughan. They arrived on a cold, dreary day in late September. Doctor Cole was aghast at the scene, as he later reported:

> We found the hospital crowded, there were very few nurses, and soldiers were coming from all parts of the camp bringing their blankets with them and putting themselves to bed in cots placed on the porches. We were at once struck by the cyanosis which most of the patients exhibited. One could pick out the infected men among those standing about by the color of their faces.[14]

They then went to the morgue, where caskets were stacked, corpses after postmortem examinations. Autopsy was a ritual centuries old—the sifting of fresh human remains for clues to the ravages of disease. In the eras before sophisticated radiography, it was the only way to inspect organs and understand mechanisms of death. One after the other, shrouds were emptied and the lifeless placed on the prosector's table. It was a grim task he had, slicing open bodies, gutting the insides, sewing them back up for burial. The routine commenced and repeated again and again. These cadavers all had a peculiar cyanotic tinge, as if rich red blood had turned a sour blue for lack of air. Without delay, large knives cut through flesh, bone cutters crunched ribs, gloved hands pulled them apart. As the chest cavities were entered, thin bloody fluid spilled out like overflowing gutters. Lungs, the apparent target for the illness, lay within. They were pulled up, chiseled out, and sliced open. The ordinarily light and spongy tissue was weighty and no longer air-filled. Instead, sodden lung looked like the consistency of beef liver. Hemorrhage oozed from the cut surface as the pathologist's blade separated matter no longer porous and alveolar but soggy. In some areas obvious pneumonia had occurred, rendering tissue consolidated—a condensing inflammation that left air sacs obliterated and lung dense, unyielding. How could one in a living state extract oxygen, the molecule of life itself, from those organs?

These were not the typical lungs of bronchopneumonia. Doctors were familiar with that: thick, inflammatory exudates spreading out from small air passageways but leaving some normal tissue between. It was a common cause of death, particularly in the elderly. This epidemic was different. Findings of lobar or bronchopneumonia were infrequent. More often lungs had not condensed. Instead, just like at Camp Lee, pathologists found:

> The first feature of the lungs in influenza to attract attention was the relatively small amount of lung tissue solid with grossly demonstrable pneumonia . . . Entitled to first place [in importance] as a conspicuous feature, is the huge, often thin and watery bloody exudate in the lung tissue and bronchioles . . . It is difficult to believe that a disease with so many distinctive features and affording, as it has, so much of a novelty in pathologic anatomy can fail to possess a correspondingly definite etiology. [15]

Academicians had no ready answers. "In the autumn of 1918, this respiratory infection passed over the United States like a huge wave, taking a tremendous toll in human lives." So said pathologists of the Brady Laboratory of Yale University in 1920. Clinicians and pathologists were puzzled by the etiology, even the mode of transmission. It was a respiratory illness, to be sure, the trachea, bronchi, and lung tissue itself affected by an inflammatory disorder of a magnitude that exchange of respiratory gases became almost impossible. Later, pneumonia then often set in, complicating the picture. In the age of chemical warfare, pathologists were quick to point out that "a basis for the interpretation of the respiratory lesions of influenza is offered by the analogous changes in the respiratory tract initiated by the inhalation of poisonous gases." [16]

Well, poison gas it was not. Such febrile illnesses as influenza, though, had plagued mankind since the dawn of time. In ages past, pestilences were readily blamed on atmospheric vapors (bad air) or even supernatural punishments—those malevolent humors of old. In fact, the ancient disease of malaria, was derived from *mal aria*, medieval Italian for "bad air."

In the 20th century, the age of microbiology, it was clear from the start that this influenza, this epidemic respiratory disorder, was a disease unto itself, with a definite but as yet invisible malevolent agent. Transmission was not bad air itself but what was carried in it, human exhalations and spittle. The mere activity of talking and laughing was enough, let alone sneezing and coughing. With a relative short incubation time—probably at most two or three days—spread and infectivity were rapid.

Before 1918, the most recent pandemic was the "Russian epidemic" of 1889–90. At that time, microbiology was in its ascendancy. Bacteriologists scurried to their microscopes and culture media looking at secretions from affected subjects. Notable among these investigations was the work of the German bacteriologist Richard Pfeiffer (1858–1945), a protégé of the illustrious microbiologist Robert Koch. In a series of 1892 experiments, Pfeiffer cultivated a peculiar rod-shaped bacterium from the nose and throat swabs of patients with the Russian influenza. These, he was convinced, were the microbes responsible, even though transmission to rabbits and other experimental animals had produced inconsistent pathologic findings.[17] Nevertheless, the scientific community embraced his theory and soon, influenza was a disease of this imperfectly proven bacterium, Pfeiffer's bacillus.

His claims were unchallenged for many years. Now, in 1918, the rising tide of influenza led clinicians to quickly implicate Pfeiffer's bacillus. One enthusiast was navy pathologist Paul Lewis. Lewis, a researcher of some renown, was doing experimental work at the Phipps Institute in Philadelphia. He shared his belief in Pfeiffer's German-borne agent with the *Philadelphia Evening Bulletin* for September 20, 1918. It fit perfectly with anti-German sentiment of the time. "German Bug Causes Influenza Physician Here Discovers," the paper declared, implying Huns across the ocean were responsible.[18] But alas, it was not to be. Skeptics never really bought into Pfeiffer's hypotheses and by 1920, the myth had been dispelled. To a large extent, the work of Peter Olitsky and Frederick Gates at the Rockefeller Institute was the death knell. They showed that secretions from influenza patients that had been filtered to remove bacteria (and presumably Pfeiffer's bacteria) still caused the illness in rabbits. "The essential effects were produced by a substance wholly unrelated to these

[Pfeiffer] bacteria," they concluded. The agent was obviously smaller than a bacterium.[19] Thus began the search for a smaller, filterable substance capable of such terrible respiratory damage—the bundles of nucleic acid to be known as the human virus.

Pfeiffer's bacterium was out. "*B. Pfeiffer* . . . did not play any more important part than the ubiquitous diplo-streptococcus. The real virus, classified *faute de mieux* as 'invisible' or a 'filter-passer' . . . remains to be discovered," quoted the British medical journal *The Lancet* on January 4, 1919. Common belief at that point was that the as yet undiscovered filter passer of Olitsky and Gates was the initial culprit setting the stage for superimposed bacterial infection with agents such as Pfeiffer's bacillus. Pfeiffer, convinced as he had been about his work, remained silent now.[20]

Back at Camp Funston, where it all may have begun, cases of this new filter passer filled the camp hospital so rapidly that three auditoriums were requisitioned. Each was the size of a cavernous warehouse with eight or more rows of cots set up so as to accommodate over two hundred patients. As fast as they were prepared there were patients to occupy them. But such arrangements hardly provided the needed one hundred square feet per patient. Isolation precautions, other than masks, were nonexistent.[21] Doctors on site found it impossible to care for so many. Calls went out for medical workers at nearby Fort Riley. But there, too, influenza had struck. The large base hospital soon filled to capacity, and by October 15 held 1,300 cases. In and around Camp Funston and Fort Riley, over fifteen thousand patients sought admission. The division surgeon reported such an urgency that barely could he outfit a building before men lined up to fill it. "Some of the pneumonia developed so quickly after the onset of the symptoms of influenza that the men were toxic by the time they reported at the regimental infirmaries." Officers forbade troops to attend any mass meetings such as movies. Care was taken to reduce crowding on streetcars. Tents were furled, and all bedding and clothing sunned and aired daily.[22]

By September 26, influenza inundated eighteen army camps across the United States. Draft calls for these places were stopped, and further efforts were made to restrict movement of troops from one camp to another. At Camp Taylor outside of Louisville, Kentucky, one young artillery officer remembered that most, 90 percent he said, of the men at the camp came down with influenza. The death rate was alarmingly high. Several hundred coffins piled up outside the hospital in the mornings. [23]

Navy bases were not exempt. In March 1918, the navy yard in Mare Island, California, reported a sharp jump in admissions for influenza. By July, even more. Billeted men seemed particularly susceptible. "Practically all cases of pneumonia developed among those confined to barracks."[24] Numbers of afflicted rose sharply at the United States Naval training station in Newport, Rhode Island, beginning September 10. The Philadelphia naval yard and marine barracks in Quantico, Virginia, saw the same. Most worrisome, by late August there had been a noticeable downturn in the disease. The percentage of pulmonary complications jumped "beyond comparison with regard to earlier epidemics."[25] Men took ill, fevers raged, and breathing worsened. Case fatality rates soared above 10 percent. Soon, seventeen navy training stations and over twenty-nine thousand men would contract the disease and almost two thousand would die. Seaborne troops were not immune. Among navy forces afloat and the expeditionary marine forces, an additional 1,200 men died of influenza. For the entire navy that autumn there would be diagnosed 91,656 cases of influenza with 4,136 deaths.[26] The surgeon general of the navy, Rear Admiral William Braisted, in his annual report for 1918 and 1919, commented that "the rate of spread during the autumn months of 1918 was so rapid indeed as to revive the old discussion as to the possibility of air-borne infection . . . [but] the disease cannot spread faster than human beings travel."[27]

Curiously, not all troops were equally susceptible. Those camps located in the middle of America and the Southeast, largely rural in their draw of draftees, fared worse. A later scientific study showed it: "in mobilization camps, communicable diseases have produced the least admission and death rates in those camps which drew from areas that were prevailingly urban." Urban recruits hailing from the East Coast did better. In their upbringing, they dealt with other communicable disease by virtue of neighborhood density. Maybe they had already contracted something similar to this contagion and were now immune. Rural counterparts, living miles from one another, may not have had that advantage. [28]

As quickly as the disease had surged in the United States that autumn, it was also appearing in France, transported on the many ships stowing those camp draftees and their resident virus. The converted steamship USS *Leviathan*, carrying over nine thousand soldiers, left Hoboken, New Jersey, on September 29, 1918, for her ninth transatlantic voyage. It did not go unnoticed that, while troops were lined up for embarkation, some men "dropped helpless on the dock." These were but the latest of numbers of men who had fallen out during their march from camp, almost surely from influenza. The next day, at sea, *Leviathan* recorded her first death, a young sailor with the Hospital Corps. His death was so sudden that he was dead by the next morning. Also by the next morning, the sick bay was full. As troops bunked up and down and side by side into spaces with poor ventilation, it was no surprise that sickness spread with stunning speed. By that night an estimated seven hundred cases had developed. Despite efforts to isolate and quarantine, during those eleven days of crossing it was estimated that two thousand fell victim of the epidemic—including the chief army surgeon and two other medical officers—and a total of ninety-six died. A number of army nurses were also onboard and were "like ministering angels during that dreadful scourge . . . brave American girls who had left home and comfort in order to undergo peril and sacrifice abroad."[29]

The major French ports of Saint-Nazaire and Bordeaux were a primary debarkation points for American troops. Many soldiers heading down those gangways were already infected, colonized during their transatlantic voyage. Soon symptoms developed as the illness worsened. Cases appeared at Base Hospital No. 8, in Savenay, located in the Bordeaux region. At neighboring Base Hospital No. 6, an epidemic of "short fevers" seen over the summer worsened sharply in September, now more severe and protracted, lasting more than a week. Over three thousand patients were hospitalized that month, and one in ten died. October was little better but then, unexplainably, numbers sharply declined. It was a good thing. Beds just occupied by flu victims opened up for a rush of battle casualties from America's large Argonne offensive, which began in late September.[30]

Yet, this had proved to be a virulent illness. Flu epidemics came and went with the seasons. Ordinarily, among healthy young men, no more than a few days' rest sufficed. The malady doctors witnessed that autumn of 1918 was vastly different. The disease struck quickly and worsened rapidly. Some looked septic, as if overwhelmed by some bacterial pathogen. Others turned blue as their blood struggled to snatch enough oxygen from lungs drenched in hemorrhagic fluid. Pneumonia sometimes followed, which destroyed more lung tissue. For too many, it was unsurvivable. Before later detective work brought out the truth, many wondered where it had all started. Asia? Europe? Some quickly blamed the French or the Spanish for somehow spreading the disease to Americans on returning ships, and that "inadequate nourishment, poor ventilation, inhalation of dust and general physical discomfort [endured by troops, which had] diminished the natural resistance to the disease."[31]

Meanwhile, at Saint-Nazaire, precautions quickly went into effect. There already was little question that this influenza was transmitted by the breath of its victims. In so thinking, just as at Camp Devens, social distancing was a priority. Individual personal space was enlarged to forty square feet in barracks and tents. Gauze masks "chemically prepared" with a solution of iodine in albolene were given on arrival and worn by everyone on the motor transports leaving the port. In and around the Bellevue Hospital unit, Base Hospital No. 1 at Vichy, further inland, a special "pneumonia hospital" had been set up in a local hotel. With appearance of numbers of influenza victims in late September another hotel was converted. Attendants garbed as if for surgery, wearing white gowns and face masks. Efforts at sanitation and asepsis doubled. For good reason. Word had spread that, in neighboring base hospitals, two nurses had died. And at nearby Base Hospital No. 76, over 40 percent of the staff were stricken and five were to die.[32]

Even closer to the front, influenza swept over American troops in the field. In the Argonne area in September, supplies to frontline soldiers were hopelessly stalled. Food and water quickly became a premium. Doughboys, desperate to quench their thirst, filled canteens from streams and shell holes littered with corpses of men and horses. The food they did get was moldy and dirty. Summer clothing was inadequate with the coming cold of autumn—there were no blankets or overcoats. Men were under constant attack from artillery and gas. They became easy prey for the looming influenza.[33] Evacuation Hospital No. 6, designed as a surgical hospital for battle casualties and located a few miles south of Verdun, began seeing more cases of influenza in late August. By September, just before the jump-off, flu cases skyrocketed. With wounded streaming in from the front, this completely overwhelmed doctors and nurses. From mid-September to early December, almost 70 percent of cases admitted were respiratory ailments. There were special wards set aside just for influenza and pneumonia patients. Any patient with fever or rapid breathing immediately transferred there. In those wards, the bronchopneumonia that was developing "was one of the most distressing conditions with which we had to deal." Almost half would die of that complication. In desperation, various remedies were tried—even including bloodletting—without benefit. The only drug that seemed to help was morphine, which arrested coughing fits and allayed the anxiety of air hunger.[34]

Soon it was called the "Spanish Influenza," although it almost certainly did not begin there. Perhaps, Spain being a neutral country in the First World War, freedom of the press produced honest and frank reporting of this new illness.[35] The virus knew no borders, yet the focus had become the crowded combatant camps and fortresses of Europe. Influenza would eventually kill almost twenty-four thousand American boys: enlisted and officers, black and white. That figure would be well over forty-two thousand if those dying of "pneumonias" were included. This, of course, does not consider affected navy or marine personnel.[36] During the World War exactly 4,128,479 people served in the armed forces. Eighteen percent contracted influenza, or roughly one in five servicemen and women.[37]

❖

Influenza spared no one. The illness soon infected armies of both sides—Allies and Central Powers. In France, the first cases appeared in April 1918, possibly coinciding with the vanguard of the AEF. French called it "grippe," an old term for an influenza-like contagion. As in America, at first pass symptoms were mild and disability short. The second surge of September and October was much worse, described by some as similar to the respiratory form of anthrax. It struck suddenly with high fevers, aches, and cough. Shortness of breath was a hallmark feature. In some cases pneumonia followed, which complicated recovery and much too often "led to the cemetery." Doctors and researchers were amazed at the disease's virulence and contagiousness. Noted scientist Francis Heckel admitted to the public that "the current flu is not only formidable by its virulence, it is also formidable by its insidious nature and its treacheries."[38] Despite precautions, deaths climbed throughout France in October, spreading to civilian populations. In typical French fashion, rampant spread was blamed on promiscuity, but there was little evidence for it. Mostly, it seemed a logical explanation—God's retribution on the sinner—just as in medieval times. But the civilian impact was substantial. One Parisian housewife lamented that influenza was worse than the "Berthas" (huge German siege cannon) and the "Gothas" (German heavy aerial bombers).[39] It was particularly lethal to those over sixty. Eventually, almost a quarter of a million of all ages succumbed to the malady.[40]

French troops suffered just like the Americans.[41] An estimate of 230,000 military cases was reported for September through November. Influenza was blamed for the deaths of over fifty thousand French soldiers, over twenty thousand before the Armistice. Thirteen of every one hundred poilu were stricken, and one in ten died. Doctors of the Service de santé recoiled at the numbers. Their only recourse was prevention: restriction of human interaction, hand washing, wearing of masks, disinfecting, quarantine. Every conveyance possible was washed down with carbolic acid: troop trains, lorries, tents, bedsheets.[42] As for mask wearing, scientists like Heckel advised: "the gauze mask aims to protect against cough and breath, containing salivary particles or highly contagious bronchial secretions. It will be worn by any patient, from the start, and especially by the nursing staff, or by family members."[43] Despite precautions, the cases for that autumn were staggering. Doctor Joan Freixas said, before a conference of the Faculté de médecine in Paris that December, "the epidemic that has struck terror in our city," and had on many occasions been so terrible that the victim had no time to mount the most basic defenses before the toxic and infectious nature of the illness completely took over.[44] It was a further drain on manpower for a country that had lost so many already. In a fortunate way, the Armistice intervened just as the pandemic hit its fall peak in October.

Face coverings proved to be the most effective preventative measure. The wearing of masks was a German design, introduced by Polish surgeon Johann von Mikulicz-Radecki in Breslau at the turn of the century. One of his colleagues, Carl Flügge, already showed how air currents could carry fine specks of contagions—such as those of diphtheria, influenza, and pneumonia—flung forth by coughing and expectoration. These liquid droplets could be like bacteria-laden dust, spreading disease from one respiratory tract to another.[45] Mikulicz was aware of this and how pathogens could project from the mouth by simply speaking, clearing the throat, and sneezing. This was especially worrisome in the operating room, where surgical infections were still a feared complication, too often ending fatally. To him it was vital that his operations be kept as sterile as possible. He forbade conversation in his operating room as a result, but then went one step further, wearing a *Mundbinde*, literally a "mouth bandage," during cases. It was not an inconvenience at all, he claimed. "Wir athmen dadurch eben so anstandslos wie eine Dame, die auf der Straße den Schleier trägt" ("We breathe as easily as a lady wearing a veil on the street"). The surgical mask, a simple layer of gauze, was sterilized and attached to the surgical cap.[46] By 1918, wearing of masks in the operating room was common practice. It took little imagination that masks would be important for this influenza pandemic. Army researchers at the Rockefeller Institute soon had convincing evidence that a close-knit cloth covering could prevent the spread of respiratory particles. Ordinarily, respiratory droplets could project ten feet or more. Masks held them in check.[47] The entire European continent, Great Britain, and America were masking up, scrubbing down, laundering, and spraying to ward off Flügge's poisonous air vapors.

Out in the front lines, no-man's-land presented no barrier. The tiny flu virus was able to do in weeks what millions of infantry could not do in years—cripple the enemy. German general Erich Ludendorff blamed the sickness on failure of his troops to overwhelm Allied forces in their spring offensive of 1918. In March, prior to the initial push, he remarked that there had been some cases of influenza but that his medical officers classified them as slight. Then, in April, the first German soldiers came down with a more severe influenza-like illness. They called it by an old nickname: *Blitzkatarrh* (lightning cold).[48] By the Marne-Rheims offensive of July, there were serious problems. The attacks fizzled out because, by then, influenza—and a voracious variety—was depleting Ludendorff's ranks. "It was a grievous business having to listen every morning," he later recalled, "to the Chiefs of Staff recital of the number of influenza cases, and their complaints about the weakness of their troops if the English attack again."[49] Sickness had indeed swept over all German divisions. For instance, seasoned Prussians of his Fifteenth Division, poised on the Marne, at one time counted 1,200 men, almost 10 percent of their strength, disabled because of influenza.[50] One German officer, Rudolf Binding, who kept a detailed journal of his war experiences, wrote in mid-August 1918:

> I have been having extraordinary attacks of fever, with such general neuralgia that I can only manage to exist in an artificial condition of tottering weakness with the help of aspirin and pyramidon [amidopyrine, an antipyretic]. This was followed by a nasty attack of champagne-fever, something like typhoid, with ghastly symptoms of intestinal poisoning which laid me out. I'm simply collapsing.[51]

His illness, most likely influenza, lasted more than two weeks, accompanied by recurrent fever and disabling fatigue. Binding blamed it as much on the lousy rations given his troops as the flu bug. He was certainly not alone in his sickness. A letter found in the pocket of a German prisoner on July 4 of that year admitted, "I feel so ill that I should like to report sick. Fever is rampant among us and already a whole lot of men are in the hospital. Every day more go in."[52] Germans, it was claimed, were affected so suddenly with influenza that they were literally dropping in their tracks. In July also, Kaiser Wilhelm himself had to leave the western front, caught in the grip of "the grippe." He was reported to have "fallen a victim to the influenza that has been so prevalent in the German army."[53]

October was a horrible month for troops. The influenza, now rampant among the American forces, had become as much a participant in the ravaging of soldiers as enemy fire. Of course, none of this was shared with the American public. For propaganda purposes, the true impact of influenza received little play in newspaper communiqués. Surgeon General Ireland told the *New York Times* in late October that:

> The American Army in Europe is the healthiest that the world has ever seen . . . There were some cases of Spanish influenza . . . but not with the after attack of pneumonia. This was due chiefly . . . to the fact that the soldiers led healthy outdoor lives.[54]

In reality, all was not quite so cheery. During the Meuse-Argonne campaign, the first and only pure offensive effort by a United States force, the First American Army, over seventeen thousand doughboys were killed and almost seventy thousand wounded. Along with these numbers, over sixty-eight thousand suffered from medical illnesses, "largely influenza." The disease had stripped the First Army of manpower sorely needed to rid their battlefield of determined German resistance.[55] Chief surgeon Alexander Stark gave a different view of combat readiness than that espoused by Ireland:

> the wave of influenza that was sweeping over the continent engulfed the First Army that already had as much to bear as it could sustain, and for a time it appeared as though its ravages would seriously affect the military operations by overwhelming the sanitary formations.[56]

Medical officers in the field immediately saw the effect of the flu. Richard Derby, surgeon for the Second Division, remarked that a number of his men were falling out with the sickness, even more often than from

bullet wounds. His evacuations from the front from influenza amounted
to three or four hundred per day. Derby blamed it on lousy conditions for
the troops: scarce food, wet weather, and little rest.[57]

No unit was free of the contagion. It assailed enlisted and officers
alike. Even brigade commanders, key figures in offensive operations
like the Meuse-Argonne, were out sick. Support troops well behind the
lines were more often affected than men in the trenches. Shortages in
these ranks affected logistics: getting food, water, and clothing to the
frontline troops. Less to eat, less to drink, and the same wet and cold
coats and blankets. Morale dwindled. "Dirty, lousy, thirsty, often hungry;
and nearly every last man is sick," as the famous Father Francis Duffy,
chaplain for the 165th Infantry, described it.[58] All in all, influenza may
have largely been responsible for the faltering offensive that almost failed
to dislodge Germans of the Hindenburg Line. Aside from the useless
waste of lives, it would have been an embarrassment for American officers
and troops.

The Armistice on November 11, 1918, brought an end to the killing
but not the dying. The entire western front was now afflicted. At Casualty
Clearing Station No. 11 near Lille, British nurse Catherine Macfie saw
no letup. Now the stricken were not battle-scarred but influenza-ridden:

> We couldn't send these young men on my ward down the
> line because they were too ill to move, and we had ever so
> many deaths. We were kept busy and it was a most depressing
> time—worse, in a way, when all the good news was coming
> through. The boys were coming in with colds and a headache
> and they were dead within two or three days. Great big, hand-
> some fellows, just came in and died. There was no rejoicing in
> Lille on the night of the Armistice. There was no rejoicing.[59]

Back in the United States, the virus continued its deadly spread among
military personnel, precariously close to civilian populations. In late
August 1918, Navy Lieutenant J. J. Keegan found a number of influenza

cases appearing at the US naval hospital on the banks of the Mystic River outside Boston. It was almost certainly brought to America's shores by Europeans and European ships, he reasoned (homegrown in America, more likely). In two weeks, he had counted more than two thousand cases, including a number of medical personnel who had treated these patients. The disease marched at lightning speed, some victims prostrate within a few hours. Patients conscious on admission soon lapsed into stupor; pulses raced, breathing quickened, and fevers raged. So little could be done other than cooling sponges, expectorants, and maybe touches of opium. Pneumonia worsened everything and hastened death. Before it receded, influenza felled over 2,500 men. Almost six in one hundred would die. Two medical officers and three nurses were in that group.[60]

Before long, cases appeared throughout Boston. That autumn and winter of 1918 and 1919, a house-to-house survey discovered that roughly one in five Bostonians had contracted the disease. Population density played a critical role. More crowded neighborhoods and tenements—those catering to the underprivileged—had higher rates of disease. Young adults, many common laborers working in close proximity to one another, had three times the rate of infection, the virus jumping from one breath to another and from dirty hand to mouth and face.[61] That sickly fall, Boston recorded over six thousand deaths.[62]

In New York, the first cases probably surfaced in mid-August and likely arrived through the port. Troopships running between Europe and America that summer carried numbers of influenza-sick passengers—and crew, as it turned out. The Cunard liner *Khiva*, shuttling soldiers back and forth, was forced to remain in New York port upon her return as there were not enough healthy sailors to handle her.[63] By September, the disease had hit the city full force. From that point until March 1, 1919, New York would see over fifteen thousand deaths from influenza and another sixteen thousand from pneumonias of all types, but many as a result of the influenza.[64]

New York City, despite its crowded streets, actually fared better than other East Coast communities. Fewer people died above the normal rate (4.4 per thousand) than in Philadelphia (7.3 per thousand) or Boston

(6.5 per thousand).[65] This was even more surprising if one considers the laxity in quarantine requirements for New York. Leland Cofer, New York State health officer, determined that first priority in deciding to quarantine vessels was their importance to the war effort. In other words, if movement of men or material was necessary for military concerns, quarantine would be lifted regardless of public risk. More positive preventative measures, though, were staggered business hours to reduce pedestrian congestion, and opening of more than 150 emergency health districts and centers to care for affected individuals. Those falling ill at home were advised to quarantine there (called home isolation), but others, living in boarding houses or tenements, were promptly removed to the emergency centers. Schools stayed open, but other, more prosaic entertainments such as sidewalk spitting (from tobacco presumably) were discouraged. In fact, spitters and rogue polluters of the kind were liable to be hauled into court and fined.[66] For the navy and the hordes of furloughed seamen prowling the city streets, advice was to steer clear of portside dalliances: "Avoid the hug / Avoid the lip, / Escape the bug / That gives the 'grippe.'"[67] Eventually, the surgeon general of the Public Health Service, Rupert Blue, issued a series of pamphlets advising citizens on measures to be taken to stop the spread of the contagion: avoid crowds, smother coughs, clean hands, open windows—breathe fresh air, and, please, "do not spit on floor or sidewalk."[68]

While the virus showed no bias, it favored tenement dwellers, the poor, the uneducated: ripe environments to shower—and share—the air with expelled particles of infection. In Chicago, predictably, disparities of class, location, and income affected death rates for the disease. Those of low literacy, low income, and in highly dense, poorly ventilated living conditions suffered disproportionately. As in Boston, manual laborers had less compunction to distance themselves—their jobs discouraged it. Masks were impractical. Transmission and infectivity was the price paid.[69] That fall of 1918, nearly eight thousand Chicagoans died of influenza and another five thousand from pneumonia.[70]

In pathologist Paul Lewis's town of Philadelphia, the scourge reached its zenith that October. By October 6, Dr. William Krusen, director of the Department of Health and Charities, announced the recording of two hundred thousand cases. And victims continued to mount, 1,300 alone on October 19. Deaths per day were well into the hundreds. Funerals had to be postponed for lack of coffins. Hospitals burst with new admissions, engulfing health-care workers with impossible numbers of ill. At the University of Pennsylvania hospital, medical students acted as full-fledged doctors and nurses. They saw patients gasping for breath as the disease rapidly progressed, their skin taking on that characteristic purplish color from lack of oxygen. Delirium soon set in as blood-tinged sputum drooled from mouth and nose, a signal that the end was near. Catholic nuns responded in droves to staff hospitals, food kitchens, and even private residences. Just like any health-care worker, their benevolence was no protection. They, too, fell ill alongside their patients. During October and November, twenty-two succumbed to the flu. In a hope to curb the pestilence, church services ceased. Theaters closed. Large gatherings were prohibited. Officials even discouraged public transportation. Calls went out for more doctors and nurses while emergency hospitals opened to provide more beds.

Meanwhile, men and women lurked warily down half-empty streets as if menacing shadows might arch over them and splash their fragile frames with dark bodings of the plague. Masks meant to shut out pestilence only convinced onlookers of the perilous nature accompanying the most elementary of human activity. Before dark, everyone scurried inside, thinking the blackness of night too inviting for the grim reaper.

Yet, just as mysterious as the autumn surge, by the end of November the death toll began falling. Sporadic cases continued to appear during November, but the ravages of September and October were not to be seen again.[71] Combined with the war it was all such a horror. A weary public was eager to put both behind. "Looking ever forward . . . they relegated the pandemic to an increasingly irrelevant past, leaving little for the retention of public memorials of its real costs."[72] The war and influenza were topics filled with too much sorrow to be visited very often.

A third surge appeared in the Northern Hemisphere the winter of 1919, more subdued than before, but it, too, abruptly retreated. As for the mysterious virus, where did it go? Nothing of modern medicine intervened. No vaccines, no antibiotics could be proffered. Perhaps it was so-called herd immunity, a collective arousal of antibodies from clinical or subclinical infection providing no soft landing place for this plague. Or mutations of the virus itself, that spontaneous rearrangement of genetic code rendering life more or less capable of existence.[73]

How did the pandemic revolutionize medicine? Maybe by not revolutionizing it at all. Maybe by teaching that the magnificent ingenuity and technology humans devised over the preceding half century was of little consequence to the whims of the tiniest of microbes. These packages of malevolent nucleic acid evaded discovery and preyed on troops and civilians alike with such voracity to equal the stupendous bombs and guns that pelted Europe's landscape for four brutal years. By showing that as much as things change, they still remain the same, that the same plague precautions preached by beaked medieval soothsayers and alchemists still carry weight today, that all the brilliance of evolving science might stand impotent in forestalling hundreds of thousands of deaths from new contagions and modern-day epidemics. That science can be uplifting—almost miraculous—and quietly humbling all at the same time. That just maybe in the grand scheme of destiny it is all a zero-sum game, that the brightest of accomplishments are offset by the simplest of defeats. Yet, medicine would indeed move forward as an inexorable force, much of it born in the First World War. The tenacity and resolve of those scientists would prevail. Viruses were to finally be categorized, even mapped, vaccines developed, suffering alleviated, death thwarted. Perhaps it was all that Rudyard Kipling said: "If you can meet with Triumph and Disaster and treat those two imposters just the same . . . yours is the Earth and everything that's in it."[74]

TWELVE

And After the Dying

"A war benefits medicine more than it benefits anybody
else. It's terrible, of course, but it does."
—Mary Merritt Crawford[1]

In many ways, the Great War was unique in its destructiveness. Among other things, it was an industrial war, a war of weaponry and technology forged by science itself, and so violent in its potential as to threaten the very existence of mankind. It destroyed forever, as political theorist John Mueller was quick to point out, the romantic and inevitable complexion of war. Armed combat now took on a repugnant nature, a detestable character shunned by a more civilized public. Perhaps not unique in its ferocity, as Mueller contended, nevertheless, in the First World War there was a certain revulsion about the whole affair that defies explanation or justification. It was simply too grim, too earthy, too murderous. Killing at a distance with volumes of artillery seemed more sterile to some but put into play a helplessness of the human element, so central to warfare in history. Soldiers only in name, they were nothing but cannon fodder for their remote, seemingly emotionless commanders eager to pummel their opponents from afar.[2]

Author Jared Diamond pointed out that 19th-century writers attempted to interpret history as a "progression from savagery to civilization." This war proved them wrong. There was no refinement of behavior.

If anything, civilization regressed, mounting a violence unheard of and subjecting combatants and civilians alike to the ravages of a senseless, pitiful conflict.[3] The contemplative French foot soldier Louis Mairet may have said it best in a letter home to his parents in December 1916. To him the war was "madness without name, stupidity without limits." "Reason is lost," he continued, "before the spectacle of a scientific struggle, where progress is used to return to barbarism, before the spectacle of a civilization that turns against itself to destroy itself."[4]

The Great War, then, heralded the advent of different societies, forms of modernity not entirely admirable or even progressive, but filled with a rearrangement of all that was once considered civilized. In the words of historian Sir Michael Howard:

> "The Great War" was widely seen as a cataclysm . . . that transformed European society and shattered its states system, destroying four great empires and provoking revolutionary upheavals whose effects are still working themselves out . . . Many, if not indeed most [historians] now interpret it as part of a general crisis—economic, social, and cultural—affecting the whole of European society at the turn of the century.[5]

Far removed from the battlefields, political transformation as radical as the new weapons of armed conflict absorbed the attention of partisan enthusiasts and gave rise to the era of nationalism, both militaristic and socialistic. The industrial age of the 19th century lent the necessary expertise to mass-produce the destructive products of science to such a degree that stockpiles of ammunition dwarfed any previous conflict and gave armies unlimited access to arsenals almost constantly replenished, and ready at the whim of leaders determined to shape a national identity. The might of industry that outstripped any 19th-century fantasies would come to characterize the aspirations of warmongers well into the future, and help spawn the atrocities of a Second World War to come. Wars that followed would incorporate the full fury of a binding government-science-industry collaboration—that may have been the lasting influence of the Great War. According to historian Jack Roth, the war, in all its brutality, aroused passions that "revealed the extraordinary energies in the masses available for collective purposes." It gave birth, in his opinion, to "the first modern effort at systematic, nationwide manipulation of collective passions."[6]

And, to Michael Howard's assessment, we should add a revolution in medical thinking. Mark Harrison argued that modern warfare as experienced in the Great War had altered the relationship between medicine and the military as a reflection of the modernization of industrialized societies over the ages. The 20th century witnessed medicine augmenting military efficiency by reducing depletion of forces from disease and from disabling injuries. It also transformed cadres of poorly trained "amateur" health-care workers into highly motivated, skilled, and dedicated professionals.[7] It was the Great War, though, that condensed the scattered medical advances of the turn of the century into heavily funded, government-sponsored efforts that spawned a new age both in the military and civilian spheres.

In June 1919, that renowned American surgeon Lewis Pilcher of Brooklyn, New York, spoke before the American Surgical Association to an international audience of former war surgeons fresh from the fields of France. "Surgeons of this war," he proclaimed, "cannot escape the higher endowment which attends the enlargement in the scope of their surgical vision; which inevitably has heightened and broadened their professional aspirations." In Pilcher's mind, the war was a revelation, not just in its brutality, but that doctors could frame a systematic attack on the medical evils of mankind this violence had exposed.[8]

Pilcher was not alone. Anthony Bowlby, in his presidential address before the Royal Society of Medicine on January 9, 1920, highlighted the impact of war wounds on civilian practice: that such a vast exposure to the vagaries of battlefield trauma could be successfully transferred to the day in and day out experiences of the civilian surgeon. In particular, traumatic shock—the bane of the seriously injured—had captivated him. It had been seen sporadically in community practice, especially in industrial accidents. But now the war had exposed its mysterious nature. Blood loss alone was not the explanation, he believed. All the extremes of weather, nutrition, and battlefield conditions played in.

Thousands of shocked casualties were the proof. Those other problems of civilian surgical practice—fractures and wound infections—were treated in abundance by countless army surgeons on the western front, and revolutionary changes in management had been made. "Surely it is evident," Bowlby went on to say, "that much of what we have learnt is applicable to civil practice . . . that surgery of the immediate future may well be expected to benefit from our recent experiences."[9]

Perhaps it is true, as author Jared Diamond pointed out, that students of human history profit from the experience of scientists.[10] And scientists flocked to this war. The muddied, cratered fields of Belgium and France became a gigantic laboratory to study the effects of Claude Bernard's *milieu extérieur* gone berserk on the human frame.[11] They could now analyze, measure, cultivate, and dissect the terrible nuances of injury created by a vast cauldron of violence—conditions they had only infrequently seen before. Adventurous researchers jumped at the chance. Historian Peter English claimed that George Crile was "supremely confident . . . that science and surgery could overcome all forms of disease." Clinical relevance, Crile believed, was essential for research—and the Great War produced this in abundance.[12] The battlefields of Europe, then, became the clinical backdrop for a metamorphosis of civilian medicine as profound as the advent of the experimental age of the 19th century. In the United States, research output increased exponentially during the war, far surpassing scientific discoveries by Germany, France, and Great Britain. Research was now a profession unto itself, not merely the idle dabbling of physician-scientists.[13] The Great War had shown the absolute necessity for laboratory-based experimentalists in the basic sciences. In the clinical arena, too, experiences were invaluable. That was certainly crystal clear to surgeon Harvey Cushing. On November 15, 1918, as he was preparing to depart for England and the United States, Cushing realized that the war had given him:

> All the advantages of a full-time university service—paid by the government—no outside responsibilities—no office hours to keep—merely undivided attention to the work at hand . . . There is nothing quite like this combination in civil life—no

comparable incentive. How can we transfer some of its good features to civil conditions?[14]

Would these transformations not have occurred without the stimulus of war? Would the understanding of wound sepsis, or early care of the injured, or the enigma of traumatic shock, the widespread use of Röntgen's rays, the splint of Thomas, and the mental anguish of traumatic neuroses linger in the back halls of medical practice, seldom visited and even less often considered? For medicine, the integration of science, government, and industry produced acts of benevolence unheard of generations before. The wealth of nations stimulated a cooperation between laboratories and clinicians far exceeding what peacetime might have fabricated.

Some academicians pleaded for an ecumenical spirit rather than more parochial endeavors of nationalism and isolationism. Albert Einstein in 1920 argued that the internationalism of culture, commerce, and industry implied a rational relationship between countries, a "sane union." Moreover, he strongly felt that scientists must be the pioneers of restoring worldwide cooperation so grievously tarnished by the war. Scientific research must not crumble, he insisted, or the intellectual life of a nation will shut down. And science had risen to the forefront in this conflict, now, more than ever, as a hallmark of a progressive society despite the butchery exhibited by more militaristic concerns.[15] Perhaps Joseph Blake of New York said it best during his lecture at the Sorbonne in Paris in 1919 when he encouraged the "perpetuation of the cordial and fruitful relations which have existed during the war between the physicians and surgeons of the different armies." It was this spirit of collaboration that must give rise to international societies and congresses, he went on to emphasize, which, coupled with the great universities in Europe and America, would provide the stimulus for progress into the future.[16]

George Crile was reported to have said, "more progress has been made in the surgery of the chest and abdomen, in the treatment of wounds, of infections, of hemorrhage and exhaustion; more knowledge has been accumulated of splints, of apparatus and of every applicable mechanism in the three brief years of war than in the past generation."[17] Without question, it was a war that ushered in a new age of medicine; one that would lay the groundwork for investigative efforts to understand the hidden principles of human biology that only such conflagrations could unmask. And as is our nature, as Mary Merritt Crawford surely believed, from the horrors of such conflicts arise new knowledge, new technology, and new incentives to benefit the health of future generations. In truth, from the evils mankind devised during this Great War came improbable but unmistakable redemption.

Acknowledgments

A work of this complexity cannot be accomplished alone. Of course, I am indebted to my literary agent Regina Ryan for recognizing the significance of the subject matter and for her talent in finding the right publisher. Similarly, I would like to thank my publisher Claiborne Hancock and Pegasus Books for choosing to assemble this manuscript and publish it in quality fashion. In so doing, I appreciated the help of Peter Kranitz and Drew Wheeler for their expert editing and Maria Fernandez in assisting me in the entire publishing process. The voices of the many personages of the Great War who filled the pages of this manuscript with their amazing stories and who dedicated their time, effort, and sanity to repair the physical and spiritual damages of this horrid conflict served as my inspiration and told their tales much more eloquently than I was capable of doing. Though long dead, their words are indelible and their legacy is eternal. They are to be venerated and their efforts commemorated. It is to them that I extend my admiration and gratitude and for them that this book is written. We must never forget those who have gone before us. Theirs are the shoulders upon which we now perch to gaze at tomorrow. In resurrecting many of those now yellowed archives, manuscripts, and memoirs to bring these figures back to life, I extend my heartfelt appreciation to Suzette Robinson and her staff at the Rowlands Medical Library of the University of Mississippi Medical Center. Their dogged tenacity unearthed long forgotten records. I would also like to thank Victor Gabella for his vital efforts in Paris to cull the French archives of the musée du Val- de-Grâce in Paris. As with all my literary exploits there is one who stands at my side, holds my hand, and lends me her strength: my wife Kelly.

Bibliography

Acton, C., J. Potter. 2012. "'These Frightful Sights Would Work Havoc with One's Brain': Subjective Experience, Trauma, and Resilience in First World War Writings by Medical Personnel." *Literature and Medicine* 30:61–85.

Adrian, E. D., L. R. Yealland. 1917. "The Treatment of Some Common War Neuroses." *Lancet* 1:867–72.

Ahreiner, G. 1917. "Ueber Behandlung der Schußwunden und den Wert der Dakin'schen Lösung." *Beiträge zur Klinischen Chirurgie* 107:286–96.

Aimone, F. 2010. "The 1918 Influenza Epidemic in New York City: A Review of the Public Health Response." *Pub Health Reports* 125:71–79.

Aitken, D. M. 1916. "The Treatment of Gunshot Fractures." *Brit Med J* 2:213–15.

"Alexander Hughes Bennett (1848–1901) and Rickman John Godlee (1849–1925)." *CA Cancer J Clin* 24 (1974):169–70.

Alvaro, G. 1896. "I Vantaggi Practici della Scoperta de Röntgen in Chirurgia." *Giornale medico del Regio Esercito* 44:385–94.

Annual Report, Navy Department. Washington, DC: Government Printing Office 1918/1919.

Archibald, E. A. 1916. "A Brief Survey of Some Experiences in the Surgery of the Present War." *Can Med Assoc J* 6:775–95.

Archibald, E. 1916. "A Note Upon the Employment of Blood Transfusion in War Surgery." *Lancet* 2:429–31.

Archibald, E. W., W. S. McLean. 1917. "Observations upon Shock, with Particular Reference to the Condition as Seen in War Surgery." *Ann Surg* 66:280–86.

Arnold, Catherine. 2018. *Pandemic 1918: Eyewitness Accounts from the Greatest Medical Holocaust in Modern History.* New York: St. Martin's Publishing Group.

Aschoff, L. 1916. "Zur Frage der Aetiologie und Prophylaxe der Gasödeme." *Deutsche Med Wochensch* 42:469–71.

Asprey, Robert B. 1996. *At Belleau Wood.* Denton: University of North Texas Press.

Audoin-Rouzeau, Stéphane. 1992. *Men At War.* Oxford: Berg.

Augerson, William. 2000. *A Review of the Scientific Literature as it Pertains to the Gulf War Illnesses.* Santa Monica, Calif.: RAND Corporation.

Auld, S. J. M. 1918. *Gas and Flame in Modern Warfare.* New York: George H. Doran Company.

Austin, R. T. 2009. "Meurice Sinclair CMG: A Great Benefactor of the Wounded of the First World War." *Injury* 40:567–70.

Aymard, J.-P., P. Renaudier. 2016. "La Tranfusion Sanguine Pendant la Grande Guerre (1914–1918)." *Hist Sci Med* 50:353–66.

Baca, V., D. Kachlik, T. Bacova, et al. 2014. "Anatomist and the Pioneer of Radiology Étienne Destot—95th Anniversary of his Death." *Clin Anat* 27:282–85.

Baguenier-Desormeaux, L. 1981. "Henry Drysdale Dakin à Compiègne en 1915." *Revue d'histoire de la pharmacie* 249:79–88.

Bamji, A. 2003. "Facial Surgery: The Patient Experience." In *Facing Armageddon: The First World War Experience*, ed. Hugh, Liddle, Peter Cecil, 490–501. Barnsley, U.K.: Pen and Sword.

Bamji, Andrew. 2017. *Faces From The Front*. Solihull: Helion and Company.

Bancroft, W. D., et al. 1926. "Medical Aspects of Gas Warfare." In *The Medical Department of the United States Army in the World War*, ed. M. W. Ireland, 25–771. Washington, DC: Government Printing Office.

Bárány, R. 1915. "Die Offene und Geschlossene Behandlung der Schussverletzungen des Gehirns." *Beiträge zur Klinischen Chirurgie* 97:397–417.

Barcroft, S. 1989. "The Hague Peace Conference of 1899." *Irish Studies in International Affairs* 3:55–68.

Barnes, Joseph K. 1883. *The Medical and Surgical History of the War of the Rebellion*, vol. 2. Washington, DC: Government Printing Office.

Barnett, R. 2019. "Influenza." *Lancet* 393:396.

Barry, J. M. 2004. "The Site of Origin of the 1918 Influenza Pandemic and its Public Health Implications." *J Translat Med* 2:1–4.

Bartlett, F. C. 1948. "Charles Samuel Myers. 1873–1946." *Obit Notices R Soc* 5:767–77.

Basford, J. R. 2001. "A Historical Perspective of the Popular Use of Electric and Magnetic Therapy." *Arch Phys Med Rehab* 82:261–69.

Battersby, J. C. 1899. "The Roentgen Rays in Military Surgery." *Brit Med J* 1:112–14.

Bayliss, W. M. 1918. *Intravenous Injection in Wound Shock*. London: Longmans, Green, and Co.

Beard, G. 1869. "Neurasthenia, or Nervous Exhaustion." *Boston Med Surg J* 3:217–21.

Beebe, Gilbert W., and Michael E. DeBakey. 1952. *Battle Casualties: Incidence, Mortality, and Logistical Considerations*. Springfield, Ill.: Charles C. Thomas.

Behring, E., Kitsato, S. 1890. "Ueber das Zustandekommen der Diphtherie-Immunität und der Tetanus-Immunität bei Thieren." *Dtsch Med Wochenscr* 16:1113–14.

Benison, S., A. C. Barger, E. L. Wolfe. 1991. "Walter B. Cannon and the Mystery of Shock: A Study of the Anglo-American Co-Operation in World War I." *Med Hist* 35:217–49.

Benison, Saul, A. Clifford Barger, and Elin L. Wolfe. 1987. *Walter B. Cannon: The Life and Times of a Young Scientist*. Cambridge, Mass.: Harvard University Press.

Bennett, A. H., R. J. Godlee. 1885. "Case of Cerebral Tumour—The Surgical Treatment." *Brit Med J* 1:988–89.

Bennett, J. P. 1986. "Henry Tonks and His Contemporaries." *Br J Plast Surg* 39:3–34.

Bergmann, E. 1890. "Surgical Treatment of Diseases of the Brain." In *Wood's Medical and Surgical Monographs*, ed. W. Wood, 767–973. New York: William Wood & Co.

Bergmann, Ernst. 1878. *Die Behandlung der Schusswunden des Kniegelenks im Kriege.* Stuttgart: Ferdinand Enke.

Bergmann, Ernst von. 1880. *Die Lehre von den Kopfverletzun.* Stuttgart: Ferdinand Enke.

Bernard, Claude. 1885. *Leçons sur les Phénomènes de la Vie, Communs aux Animaux et aux Végétaux.* Paris: J.-B. Balliere et fils.

Best, Nicholas. 2008. *The Greatest Day in History.* New York: PublicAffairs.

Bier, A. 1916. "Anaerobe Wundinfektion (Abgesehen von Wundstarrkrampf)." *Beiträge zur Klinischen Chirurgie* 101:271–335.

Bier, Auguste. 1903. *Hyperämie als Heilmittel.* Leipzig: F. C. W. Vogel.

Biernoff, S. 2010. "Flesh Poems: Henry Tonks and the Art of Surgery." *Visual Culture in Britain* 11:25–47.

Binding, Rudolf. 1929. *A Fatalist at War.* Boston: Houghton Mifflin Company.

Black, Catherine. 1939. *King's Nurse Beggar's Nurse.* London: Hurst & Blackett.

Black, Elizabeth Walker. 1919. *Hospital Heroes.* New York: Charles Scribner's Sons.

Black, J. E., T. G. Glenny, J. W. McNee. 1915. "Observations on Six Hundred and Eighty-five Cases of Poisoning by Noxious Gases Used by the Enemy." *Br Med J* 24:509–18.

Blackwood, N. J. 1920. "History of the U.S. Naval Hospital, Chelsea, Mass., 1915–1918." *US Naval Med Bull* 14:311-338.

Blake, J. A. 1919. "The Influence of War Upon the Development of Surgery." *Ann Surg* 69:453–65.

"Blessures du Cerveau: Conclusions." *Comptes Rendus de la Conference Chirurgicale Interalliee pour l'Etude des Plaies de Guerre.* Paris: Archiv de Méd et de Pharm Milit, 1917. 451–52.

Bliss, Michael. 2005. *Harvey Cushing: A Life in Surgery.* Oxford: Oxford University Press.

Blundell, J. 1818. "Experiments on the Transfusion of Blood by the Syringe." *Med Chir Trans* 9:56–92.

Boeckh, Katrin, and Sabine Rutar, eds. 2018. *The Wars of Yesterday: The Balkan Wars and the Emergence of Modern Military Conflict, 1912–13.* Oxford: Berghahn Books.

Booth, J. 1977. "A Short History of Blood Pressure Measurement." *Proc R Soc Med* 70:793–799.

Borden, W. C. 1900. *The Use of the Röntgen Ray by the Medical Department of the United States Army in the War with Spain (1898).* Washington, DC: Government Printing Office.

Bourdillon, P., C. Apra, M. Leveque. 2018. "First Clinical Use of Stereotaxy in Humans: The Key Role of X-ray Localization Discovered by Gaston Contremoulins." *J Neurosurg* 128:932–37.

Bourke, Joanna. 1996. *Dismembering the Male: Men's Bodies, Britain, and the Great War.* Chicago: University of Chicago Press.

Bourne, C. M., R. K. Chhem. 2014. "War Medicine as Springboard for Early Knowledge Construction in Radiology." *Med Studies* 4:53–70.

Bowlby, A. 1920. "On the Application of War Methods to Civil Practice." *Proc R Soc Med* 13:35–48.

———. 1915. "Wounds of War." *Lancet* 2:1385–98.

Bowlby, A., C. Wallace. 1917. "The Development of British Surgery at the Front." *Br Med J* 1:705–21.

Bradford, J. R., T. R. Elliott. 1915. "Cases of Gas Poisoning among the British Troops in Flanders." *Br J Surg* 3:234–46.

Bradley, J., M. Dupree, A. Durie. 1997. "Taking the Water-Cure: The Hydropathic Movement in Scotland, 1840–1940." *Bus Econ Hist* 26:427–37.

Brauer, L., F. Haenisch. 1915/1916. "Eins selbständige, transportable Feldröntgenanlage fiir interne und chirurgische Untersuchungen." *Fortschritte auf dem Gebiete der Röntgenstrahlen [RöFo]* 23:38–46.

Breakey, W. F., J. B. Mulliken. 2015. "Sir William Arbuthnot Lane and His Contributions to Plastic Surgery." *J Craniofac Surg* 26:1504–07.

Brennecke, Ernest. 1925. *The Life of Thomas Hardy.* New York: Greenberg Publisher.

Bresalier, M. 2013. "Fighting Flu: Military Pathology, Vaccines, and the Conflicted Identity of the 1918–19 Pandemic in Britain." *J Hist Med Allied Sci* 68:87–128.

Breton, D. L. 1991. "Handicap d'Apparence: Le Regard de l'Autre." *Ethnologie française* 21:323–30.

Breuer, Joseph, and Sigmund Freud. 2000. *Studies on Hysteria*, trans. James Strachey. New York: Basic Books.

Brewer, Madison M. 1898. *Report to Adjutant Tenth Cavalry, camped near Santiago de Cuba.* Field communication. Washington, DC: U.S. Army Center for Military History.

Bristow, Nancy K. 2012. *American Pandemic: The Lost Worlds of the 1918 Influenza Epidemic.* Oxford: Oxford University Press.

Brophy, L. P. 1956. "Origins of the Chemical Corps." *Military Affairs* 20:217–26.

Brophy, Leo P., Wyndham D. Miles, and Rexmond C. Cochrane. 1959. *The Chemical Warfare Service: From Laboratory to Field.* Washington, DC: Office of Military History.

Bruhn, Charles. 1915–17. *Die Gegenwärtigen Behandlungswege der Kieferschussverletzungen.* Wiesbaden: J. F. Bergmann.

Buchholtz, Arend. 1913. *Ernst von Bergmann.* Leipzig: C. W. Vogel.

Budd, William. 1873. *Typhoid Fever: Its Nature, Mode of Spreading, and Prevention.* London: Longmans, Green, and Co.

Buguet, A., A. Gascard. 1896. "Détermination à l'aide des rayons X de la profondeur où siège un corps étranger dans les tissus." *Comptes Rendus de l'Acad Sci* 122:786–87.

Bullard, Robert Lee. 1925. *Personalities and Reminiscences of the War.* New York: Doubleday, Page & Company.

Cale, H. 1919. "The American Marines at Verdun, Chateau Thierry, Bouresches, and Belleau Wood." *Indiana Magazine of History* 15:179–91.

Cramp, W. C. 1912. "A Consideration of Gas Bacillus Infection with Special Reference to Treatment." *Ann Surg* 56:544–64.

Cannon, W. B. 1918. "A Consideration of the Nature of Wound Shock." In *The Nature and Treatment of Wound Shock and Allied Conditions*, ed. W. B Cannon, E. M. Cowell, J. Fraser and A. N. Hooper, 71–92. Chicago: American Medical Association.

———. 1919. "The Course of Events in Secondary Wound Shock." *JAMA* 73:174–81.

Cannon, Walter Bradford. 1945. *The Way of an Investigator.* New York: W. W. Norton & Company.

Carden-Coyne, Ana. 2009. *Reconstructing the Body: Classicism, Modernism, and the First World War.* Oxford: Oxford University Press.

Carrel, A. 1902. "La Technique Opératoire des Anastomoses Vasculaires et la Transplantation des Viscères." *Lyon Médical* 98:859–64.

———. 1915. "Science Has Perfected the Art of Killing—Why Not of Saving?" *Surg Gynecol Obstet* 20:710–11.

———. 1932. "Tuffier." *Revue de Paris* 39:347–59.

Carrel, A., H. Dakin, M. Daufresne, et al. 1915. "Traitement Abortif de l'Infection des Plaies." *Bull l' Académie Natl Med* 74:361–68.

Carrel, A., and G. Dehelly. 1917. *The Treatment of Infected Wounds.* Toronto: The Macmillan Company.

Carrel, Alexis. 1935, 1939. *Man the Unknown.* New York: Harper & Brothers.

Carrel, Alexis, and Virgilia Peterson. 1950. *The Voyage to Lourdes.* New York: Harper & Brothers.

Carter, A. J. 1991. "Hugh Owen Thomas: The Cripple's Champion." *Brit Med J* 303: 1578–81.

Carter, K. C. 1988. "The Koch-Pasteur Dispute on Establishing the Cause of Anthrax." *Bull Hist Med* 62:42–57.

Catlin, A. W. 1919. *"With the Help of God and a Few Good Marines."* New York: Doubleday, Page & Company.

Cernak, I. 2017. "Understanding Blast-Induced Neurotrauma: How Far Have We Come?" *Concussion* 2:1–19.

Chalier, A., R. Glenard. 1916. "Les Grandes Blessures de Guerre." *Revue de Chirurgie* 51:210–73.

Chambers, J. A., P. D. Ray. 2009. "Achieving Growth and Excellence in Medicine." *Ann Plast Surg* 63:473–78.

Nélaton, Charles and Louis Ombrédanne. 1907. *Les Autoplasties.* Paris: G. Steinheil.

Chisolm, J. Julian. 1864. *Manual of Military Surgery.* Columbia: Evans and Cogswell.

Clayton, Ann. 2006. *Chavasse: Double VC.* Barnsley, U.K.: Pen and Sword.

Cochrane, Rexmond C. 1957. *Gas Warfare at Belleau Wood, June 1918.* Washington, DC: US Army Chemical Corps Historical Office.

Coenen, H. 1916. "Ein Rückblick auf 20 Monate Feld Ärztlicher Tätigkeit, mit Besonderer Berflicksichtigung der Gasphlegmone Beiträge zur klinischen Chirurgie." *Beiträge zur Klinischen Chirurgie* 6:397–464.

Colebrook, L. 1956. "Alexander Fleming 1881–1955." *Bio Mem Royal Soc* 2:117–26.

Conradi, H., R. Bieling. 1916. "Zur Aetiologie und Pathogenese des Gasbrands." *Münchener Med Wochenschrift* 63:133–78, 1023–68, 1561–1608.

Cooper, Astley. 1825. *The Lectures: Principles and Practice of Surgery*, vol. 1. Boston: Wells and Lilly.

Cooter, R. 1990. "Medicine and the Goodness of War." *CBMH/BCHM* 7:147–59.

Cope, V. Z. 1961. "The Medical Balance-Sheet of War." In *Some Famous General Practitioners and Other Medical Historical Essays*, 169–83. London: Pitman Medical Publishing.

Corner, George W. 1964. *A History of the Rockefeller Institute: 1901–1953, Origins and Growth*. New York: The Rockefeller Institute Press.

Corryllos, P. 1915. "Le Traitement des Plaies du Crane par Projectiles de Guerre." *Arch Chir (Le Mans)* 50:1–49.

Couthamel, Jason, and Peter Leese. 2017. *Psychological Trauma and the Legacies of the First World War*. New York: Palgrave Macmillan.

Cowell, E. M. 1919. "A Method of Teaching the Front Line Application of Thomas's Splint by Numbers." *J R Army Med Corps* 33:175–78.

Cowell, E. 1928. "The Pathology and Treatment of Traumatic (Wound) Shock." *Proc Royal Soc Med* 21:1611–18.

Crile, G. W. 1915. "Notes on Military Surgery." *Ann Surg* 62:1–10.

———. 1907. "On the Direct Transfusion of Blood—An Experimental and Clinical Research." *Canada Lancet* 60:1057–68.

Crile, George. 1947. *An Autobiography*. Philadelphia: J. B. Lippincott.

Crile, George W. 1899. *An Experimental Research into Surgical Shock*. Philadelphia: J. B. Lippincott Company.

———. 1903. *Blood-Pressure in Surgery: An Experimental and Clinical Research*. Philadelphia: J. B. Lippincott Company.

———. 1909. *Hemorrhage and Transfusion: An Experimental and Clinical Research*. New York: D. Appleton and Company.

Crile, George W., and William E. Lower. 1914. *Anoci-Association*. Philadelphia: W. B. Saunders Company.

Crosby, Alfred W. 2003. *America's Forgotten Pandemic: The Influenza of 1918*. Cambridge, Mass.: Cambridge University Press.

Crouthamel, Jason, and Peter Leese. 2017. *Psychological Trauma and the Legacies of the First World War*. London: Palgrave Macmillan.

Cruse, W. P. 1987. "Auguste Charles Valadier: A Pioneer in Maxillofacial Surgery." *Mil Med* 152:337–341.

Curie, Ève. 1938. *Madame Curie*. London: William Heinemann.

Curie, Marie. 1923. *Pierre Curie*, trans. Charlotte Kellogg and Vernon Kellogg. New York: Macmillan Company.

Curie, Marie, and Pierre. 1921. *La Radiologie et la Guerre*. Paris: Felix Alcan.

Cushing, H. 1918. "A Study of a Series of Wounds Involving the Brain and Its Enveloping Structures." *Brit J Surg* 5:558–684.

———. 1916. "Concerning Operations for the Cranio-Cerebral Wounds of Modern Warfare." *Mil Surg* 38:601–15.

———. 1927. "Neurosurgery." In *The Medical Department of the United States Army in the World War*, ed. Charles Lynch, Frank W. Weed, and Loy McAfee Ireland, 749–758. Washington, DC: Government Printing Office.

———. 1918. "Notes on Penetrating Wounds of the Brain." *Brit Med J* 1:221–26.

———. 1902. "On the Avoidance of Shock in Major Amputations by Cocainization of Large Nerve-Trunks Preliminary to Their Division. With Observations on Blood-Pressure Changes in Surgical Cases." *Ann Surg* 36:321–45.

———. 1908. "Technical Methods of Performing Certain Cranial Operations." *Surg Gynecol Obstet* 6:227–46.

———. 1905. "The Special Field of Neurological Surgery." *Bull Johns Hopkins Hosp* 16:77–87.

———. 1920. "The Special Field of Neurological Surgery After Another Interval." *Arch Neurol Psych* 4:603–36.

Cushing, Harvey. 1936. *From a Surgeon's Journal*. Boston: Little, Brown, and Company.

———. 1908. "Surgery of the Head." In *Surgery: Its Principles and Practice*, ed. William Williams Keen, 17–276. Philadelphia: W. B Saunders Company.

———. 1917. *Tumors of the Nervus Acusticus and the Syndrome of the Cerebellopontine Angle*. Philadelphia: W. B. Saunders Company.

Cutler, Elliot Carr. 1915. *A Journal of the Harvard Medical School Unit to the American Ambulance Hosspital in Paris: Spring of 1915*. New York: Evening Post Job Printing Office.

Dakin, H. D. 1915. "On the Use of Certain Antiseptic Substances in the Treatment of Infected Wounds." *Br Med J* 2:318–20.

———. 1915. "The Antiseptic Action of Hypochlorites: The Ancient History of the 'New Antiseptic.'" *Br Med J* 2:809–10.

Darmon, P. 2003. "La Grippe Espagnole Submerge la France." *L'Histoire* 281:79–85.

d'Aubigny, M. 1921. "Rapport sur les Armements." *Les Archives de la Grande Guerre* 8:487–538.

Davidson, S. A. 1988. "Dr. Robert Tait McKenzie: A Man for All Seasons." *CMAJ* 138:70–72.

de Bassompierre, Alfred. 1916. *The Night of August 2–3, 1914, at the Belgian Foreign Office*. London: Hodder & Stoughton.

Debré, Patrice. 1994. *Louis Pasteur*. Baltimore: Johns Hopkins University Press.

DeKosky, R. K. 1976. "William Crookes and the Fourth State of Matter." *Isis* 67:36–60.

Delaporte, S. 1994. "Les Défigurés de la Grande Guerre." *Guerres Mondiales et Conflits Contemporains* 175:103–21.

Delbert, P. 1916. "Actions de Certains Antiseptiques sur le Pus." *Bull et Mem Société Chir* 42:92–110.

Delorme, E. 1914. "Considérations Générales sur le Traitement des Blessures de Guerre." *Compte rendus de l'Academie des Sciences* 159:543–55.

Delorme, Edmond. 1914. "Blessures de guerre, Conseils aux chirurgiens." *Comptes Rendus, Des Seances de Academie des Sciences*. Paris. 394–99.

———. 1919. *Les Enseignements Chirurgicaux de la Grande Guerre (Front Occidental)*. Paris: A. Maloine et Fils.

———. 1888. *Traite de Chirurgie de Guerre Tome I*. Paris: Felix Alcan.

del Regato, J. A. 1978. "Antoine Béclère." *Int J Radiation Oncology Biol Phys* 4:1069–79.

Depage, A. 1914. "War Surgery." *Ann Surg* 60:137–42.

Depage, A., G. Maloens. 1917. "L'Ambulance de l'Océan à La Panne Aperçu Clinique sur les Effets Comparés de Divers Traitements des Plaies de Guerre." *Trans Ambul Océan La Panne* 2:1–19.

Derby, Richard. 1919. *"Wade in, Sanitary!": The Story of a Division Surgeon in France.* New York: G. P. Putnam's Sons.

Derquenne, F. 2015. "Deux Pionniers Français de la Chirurgie Esthétique: François Dubois et Raymond Passot." *Hist Sci Med* 49:29–40.

Diamantis, A., E. Magiorkinis. 2016. "Mobile Radiography Units in Balkan Wars." *J R Army Med Corps* 162:78–80.

Diamond, Jared. 1997. *Guns, Germs, and Steel: The Fates of Human Societies.* New York: W. W. Norton & Company.

Dineur, T. 1896. "Balle de Revolver Perdue dans la Jambe et Découverte par la Radiographie." *Arch Med Belges* 21:330–35.

Dolamore, W. H. 1918. "The Treatment of Injuries of the Face and Jaws at Dusseldorf." *J Assoc Mil Dental Surg* 2:137–46.

Doughty, W. H. 1867. "Report of Two Cases of Ligation of the Subclavian Artery." *South Med Surg J* 21:30–36.

Doust, B. C., A. B. Lyon. 1918. "Face Masks in Infections of the Respiratory Tract." *JAMA* 71:1216–19.

Dowdeswell, T. L. 2017. "The Brussels Peace Conference of 1874 and the Modern Laws of Belligerent Qualification." *Osgood Hall Law Journal* 54:805–50.

Duchess of Sutherland, Millicent. 1914. *Six Weeks at the War.* London: The Times.

Duckett, M. W. 1876. *Dictionnaire de la Conversation et de la Lecture.* Paris: Dirmin-Didot.

Duclaux, Émile. 1920. *Pasteur: The History of a Mind.* Philadelphia: W. B. Saunders Company.

Duffy, Francis P. 1919. *Father Duffy's Story.* New York: George H. Doran Company.

Dugas, L. A. 1867. "A Lecture on Suppuration." *South Med Surg J* 21:36–55.

Duhamel, Georges. 1917. *Vie des Martyrs, 1914–1916.* Paris: Mercure de France.

Eckart, Wolfgang U., and Christoph Gradmann. 2017. *Die Medizin und der Erste Weltkrieg.* Herbolzheim: Springer-Verlag.

Edmonds, James E. 1935. *Military Operations France and Belgium 1918.* London: Macmillan and Co.

———. 1932. "Military Operations France and Belgium, 1916: Sir Douglas Haig's Command to the 1st July: Battle of the Somme." In *History of the Great War Based on Official Documents by Direction of the Historical Section of the Committee of Imperical Defence,* ed. Imperial War Museum, 483. London: Battery Press.

Edwards, D. S., E. R. Mayhew, A. S. C. Rice. 2014. "'Doomed to go in Company with Miserable Pain': Surgical Recognition and Treatment of Amputation-Related Pain on the Western Front during World War 1." *Lancet* 384:1715–19.

Ehrlich, P. 1891. "Experimentelle Untersuchungen über Immunität." *Dtsch Med Wochenschr* 17:1218–19.

Eksteins, Modris. 1989. *Rites of Spring: The Great War and the Birth of the Modern Age.* New York: Doubleday.

Elliot, T. R. 1914. "Transient Paraplegia from Shell Explosion." *Brit Med J* 2:1005–06.

Elliott, L. P. 1979. "William Henry Welch: Pioneer American Microbiologist and Physician." *Bios* 50:73–77.

Emling, Shelley. 2012. *Marie Curie and Her Daughters*. New York: Palgrave Macmillan.

Engerand, Fernand. 1918. *Le Secret de la Frontière 1815—1871—1914 Charleroi*. Paris: Editions Bossard.

English, Peter C. 1980. *Shock, Physiological Surgery, and George Washington Crile*. Westport, Conn.: Greenwood Press.

Estes, W. L. 1912. "End Results of Fractures of the Shaft of the Femur." *Ann Surg* 56:162–84.

Evans, B. 1982. "A Doctor in the Great War—An Interview with Sir Geoffrey Marshall." *Brit Med J* 285:1780–83.

Evans, Thomas W. 1873. *History of the American Ambulance Established in Paris during the Siege of 1870–71*. London: Chiswick Press.

Ferrandis, J.-J., A. Segal. 2009. "L'Essor de la Radiologie Osseuse Pendant la Guerre de 1914–1918." In *Journées d'Histoire des Maladies des Os et des Articulations*, ed. B.-P. Amor, P. Bonnichon, D. Gourivitch, 48–50. Paris: Rhumatologie Pratique.

Finger, S., P. J. Koehler, C. Jagella. 2004. "The Monakow Concept of Diaschisis: Origins and Perspectives." *Arch Neurol* 61:283–88.

Finucane, M. I. 1900. "General Nervous Shock, Immediate and Remote, After Gunshot and Shell Injuries in the South African Campaign." *Lancet* 2:807–09.

Finzi, Kate John. 1916. *Eighteen Months in the War Zone*. London: Cassell and Company.

Fischer, H. 1870. "Ueber den Shok." *Sammlung klinischer Vortage* 10:69–82.

Fishman, R. S. 1997. "Gordon Holmes, the Cortical Retina, and the Wounds of War." *Documenta Ophthal* 93:9–27.

Flamm, H. 2012. "Das Österreichische Rote Kreuz und österreichische Bakteriologen in den Balkankriegen 1912/13—Zentennium des ersten Einsatzes der Bakteriologie auf Kriegsschauplätzen." *Wien Med Wochenschr* 162:132–47.

Fleming, A. 1915. "On the Bacteriology of Septic Wounds." *Lancet* 2:638–43.

Flügge, C. 1897. "Ueber Luftinfection." *Zeitschriff Hygiene Inf* 25:179–224.

Foray, N., M. Amiel, R. Mornex. 2017. "Étienne Destot (1864–1918) ou l'Autre Père de la Radiologie Française." *Cancer/ Radiothérapie* 21:138–47.

Foveaux, Jessie Lee Brown. 1997. *Any Given Day: The Life and Times of Jessie Lee Brown Foveaux*. New York: Warner Books.

Fox, P. 2006. "Confronting Postwar Shame in Weimar Germany: Trauma, Heroism and the War Art of Otto Dix." *Oxford Art J* 29:249–67.

Fraenkel, E. 1893. "Ueber die Aetiologie der Gasphlegmonen (Phlegmone Emphysematosa)." *Centralbl f Bakteriol u Parasitenk* 13:13–16.

———. 1916. "Ueber Gasbrand." *Deutsche Medizinische Wochenschrift* 42:1533–35.

Fraenkel, Eugen. 1893. *Ueber Gasphlegmonen*. Hamburg und Leipzig: Leopold Voss.

François, B, G. Sternberg, E. Fee. 2014. "The Lourdes Medical Cures Revisited." *J Hist Med Allied Sci* 69:135–62.

Franz, Carl. 1920. "Die Wundinfektionskrankheiten." In *Kriegschirurgie*, 43–100. Leipzig: Werner Klinkhardt.

Freeman, J. 1985. "Professor Tonks: War Artist." *Burlington Magazine* 127:284-293.

Freixas, Joan. 1919. *Traitement de la Grippe*. Paris: J.-D. Baillière et Fils.

Fries, A. A. 1923. "Chemical Warfare Service." *Infantry Journal* 21:524–34.

Fries, Amos A., and Clarence J. West. 1921. *Chemical Warfare*. New York: McGraw-Hill Book Company.

Galvez-Behar, G. 2005. "Le Savant, l'Inventeur et le Politique: Le Rôle du Sous-Secrétariat d'État aux Inventions Durant la Première Guerre Mondiale." *Vingtième Siècle. Revue d'histoire* 85:103–17.

Garrison, Fielding H. 1929. *An Introduction to the History of Medicine*. Philadelphia: W. B. Saunders Company.

Gaupp, R. 1915. "Hysterie und Kriegsdienst." *Münchener Med Wochenschrift* 62:361–63.

———. 1916. "Kriegsneurosen." *Zeitschrift f Neurologie und Psych* 34:357–90.

Gavin, Lettie. 1997. *American Women in World War 1: They Also Served*. Niwot: University Press of Colorado.

Gehrhardt, M. 2018. "La Greffe Générale: The Voice of French Facially Injured Soldiers." *Modern Contemp France* 26:353–68.

Gehrhardt, Marjorie. 2015. *The Men with Broken Faces*. Oxford: Peter Lang.

Gehrhardt, Marjorie. 2013. *The Destiny and Representation of Facially Disfigured Soldiers During the First World War and the Interwar Period in France, Germany, and Great Britain*. Doctoral Thesis, Exeter: University of Exeter.

George, David Lloyd. 1934. *War Memoirs 1917*. Boston: Little, Brown, and Company.

Gergö, Emerich. 1914/1915. "Neue Type eines Feldröntgenautomobils." *Fortschritte auf dem Gebiete der Röntgenstrahlen [RöFo]* 22:400–05.

Gilchrist, Harry L. 1928. *A Comparative Study of World War Casualties from Gas and Other Weapons*. Edgewood, Md.: Chemical Warfare School.

Gilchrist, Harry L., and Philip B. Matz. 1933. *The Residual Effects of Wartime Gases*. Washington, DC: Government Printing Office.

Gillies, H. D. 1920. *Plastic Surgery of the Face*. Oxford: Oxford University Press.

Gillies, H. D. and D. R. Millard. 1957. *The Principles and Art of Plastic Surgery*. Boston: Little, Brown and Company.

Gilman, S. L. 2008. "Electrotherapy and Mental Illness: Then and Now." *Hist Psychiatry* 19:339–57.

Girard, Marion Leslie. 2008. *A Strange and Formidable Weapon*. Lincoln: University of Nebraska Press.

Glasser, Otto, and Margret Boveri. 2013. *Wilhelm Conrad Röntgen und Die Geschichte der Röntgenstrahlen*. Berlin: Springer-Verlag.

Glasser, Otto. 1993. *Wihelm Conrad Röntgen and the Early History of the Roentgen Rays*. Springfield, Ill.: Norman Publishing.

Glicenstein, J. 2015. "Louis Ombrédanne (1871–1956), Chirurgien Pédiatre et Plasticien." *Ann Chir Plastique Esthétique* 60:87–93.

Glynn, T. R. 1910. "The Traumatic Neuroses." *Lancet* 2:1332–36.

Gram, H. C. 1884. "Über die isolierte Färbung der Schizomyceten in Schnitt-und Trockenpräparaten." *Fortschritte der Medizin* 2:185–89.

Grantz, K. H., M. S. Rane, H. Salje, et al. 2016. "Disparities in Influenza Mortality and Transmission Related to Sociodemographic Factors Within Chicago in the Pandemic of 1918." *Proc Natl Acad Sci USA* 113:13839–44.

Graves, Robert. 1929. *Good-bye To All That*. New York: Doubleday.

Gray, H. M. W. 1919. *The Early Treatment of War Wounds*. London: Hodder & Stoughton.

Greenblatt, S. H. 2003. "Harvey Cushing's Paradigmatic Contributions to Neurosurgery and the Evolution of His Thoughts about Specialization." *Bull Hist Med* 77:789–822.

Greenblatt, Samuel H. 1997. *A History of Neurosurgery in its Scientific and Professional Contexts*. Park Ridge, Ill.: American Association of Neurological Surgeons.

Greenough, R. B. 1915. "The American Hospital of Paris." *Bost Med Surg J* 172:954–55.

Gross, Samuel David. 1882. *A System of Surgery: Pathological, Diagnostic, Therapeutic, and Operative*, vol. 1. Philadelphia: Henry C. Lea's Sons & Company.

Groves, E. W. H. 1940. "The Life and Work of Moynihan." *Brit Med J* 1:649–51.

Guiou, N. 1918. "Blood Transfusion in a Field Ambulance." *Br Med J* 1:695–96.

Guthrie, G. J. 1820. *Observations on Gun-Shot Wounds and on Injuries of Nerves*. London: Burgess and Hill.

———. 1827. *Treatise on Gun-Shot Wounds*. London: Charles Woods.

Haber, Fritz. 1924. *Fünf Vorträge aus den Jahren 1920–1923*. Berlin: Julius Springer.

Haber, L. F. 1986. *The Poisonous Cloud*. Oxford: Clarendon Press.

Haggard, W. D. 1918. "The Medical Profession and the Great War." *Trans Southern Surg Assoc* 30:1–11.

Haldane, J. B. S. 1925. *Callinicus: A Defence of Chemical Warfare*. New York: E. P. Dutton & Company.

Hall, M. W. 1928. "Communicable and Other Diseases." In *The Medical Department of the United States Army in the World War*, ed. M. W. Ireland, 61–169. Washington, DC: Government Printing Office.

Hamilton, David. 2017. *First Transplant Surgeon: The Flawed Genius of Nobel Prize Winner, Alexis Carrel*. Singapore: World Scientific Publishing.

Hamilton, Douglas T. 1916. *High-Explosive Shell Manufacture*. New York: The Industrial Press.

Hansbury-Sparrow, Arthur Alan. 1932. *The Land-Locked Lake*. London: Arthur Barker.

Hardy, Thomas. 1920. *The Works of Thomas Hardy in Prose and Verse*. London: Macmillan and Company.

Haret, M. 1915. "Le Role de la Voiture Radiologique du Service de Santé aux Armées." *J de Radiol et d'Electrol* 1:497–99.

Harries, Meiron, and Susie Harries. 1997. *The Last Days of Innocence*. New York: Vintage Press.

Harrison, M. 1999. "Medicine and the Management of Modern Warfare: An Introduction." In *Medicine and Modern Warfare*, ed. Roger Cooter, Mark Harrison, and Steve Sturdy, 1–27. Amsterdam: Rodopi.

Hart, C. W. 2014. "Harvey Cushing, M.D., in His World." *J Rel Health* 53:1923–29.

Heller, Charles E. 1984. *Chemical Warfare in World War I: The American Experience, 1917–1918*. Fort Leavenworth, Kan.: Combat Studies Institute.

Heller, H. H. 1922. "Classification of the Anaerobic Bacteria." *Bot Gazette* 73:70–79.

———. 1920. "Etiology of Acute Gangrenous Infections of Animals: A Discussion of Blackleg, Braxy, Malignant Edema and Whale Septicemia: Studies on Pathogenic Anaeerobes. I." *J Infect Dis* 27:385–451.

Helling, T. S., W. S. Marble. 2019. "Surgeons to the Front: Twentieth-Century Warfare and the Metamorphosis of Battlefield Surgery." In *The Last 100 Yards: The Crucible of Close Combat in Large-Scale Combat Operations*, ed. Paul E. Berg, 191–210. Fort Leavenworth, Kan.: Army University Press.

Helling, T. S., E. Daon. 1998. "In Flanders Fields: The Great War, Antoine Depage, and the Resurgence of Debridement." *Ann Surg* 228:173–81.

Hemmings, Robert. 2008. "Rivers, Myers and the Culture of War Neuroses." In *Modern Nostalgia*, 28–53. Edinburgh: Edinburgh University Press.

Henrard, M., M. Janssen. 1917. "Extraction des Projectiles Magnétique Intracérébraux au Moyen de l'Electro-aimant et de l'Appareil Téléphonique de Hedley." *Bull et Mem Soc Chir (Paris)* 43:1850–58.

Henry, H. 1920. "On the Antitoxin Content of some Gas Gangrene Sera used in the Later Stages of the War." *J Path* 23:270–72.

Heraclitus. 2016. "Testimonia." In *Early Greek Philosophy*, vol. 3, ed. André Laks and Glenn W. Most, 168. Cambridge: Loeb Classical Library.

Hermann, R. E. 1994. "George Washington Crile (1864–1943)." *J Med Bio* 2:78–83.

Herwig, Holger H. 2011. *The Marne, 1914: The Opening of World War I and the Battle that Changed the World*. New York: Random House.

Hildanus, Guilhelmus Fabricus. 1617. *Gangraena et Sphacelo*. Oppenheimii: Typis Hieronymi Galleri.

Hildebrandt, August. 1905. *Die Verwundungen durch die modernen Kriegsfeuerwaffen ihre Prognose und Therapie im Felde*. Berlin: August Hirschwald.

Hill, L., H. Barnard. 1897. "A Simple and Accurate Form of Sphygmomanometer or Arterial Pressure Gauge Contrived for Clinical Use." *Brit Med J* 2:904.

History of the U.S.S. Leviathan. Brooklyn: Brooklyn Eagle Job Department, 1919.

Hoehling, Adolph A. 1961. *The Great Epidemic: When the Spanish Influenza Struck*. New York: Little, Brown.

Holdorff, B., T. Dening. 2011. "The Fight for 'Traumatic Neurosis,' 1889–1916: Hermann Oppenheim and his Opponents in Berlin." *Hist Psych* 22:465–76.

Holls, Frederick W. 1900. *The Peace Conference at The Hague*. New York: The Macmillan Company.

"Home Hospitals and the War." *Brit Med J* 1 (1915):39–42.

Homer. 1925. *Iliad*. Cambridge, Mass.: Harvard University Press.

Hone, Joseph M. 1939. *The Life of Henry Tonks*. London: M. Joseph.

Howard, M. 1993. "World War One: The Crisis in Euopean History—The Role of the Military Historian." *J Mil Hist* 57:127–38.

"Hugh Owen Thomas, M.D., M.R.C.S. [obituary]." *Lancet* 1 (1891):174–75.

Hulbert, H. S. 1920. "Gas Neurosis Syndrome." *Am J Insanity* 77:213–16.

Hustin, A. 1914. "Note sur une Nouvelle Méthode de Transfusion." *Ann Bull Soc Med et Nat Bruxelles* 72:104–11.

Hutchinson, Woods. 1918. *The Doctor in War.* Boston: Houghton Mifflin Company.

Hutto, Richard Jay. 2006. *Their Gilded Cage: The Jekyll Island Club Members.* Macon, Ga.: Henchard Press.

Hutyra, Franz, and Josef Marek. 1913. *Spezielle Pathologie und Therapy der Haustiere.* Jena: Gustav Fischer.

Influenza. Annual Report. Washington, DC: United States Public Health Service, 1918.

Ireland, M. W. 1930. "A Fighter for the Cause of Health: The Military Record of Colonel Victor C. Vaughan." *J Lab Clin Med* 15:878–84.

Ireland, Merritte W. 1919. *Report of the Surgeon General of the Army.* Annual Report. Washington, DC: Government Printing Office.

Ivy, R. H. 1971. "The Mysterious A. C. Valadier." *Plast Reconstr Surg* 47:365–70.

Janeway, H. H., E. M. Ewing. 1914. "The Nature of Shock. Its Relation to Acapnia and to Changes in the Circulation of the Blood and to Exhaustion of the Nerve Centres." *Ann Surg* 59:158–75.

Johnson, L. W. 1920. "Queen's Hospital for Facial and Jaw Injuries, Frognal, Sidcup, Kent, England." *US Naval Med Bull* 14:17–65.

Jones, E. 2014. "Terror Weapons: The British Experience of Gas and Its Treatment in the First World War." *War Hist* 21:355–75.

Jones, E., S. Rahman, R. Woolven. 2007. "The Maudsley Hospital: Design and Strategic Direction." *Med Hist* 51:357–78.

Jones, John. 1775. *Plain Concise Practical Remarks on the Treatment of Wounds and Fractures.* New York: John Holt.

Jones, Joseph. 1871. *Surgical Memoirs of the War of the Rebellion: II: The Nature, Causes, and Treatment of Hospital Gangrene, as it Prevailed in The Confederate Armies 1861–1865.* Cambridge: Hurd and Hougton.

Jones, R. 1914. "Treatment of Fractures of the Thigh." *Brit Med J* 2:1086–87.

Jones, R., O. Lodge. 1896. "The Discovery of a Bullet Lost in the Wrist by Means of the Roentgen Rays." *Lancet* 1:476–77.

Jones, Simon. 2007. *World War I Gas Warfare Tactics and Equipment.* Oxford: Osprey Publishing.

Joy, R. J. T. 1954. "The Natural Bonesetters with Special Reference to the Sweet Family of Rhode Island." *Bull Hist Med* 28:416–41.

Judd, James R. 1919. *With the American Ambulance in France.* Honolulu: Star Bulletin Press.

Kausch, W. 1915. "Ueber die Gasphlegmone." *Beiträge zur klinischen Chirurgie* 2:7–31.

Kazanjian, V. H. 1965. "Remembrance of Things Past." *Plast Reconstr Surg* 35:5–13.

Keegan, J. J. 1918. "The Prevailing Pandemic of Influenza." *JAMA* 71:1051–55.

Keegan, John. 1976. *The Face of Battle.* New York: Penguin Books.

Keen, W. W. 1918. "Military Surgery in 1861 and 1918." *Ann Am Acad Pol Sol Sci* 80:11–22.

Keith, Arthur. 1919. *Menders of the Maimed.* London: Oxford University Press.

Kennedy, P. M. 1971. "Imperial Cable Communication and Strategy, 1870–1914." *English Historical Review* 86:728–52.

Kimpton, A. R., J. H. Brown. 1913. "A New and Simple Method of Transfusion." *JAMA* 61:117–18.

King, Ross. 2006. *The Judgment of Paris*. New York: Walker and Company.

Kipling, Rudyard. 1918. *Twenty Poems*. Toronto: The Macmillan Company.

Klose, F. 1918. "Gasödemschutz und–Bekämpfung." *Beiträge zur Klinischen Chirurgie* 113:76–98.

———. 1916. "Ueber Toxin-und Antitoxinversuche mit dem Fränkelschen Gasbrandbazillus." *Feldarztliche Beilage zur Münch. Med. Wochenschrift* 63:723–26.

Koch, R. 1877. "Die Ätiologie der Milzbrand-Krankheit, begründet auf die Entwicklungsgeschichte des Bacillus Anthracis." *Beitrage zur Biologie der Pflanzen* 2:277–310.

Kocher, Theodor. 1901. *Hirnerschütterung Hirndruck und Chirurgische Eingriffe bei Herzkrankheiten*. Wien: Alfred Holder.

Krause, J. 2013. "The Origins of Chemical Warfare in the French Army." *War in History* 20:545–56.

Kriegsministeriums, Sanitäts-Department des Königlich Preussischen. 1918. *Veröffentlichungen aus dem Gebiete des Militär-Sanitätswesens*. Militär-Sanitätswesens. Berlin: Springer-Verlag.

Kuhn, Thomas S. 1962. *The Structure of Scientific Revolutions*. Chicago: University of Chicago Press.

Kumar, D. R., F. Aslinia, S. H. Yale, J. J. Mazza. 2011. "Jean-Martin Charcot: The Father of Neurology." *Clin Med Res* 9:46–49.

Kümmell, H. 1915. "Wundinfektion insbesondere Wundstarrkrampf und Gasbrand." *Beiträge zur Klinischen Chirurgie* 1:421–39.

Küttner, H. 1898. "Ueber die Bedeutung der Röntgenstrahlen für die Kriegschirurgie: Nach Erfahrungen im Griechisch-Türkischen Krieg 1897." *Beitr Klinische Chir* 20:167–229.

La Motte, E. N. 1915. "An American Nurse in Paris." *Survey* 34:333–36.

La Motte, Ellen N. 1916. *The Backwash of War*. New York: Knickerbocker Press.

Laborit, H., P. Huguenard. 1951. "L'Hibernation Artificielle par Moyens Pharmacodynamiques et Physiques." *Press Med* 59:1329.

Lahaie, O. 2011. "L'Épidémie de Grippe Dite 'Espagnole' et sa Perception par l'Armée Française (1918–1919)." *Revue Historique des Armées* 262:1–10.

Lalardrie, J. P. 1972. "Hippolyte Morestin 1869–1918." *Brit J Plast Surg* 25:39–41.

Landsteiner, K. 1900. "Zur Kenntnis der Antifermentativen, Lytischen und Agglutinierenden Wirkungen des Blutserums und der Lymphe." *Centralblatt für Bakteriologie, Parasitenkunde* 27:357–62.

Lane, N. 2015. "The Unseen World: Reflections on Leeuwenhoek (1677) 'Concerning Little Animals.'" *Phil Trans R Soc B* 360:1–10.

Langdon-Brown, W. 1936. "To a Very Wise Man." *St. Bartholomew's Hosp J* 49:29–30.

Larrey, D. J. 1829. *Clinique Chirurgical*. Paris: Gabon.

Latta, T. 1832. "Malignant Cholera: Letter from Dr. Latta." *Lancet* 2:274–77.

Le Breton, D. 1991. "Handicap d'Apparence: Le Regard des Autres." *Ethnologie française* 21:323–30.

Le Dran, Henri-François. 1738. *Traité ou Réflexions Tirées de la Pratique sur les Playes d'Armes à Feu*. Paris: Charles Osmont.

Le Dran, Henry-Francis. 1740. *Observations in Surgery*, trans. J. S. Sparrow. London: James Hodges.

Lecène, P., H. Mondor. 1920. "L'Oeuvre Chirurgicale de H. Morestin." *J Chir* 16:1–8.

LeCount, E. R. 1919. "The Pathologic Anatomy of Influenzal Bronchopneumonia." *JAMA* 72:650–52.

Lee, R. I. 1917. "A Simple and Rapid Method for the Selection of Suitable Donors for Transfusion by the Determination of Blood Groups." *Br Med J* 2:684–85.

Lemaitre, R. 1918. "A Propos de 2537 Cas de Sutures Primitives pour Plaies de Guerre." *Lyon Chir* 15:65–108.

Lengel, Edward G. 2008. *To Conquer Hell*. New York: Henry Holt and Company.

Lepick, Olivier. 2017. "France's Political and Military Reaction in the Aftermath of the First German Chemical Offensive in April 1915: The Road to Retaliation in Kind." In *One Hundred Years of Chemical Warfare: Research, Deployment, Consequences*, ed. B. Friedrich et al., 69–76. Berlin: Springer.

"Lessons of a Great Epidemic: The Pathology of Influenza." *Lancet* 1 (1919):25–26.

LeVot, J. 2015. "La Radiologie Militaire au Cours du Premier Conflit Mondial." *Médecine et Armées* 44:55–61.

Lindeman, E. 1913. "Simple Syringe Transfusion with Special Cannulas." *Am J Dis Children* 6:28–32.

Linden, S. C., E. Jones. 2013. "German Battle Casualties: The Treatment of Functional Somatic Disorders during World War I." *J Hist Med Allied Sci* 68:627–58.

Linton, D. S. 2000. "The Obscure Object of Knowledge: German Military Medicine Confronts Gas Gangrene during World War I." *Bull Hist Med* 74:291–316.

Liston, Robert. 1892. "On Fracture of the Neck of the Femur." In *Dissertations by Eminent Members of the Royal Medical Society*, ed. Douglas Maclagan, 95–103. Edinburgh: David Douglas.

Long, F. X. 2002. "Les Blessés de la Face Durant la Grande Guerre: Les Origines de la Chirurgie Maxillo-Faciale." *Hist Sci Med* 36:175–83.

Loughran, T. 2010. "Shell Shock, Trauma, and the First World War: The Making of a Diagnosis and Its Histories." *J Hist Med Allied Sci* 67:94–119.

Love, A. G. 1925. "Medical and Casualty Statistics." In *The Medical Department of the United States Army in the World War*, vol. 15, part 2, ed. M. W. Ireland, 670–74. Washington, DC: Government Printing Office.

Love, A. G., C. B. Davenport. 1919. "Immunity of City-Bred Recruits." *Arch Int Med* 24:129–53.

Lower, R. 1667. "An Account of the Experiment of Transfusion Practiced upon a Man in London." *Philos Trans R Soc* 30:557–59.

Ludendorf, Erich. 1919. *My War Memories, 1914–1918*. London: Hutchinson & Co.

Ludendorff, Eric. 1921. *My War Memories, 1914–1918*, vol. 2. London: Hutchinson & Co.

Ludmerer, Kenneth M. 1999. *Time to Heal*. New York: Oxford University Press.

Lynch, Charles, Joseph H. Ford, Frank W. Weed. 1925. "Evacuation Hospitals, Mobile Hospitals, Mobile Surgical Units, Professional Teams, Convalescent

Depots, Evacuation Ambulance Companies, Mobile Laboratories." In *The Medical Department of the United States Army in the World War*, ed. M. W Ireland, 184–201. Washington, DC: Government Printing Office.

Macewen, W. 1888. "An Address of the Surgery of the Brain and Spinal Cord." *Brit Med J* 2:302–09.

MacLeod, George H. B. 1862. *Notes on the Surgery of the War in the Crimea with Remarks on the Treatment of Gunshot Wounds*. Philadelphia: J. B. Lippincott & Co.

MacLeod, Roy, and Jeffrey A. Johnson. 2007. *Frontline and Factory: Comparative Perspectives on the Chemical Industry at War, 1914–1918*. Berlin: Springer Science.

Macnab, D. S. 1941. "Hugh Owen Thomas (1834–1891)." *CMAJ* 45:448–52.

MacNeal, W. J. 1919. "The Influenza Epidemic of 1918 in the American Expeditionary Forces in France and England." *Arch Int Med* 23:657–88.

Macpherson, W. G. 1922. *Medical Services: Surgery of the War*. London: His Majesty's Stationery Office.

Mairet, Louis. 1919. *Carnet d'un Combattant*. Paris: Éditions Georges Crés.

Maisonneuve, M. 1853. "De la Gangrene Foudroyante, avec Developpement et Circulation de Gaz Putrides dans les Veines (pneumo-hemie putride)." *Comptes rendus l'Academie des Sciences* 37:425–27.

Makins, G. H. 1917. "The Development of British Surgery in the Hospitals on the Lines of Communication in France." *Br Med J* 1:789–806.

Maloney, W. J. M. A. 1919. "'The National' and Dr. F. E. Batten." *J Nerv Ment Dis* 49:91–94.

Mansell-Moullin, C. W. 1880. *On the Pathology of Shock*. London: H. G. Saunders.

Marck, K. W., R. Palyvoda, A. Bamji, J. J. van Wingerden. 2017. "The Tubed Pedicle Flap Centennial: Its Concept, Origin, Rise, and Fall." *Eur J Plast Surg* 40:473–78.

Martin, F. 1918. "Visit of Three British Surgeons to America." *Boston Med Surg J* 179:135–38.

Maudsley, H. 1909. "A Mental Hospital—Its Aims and Uses." *Arch Neurol Psych* 4:1–12.

Maudsley, Henry. 1871. *Body and Mind*. New York: Appleton and Company.

McDonald, I. 2007. "Gordon Holmes Lecture: Gordon Holmes and the Neurological Heritage." *Brain* 130:288–98.

McKenzie, R. Tait. 1918. *Reclaiming the Maimed: A Handbook of Physical Therapy*. New York: The Macmillan Company.

McMeekin, Sean. 2013. *July 1914: Countdown to War*. New York: Basic Books.

Meakins, J. 1946. "Edward William Archibald, B.A., M.D." *CMAJ* 54:194–98.

Medical Research Committee, The. 1918. *Acidosis and Shock*. Special Investigation Committee on Surgical Shock and Allied Conditions No. 7. London: The Medical Research Committee.

Medical Research Committee, The. 1917. "Memorandum upon Surgical Shock and Some Allied Conditions." *Br Med J* 1:381–83.

Méléra, César. 1925. *Verdun (Juin–Juillet 1916)*. Paris: Hachette Livre.

Micale, Mark S. 2008. *Hysterical Men*. Cambridge, Mass.: Harvard University Press.

———. 2001. "Jean-Martin Charcot and les Névroses Traumatiques: From Medicine to Culture in French Trauma Theory of the Late Nineteenth Century." In *Traumatic*

Pasts: History, Psychiatry, and Trauma in the Modern Age, 1870–1930, ed. Mark S. Micale and Paul Lerner, 115–39. Cambridge: Cambridge University Press.

Mikulicz, J. 1897. "Das Operiren in Sterilisirten Zwirnhandschuhen und mit Mundbinde." *Zentralbl f Chir* 24:713–17.

Mollison, P. I. 2000. "The Introduction of Citrate as an Anticoagulant for Transfusion and of Glucose as a Red Cell Preservative." *Brit J Haematology* 108:13–18.

Monprofit, M. 1913. "La Chirurgie dans la Guerre des Balkans." *Semaine Medicale* 33:128.

Moran, Lord. 1945. *The Anatomy of Courage*. New York: Carroll & Graf.

Morestin, H. 1917. "Des Autoplasties en Jeu de Patience." *Bull de l'Acad de Méd* 77:371.

———. 1915. "La Réduction Graduelle des Difformités Tégumentaires." *Bull Mem Soc Chir de Paris* 41:1233–53.

Mott, F. 1916. "The Effects of High Explosives Upon the Central Nervous System." *Lancet* 1:331–38; 441–49; 545–53.

———. 1922. "The Maudsley Hospital, Past and Present." *J Ment Sci* 67:319–39.

Mott, F. W. 1916. "Special Discussion on Shell Shock Without Visible Signs of Injury." *Proc R Soc Med* 9:i–xxiv.

Mott, Frederick. 1919. *War Neuroses and Shell Shock*. London: Hodder & Stoughton.

Moureu, Charles. 1920. *La Chimie et la Guerre: Science et Avenir*. Paris: Masson.

Moynihan, B. 1916. "The Treatment of Gunshot Wounds." *Brit Med J* 2879:333–37.

Mueller, J. 1991. "Changing Attitudes Towards War: The Impact of the First World War." *Brit J Political Sci* 21:1–28.

Muir, Ward. 1918. *The Happy Hospital*. London: Simpkin, Marshall, Hamilton, Kent & Co.

Myers, C. S. 1915. "A Contribution to the Study of Shell Shock." *Lancet* 1:316–20.

———. 1919. "A Final Contribution to the Study of Shell Shock." *Lancet* 1:51–54.

Myers, Charles. 1940. *Shell Shock in France 1914–1918*. Cambridge: Cambridge University Press.

Niehues, H. 1909. "Ueber den Heutigen Stand der Verwendung von Röntgenstrahlen im Kriege." *Berliner Klinische Wochenschrift* 46:2293–96.

Nitske, W. Robert. 1971. *The Life of Wilhelm Conrad Röntgen, Discoverer of the X-ray*. Tucson: University of Arizona Press.

Noël, Suzanne. 1926. *La Chirurgie Esthétique: Son Rôle Social*. Paris: Masson et Cie.

Nordmann, C. 1915. "Science et Guerre." *Revue Scientifique* 30:698–708.

Olitsky, P. K., F. L. Gates. 1921. "Experimental Studies of the Nasopharyngeal Secretions from Influenza Patients." *J Exp Med* 33:125–45.

Opie, E. L., A. W. Freeman, F. G. Blake, et al. 1919. "Pneumonia at Camp Funston: Report to the Surgeon-General." *JAMA* 72:108–16.

Oppenheim, H. 1917. "Stand der Lehre von den Kriegs-und Unfall-Neurosen." *Berliner Klinische Wochenschrift* 54:1169–72.

Oppenheim, Janet. 1991. *"Shattered Nerves."* New York: Oxford University Press.

Oudin, M., M. Barthélemy. 1896. "Communiquent une Photographie des Os de la Main Obtenue a l'aide des 'X-Strahlen.'" *Comptes Rendus de l'Acad Sci* 122:150–51.

"Owen Roberts M.D., St. Asaph." *Brit Med J* 1 (1871):409.

Pacini, Filippo. 1854. *Osservazioni Microscopiche e Deduzioni Patologiche sul Cholera Asiatico*. Firenze: Federigo Bencini.

Page, M., S. V. Appleyard. 1913. "Medical and Surgical Experience in the Balkan War." *Lancet* 182:162–64.

Pallardy, G. 1999. "La Radiologie est Entrée Avant l'Électricité dans les Hôpitaux de Paris." *Hist Sci Med* 33:333–42.

Pallardy, G., J. P. Mabille. 1999. "Antoine Béclère." *J Radiol* 80:600–03.

Pallardy, G., M.-J. Pallardy. 1995. "Georges Massiot: Ingénieur-Constructeur et Manipulateur." *1895–1995 Le Premier Siècle de la Radiologie* October:32–38.

Passot, Raymond. 1933. *Sculpteur de Visages*. Paris: Denoël et Steele.

Pasteur, L. 1933. "Étude sur la Maladie Charbonneuse." In *Oeuvres de Pasteur*, ed. L. Vallery-Radot, 164–71. Paris: Masson et Cie.

Patterson, K. D., G. F. Pyle. 1991. "The Geography and Mortality of the 1918 Influenza Pandemic." *Bull Hist Med* 65:4–21.

Payr, E. 1915. "Ueber Gasphlegmonen im Kriege." *Deutsche Med Wochensch* 2:57–58.

Pechura, Constance M., and David P. Rall. 1993. *Veterans at Risk: The Health Effects of Mustard Gas and Lewisite*. Health and Disease Prevention. Washington, DC: National Academy Press.

Pelis, K. 2001. "Taking Credit: The Canadian Army Medical Corps and the British Conversion to Blood Transfusion in WWI." *J Hist Med Allied Sci* 56:238–77.

Penfield, W. 1933. "Sir Percy Sargent 1873–1933." *Arch NeurPsych* 30:413–14.

Pershing, John J. 1919. *Final Report*. Washington, DC: Government Printing Office.

Pfeiffer, R. 1893. "Die Aetiologie der Influenza." *Zeitschr für Hyg und Infektionskr* 12:357–86.

Phillips, S.-A., L. C. Biant. 2011. "The Instruments of the Bonesetter." *J Bone Joint Surg [Br]* 93:115–19.

Pilcher, L. S. 1919. "The Influence of War Surgery upon Civil Practice." *Ann Surg* 69:565–74.

Platt, H. 1962. "Moynihan: The Education and Training of the Surgeon." *Ann R Coll Surg Engl* 30:220–28.

Porter, William Townsend. 1918. *Shock at the Front*. Boston: Atlantic Monthly Press.

Pound, Reginald. 1964. *Gillies, Surgeon Extraordinary: A Biography*. London: M. Joseph.

Powell, M. P. 2016. "Sir Victor Horsley at the Birth of Neurosurgery." *Brain* 139:631–34.

Prentiss, Augustin M. 1936. *Chemicals in War: A Treatise on Chemical Warfare*. New York: McGraw-Hill Book Company.

Primrose, A., E. S. Ryerson. 1916. "The Direct Transfusion of Blood: Its Value in Haemorrhage and Shock in the Treatment of the Wounded of War." *Br Med J* 2:384–86.

Pugh, W. S. 1919. "Education and Sanitation Aboard Ship." *US Naval Med Bull* 13:254–66.

Rand, C. W. 1940. "Doctor Cushing As I Knew Him." *Bull Los Angeles Neurological Soc* 5:1–8.

Rawlings, B. Buford. 1913. *A Hospital in the Making: A History of the National Hospital for the Paralysed and Epileptic*. London: Sir Isaac Pitman & Sons.

Reggiani, Andrés Horacio. 2007. *God's Eugenicist: Alexis Carrel and the Sociobiology of Decline.* New York: Berghahn Books.

Reich, S. G. 1987. "Harvey Cushing's Guillain-Barrè Syndrome: An Historical Diagnosis." *Neurosurgery* 21:135–41.

Reicharchiv. 1932. *Der Weltkrieg 1914 bis 1918: Die Operationen des Jahres 1915.* Berlin: E.S. Mittler & Sohn.

Remarque, Erich Maria. 1928, 1956. *All Quiet on the Western Front.* New York: Ballantine Books.

Report of the Committee of Enquiry into "Shell-Shock." Committee Report. London: His Majesty's Stationery Office, 1922.

Risien Russell, J. S. 1913. "The Treatment of Neurasthenia." *Lancet* 2:1453–56.

Ritter, C. 1916. "Ueber Gasbrand." *Beitrage zur Klinischen Chirurgie* 3:47–72.

Riva-Rocci, S. 1896. "Un Nuovo Sfigmomanometro." *Gazzetta Medical* 47:1001–17.

Rivers, W. H. R. 1920. *Instinct and the Unconsciousness.* Cambridge: Cambridge University Press.

———. 1918. "The Repression of War Experience." *Proc R Soc Med* 11:1–20.

Robertson, L. B. 1916. "The Transfusion of Whole Blood: A Suggestion for Its More Frequent Employment in War Surgery." *Brit Med J* 2:38–40.

Robertson, L. B., A. Brown. 1915. "Blood Transfusion in Infants and Young Children." *Can Med Assoc J* 5:298–305.

Robertson, L. B., C. G. Watson. 1917. "Further Observations on the Results of Blood Transfusions in War Surgery, with Special Reference to the Results in Primary Haemorrhage." *Br Med J* 2:679–83.

Robertson, O. H. 1918. "Transfusion with Preserved Red Blood Cells." *Brit Med J* 1:691–95.

Robinette, J. 2007. "The Narrative Shape of Traumatic Experience." *Lit and Med* 26:290–311.

Roland, A. 1985. "Science and War." *Osiris* 1:247–72.

Rolleston, J. D. 1939. "Dr. Antoine Béclère." *Nature* 143:591.

Rollet, M. 1914. "Extraction des Balles Allemandes et des Éclats d'Obus a l'Électro-aimant Géant." *Comptes rendus Séances de l'Académie des Sciences* 159:562–64.

Röntgen, W. C. 1895. "Uber Eine Neue Art von Strahlen." *Sitzungsberichte der Physikalische-Medizinischen Gesellschaft zu Würzburg* 137–47.

Rosenbusch, Gerd, and Annemarie de Knecht-van-Eekelen. 2019. *Wilhelm Conrad Röntgen: The Birth of Radiology.* Berlin: Springer.

Roth, Jack J. 1967. *World War I: A Turning Point in Modern History.* New York: Alfred A. Knopf.

Roubaud, Noële, and R. N. Brehamet. 1960. *Le Colonel Picot et les Gueules Cassées.* Paris: Nouvelles Éditions Latines.

Rous, P., J. R. Turner. 1916. "The Preservation of Living Red Blood Cells in Vitro: I. Methods of Preservation." *J Exp Med* 23:219–37.

Roussy, G., and J. Lhermitte. 1917. *Psychoneuroses de Guerre.* Paris: Masson et Cie.

"The First World War and Its Impact: 1914–1921." In *Einstein on Politics*, ed. David E. Rowe and Robert Schulmann, 61–92. Princeton, N.J.: Princeton University Press.

Rusca, F. 1914/1915. "Experimentelle Untersuchungen über die trauma tische Druckwirkung der Explosionen." *Deutsche Zeitschrift für Chirurgie* 132:315–73.

Russell, W. R. 1935. "Major Hysteria." *Brit Med J* 1:872–76.

Sachs, Ernest. 1958. *Fifty Years of Neurosurgery: A Personal Story.* New York: Vantage Press.

Sade, R. M. 2015. "Transplantation at 100 Years: Alexis Carrel, Pioneer Surgeon." *Ann Thorac Surg* 80:2415–18.

Salleron, M. 1858. *Compte-Rendu des Amputations Primitives et des Amputations Consécutives.* Paris: Henri et Charles Noblet.

Sargent, P., G. Holmes. 1915. "The Treatment of the Cranial Injuries of Warfare." *Brit Med J* 1:537–41.

Sassoon, Siegfried. 1936. *Sherston's Progress.* London: Faber and Faber.

Savory, W. S. 1870. "Collapse." In *A System of Surgery,* ed. T. Holmes, 746–65. London: Longmans, Green, and Co.

Schindler, Dietrich, and Jiri Toman. 1988. *The Laws of Armed Conflict.* Leiden: Martinue Nijhoff Publishers.

Scott, James Brown. 1920. "The Conference of 1899." In *The Proceedings of the Hague Peace Conferences,* 260–262. New York: Oxford University Press.

Sebald, M., D. Hauser. 1995. "Pasteur, Oxygen and the Anaerobes Revisted." *Anaerobe* 1:11–16.

Selcer, P. 2008. "Standardizing Wounds: Alexis Carrel and the Scientific Management of Life in the First World War." *Brit J Hist Sci* 44:73–107.

Senn, N. 1898. "Recent Experiences in Military Surgery After the Battle of Santiago." *J Mil Service Institute* 23:309–23.

Shephard, Ben. 2003. *A War of Nerves: Soldiers and Psychiatrists in the Twentieth Century.* Cambridge, Mass.: Harvard University Press.

Sherman, George William. 1976. *The Pessimism of Thomas Hardy.* Madison, N.J.: Fairleigh Dickinson University Press.

Shorvon, Simon, and Alastair Compston. 2019. *Queen Square: A History of the National Hospital and Its Institute of Neurology.* Cambridge: Cambridge University Press.

Showalter, Elaine. 1987. *The Female Malady: Women, Madness and English Culture 1830–1980.* London: Virago.

Simonds, J. P. 1915. "Studies in Bacillus Welchii with Special Reference to Classification and to its Relation to Diarrhea." *Rockefeller Institute Monograph* 5:1–130.

Sked, A. 1987. "Epochenwende Erster Weltkrieg: The Historical Significance of the First World War." In *Die Habsburgermonarchie 1848–1918,* ed. Helmut Rumpler and Ulrike Harmat, 21–47. Wein: Austrian Academy of Sciences Press.

Slobodin, Richard. 1978. *W. H. R. Rivers.* New York: Columbia University Press.

Smith, G. Elliot, and T. H. Pear. 1917. *Shell Shock and Its Lessons.* London: Longmans, Green & Co.

Soltau, A. B. 1919. "Discussion on Influenza." *Proc R Soc Med* 12:27–28.

Somervell, T. Howard. 1936. *After Everest.* London: Hodder and Stoughton.

Soper, G. A. 1918. "The Pandemic in the Army Camps." *JAMA* 71:1899–1909.

Soupault, Robert. 1952. *Alexis Carrel 1873–1944.* Paris: Librairie Plon.

Stark, A. N. 1920. "Medical Activities of the American Expeditionary Forces in the Zone of the Armies." *Mil Surg* 47:154–76.

Starr, C. L. 1923. "Lawrence Bruce Robertson, B.A., M.B." *Can Med Assoc J* 13:216–17.

Stetler, C. M. 2017. "The 1918 Spanish Influenza: Three Months of Horror in Philadelphia." *Pennsylvania History* 84:462–87.

Stevenson, David. 2005. *1914–1918: The History of the First World War.* New York: Penguin Books.

Stoltzenberg, Dietrich. 2004. *Fritz Haber: Chemist, Nobel Laureate, German, Jew.* Philadelphia: Chemical Heritage Press.

Strohl, E. L. 1962. "Crazy Sally of Epsom." *JAMA* 182:268.

Sutherland, Millicent. 1914. *Six Weeks at the War.* London: The Times.

Tatu, L. 2018. "Edgar Adrian (1889–1977) and Shell Shock Electrotherapy: A Forgotten History?" *Eur Neurol* 79:106–07.

Taubenberger, J. K., D. M. Morens. 2006. "1918 Influenza: The Mother of all Pandemics." *Emerg Inf Dis* 12:15–22.

Taubenberger, J. K., A. H. Reid, T. A. Janczweski, T. G. Fanning. 2001. "Integrating Historical, Clinical and Molecular Genetic Data in order to Explain the Origin and Virulence of the 1918 Spanish Influenza Virus." *Phil Trans R Soc Lond* B:1829–39.

The German Offensive of July 15, 1918. After Action Report. Leavenworth, Kan.: The General Service Schools, 1923.

"The Influenza Epidemic of 1918–1919." *Brit Med J* 2 (1920):211–12.

"The Military Medical Services in 1918." *Brit Med J* 1 (1919):131–33.

Théodoridès, J. 1966. "Casimir Davaine (1812–1882) A Precursor of Pasteur." *Med Hist* 10:155–65.

1917. "The Queen's Hospital, Frognal, Sidcup." *Lancet* 2:687–89.

Thies, A. 1917. "Die Behandlung der Gasphlegmone mit der Rhythmischen Stauung." *Beiträge zur Klinischen Chirurgie* 105:595–636.

———. 1918. "Ueber Zwei Hauptformen der Gasinfektion." *Beiträge zur Klinischen Chirurgie* 109:157–93.

Thomas, Hugh Owen. 1887. *Contributions to Surgery and Medicine,* vol. 3. London: H. K. Lewis.

———. 1875. *Diseases of the Hip, Knee, and Ankle Joints.* London: H. K. Lewis.

Thomson, A. Landsborough. 1987. *Half a Century of Medical Research, Volume One: Origins and Policy of The Medical Research Council (UK).* London: Medical Research Council.

Tissier, H. 1916. "Recherches sur la Flore Bactérienne des Plaies de Guerre." *Ann d'Institut Pasteur* 30:681–90.

Tjomsland, Anne. 1941. *Bellevue in France.* New York: Froben Press.

Tolhurst, David. 2015. *Pioneers in Plastic Surgery.* Berlin: Springer.

Toombs, Robert. 1981. *The War Against Paris, 1871.* Cambridge: Cambridge University Press.

Trilla, A., C. Trilla, C. Daer. 2008. "The 1918 'Spanish Flu' in Spain." *Clin Inf Dis* 47:668–73.

Trumpener, U. 1975. "The Road to Ypres: The Beginning of Gas Warfare in World War I." *J Modern Hist* 47:460–80.

Tuffier, T., A. Carrel. 1914. "Patching and Section of the Pulmonary Orifice of the Heart." *J Exp Med* 20:3–8.

Turner, W. A. 1916. "Arrangements for the Care of Cases of Nervous and Mental Shock Coming from Overseas." *Lancet* 1:1073–75.

———. 1915. "Remarks on Cases of Nervous and Mental Shock Observed in the Base Hospitals in France." *Brit Med J* 1:833–35.

Turner, William Aldren, and Thomas Grainger Stewart. 1910. *A Textbook of Nervous Diseases*. Philadelphia: P. Blakiston's Son & Co.

Uff, C., D. Frith, C. Harrison, et al. 2011. "Sir Victor Horsley's 19th Century Operations at the National Hospital for Neurology and Neurosurgery, Queen Square." *J Neurosurg* 114:534–42.

Valadier, A. C. 1916. "A Few Suggestions for the Treatment of Fractured Jaws." *Brit J Surg* 4:64–73.

Van Hee, R. 2012. "Antoine Depage's Relationship with Queen Elisabeth of Belgium." *Acta Chir Belg* 112:170–81.

Varaschin, Denis, and Lodovic Laloux. 2006. *10 Mars 1906, Courrières, aux Risques de l'Histoire*. Paris: Éditions GRHEN.

Vaughan, W. T. 1921. "Influenza: A Epidemiologic Study." *Am J Hygiene* 127–73.

Velpeau, A-A-L-M. 1832. *Nouveaux Elements de Medecine Operatoire*. Paris: J.-B. Bailliere.

Vierordt, Karl. 1855. *Die Lehre vom Arterienpuls in Gesunden und Kranken Zuständen*. Braunschweig: Friedrich Vieweg und Sohn.

Vilensky, J. A., P. R. Sinish. 2004. "The Dew of Death." *Bull Atomic Scientists* 60:54–60.

Vincent, B. 1912. "Blood Transfusions: Indications, Methods, and Results." *Boston Med Surg J* 147:239–42.

Vinet, E. 1919. "La Guerre des Gaz et les Travaux des Services Chimiques Français." *Chimie & Industrie* 2:1377–1415.

Volkart, W. 1926. "Der Giftgaskrieg und seine Entstehung." *Allgemeine schweizerische Militärzeitung* 72:69–78.

von Basch, Karl. 1880. "Ueber die Messung des Blutdrucks am Menschen." *Zeitschrift für Klinische Medizin* 2:79–96.

von Rothe, A. 1915. "Chirurgie im Kriegslazarette." *Beitrage zur Klinischen Chirurgie* 96:181–209.

Wallace, Cuthbert, and John Fraser. 1918. *Surgery at a Casualty Clearing Station*. London: A. & C. Black.

War Department. 1919. *Annual Report 1918, Director Chemical War Service*. Annual Report. Washington, DC: Government Printing Office.

War Plans Division. 1918. *A Survey of German Tactics, 1918*. Monograph No. 1. Washington, DC: War Department.

Warren, John Collins Jr. 1895. *Surgical Pathology and Therapeutics*. Philadelphia: W. B. Saunders.

Warthin, A. S., C. V. Weller. 1919. "The Lesions of the Respiratory and Gastrointestinal Tracts Produced by Mustard Gas (Dichlorethylsulfide)." *J Lab Clin Med* 4:229–64.

Watson, Frederick. 1934. *The Life of Sir Robert Jones*. London: Hodder & Stoughton, Ltd.

Webb, T. E. F. 2006. "'Dottyville'—Craiglockhart War Hospital and Shell-Shock Treatment in the First World War." *J R Soc Med* 99:342–46.

Wehberg, Hans. 1920. *Wider den Aufruf der 93!*. Berlin: Deusche Verlagsgesellschaft für Politik u. Geschichte.

Weinberg, M. 1916. "Bacteriological and Experimental Researches on Gas Gangrene." *Proc Roy Soc Med* 9:119–44.

———. 1914. "Recherches Bactériologiques sur la Gangrène Gazeuse." *Compte rendus Société Biologie* 77:506–08.

Welch, W. H. 1900. "Morbid Conditions Caused by Bacillus Aerogenes Capsulatus." *Bull Johns Hopkins Hosp* 11:185–204.

Welch, W. H., G. H. F. Nuttall. 1892. "A Gas-Producing Bacillus (Bacillus Aerogenes Capsulatus, Nov. Spec.) Capable of Rapid Development in the Blood-Vessels After Death." *Bull Johns Hopkins Hosp* 3:81–91.

Wells, H. G. 1914. *The War That Will End War*. London: Frank & Cecil Palmer.

Westmore, A., C. Hunter. 2013. "Introduction: World War II and Medical Research in Australia." *Health and History* 15:1–10.

Wever, P., L. van Bergen. 2012. "Prevention of Tetanus During the First World War." *Med Humanit* 38:78–82.

Whitfield, N. 2015. "Surgical Skills Beyond Scientific Management." *Med Hist* 59:421–42.

Willems, Charles. 1917. *Manuel de Chirurgie de Guerre*. Paris: A. Maloine et fils.

Wilson, A. 1914. "Notes on 150 Cases of Wounded French, Belgians, and Germans." *Brit Med J* 2:806–07.

Wilson, Jean Moorcroft. 1999. *Siegfried Sassoon: The Making of a War Poet*. New York: Routledge.

Wiltshire, H. 1916. "A Contribution to the Etiology of Shell Shock." *Lancet* 1:1207–12.

Winter, Jay. 2000. *Remembering War*. New Haven, Conn.: Yale University Press.

Winternitz, M. C., Isabel M. Wason, and Frank P. McNamara. 1920. *The Pathology of Influenza*. New Haven, Conn.: Yale University Press.

Wren, S., Ashwood, N. 2010. "The Life and Times of Hugh Owen Thomas." *Trauma* 12:197–201.

Yealland, Lewis R. 1918. *Hysterical Disorders of Warfare*. London: Macmillan and Co.

York, G. K. III, Steinberg, D. A. 2011. "Hughlings Jackson's Neurological Ideas." *Brain* 134:3106–13.

Zhang, W. Y., G. G. Hallock. 2020. "Gillies and Dunedin: The Birthplace of Modern Plastic Surgery." *J Plast Reconstr Aesthet Surg* 73:1012–17.

Endnotes

Chapter One.

1   H. G. Wells, *The War That Will End War* (London: Frank & Cecil Palmer, 1914), 7.

2   *Ibid.*, 11.

3   Alfred de Bassompierre, *The Night of August 2–3, 1914, at the Belgian Foreign Office* (London: Hodder & Stoughton, 1916), 41.

4   Sean McMeekin, *July 1914: Countdown to War* (New York: Basic Books, 2013), 375–76.

5   Barbara Tuchman, The Guns of August (New York: Dell Publishing, 1962), 149–50.

6   Edith Wharton, *Fighting France from Dunkerque to Belport* (New York: Charles Scribner's Sons, 1919), 15.

7   McMeekin, *July 1914*, 376.

8   Quote taken from C. Acton and J. Potter, "'These Frightful Sights Would Work Havoc with One's Brain': Subjective Experience, Trauma, and Resilience in First World War Writings by Medical Personnel," *Literature and Medicine* 30 (2012): 61–85.

9   Modris Eksteins, *Rites of Spring: The Great War and the Birth of the Modern Age* (New York: Doubleday, 1989), xv, 163.

10 James R. Judd, *With the American Ambulance in France* (Honolulu: Star-Bulletin Press, 1919), 108. *Poilu* was common slang for the typical French infantryman, meaning "hairy one," usually because, after days or weeks at the front there was an ample growth of facial hair. This term was akin to the American *GI*.

11 Kate John Finzi, *Eighteen Months in the War Zone* (London: Cassell and Company, 1916), 37–38.

12 César Méléra, *Verdun (Juin-Juillet 1916)* (Paris: Hachette Livre, 1925), 34–35.

13 C. Nordmann, "Science et Guerre," *Revue Scientifique* 30 (1915): 698–708.

14 George Crile, *An Autobiography*, vol. 1 (Philadelphia: J. B. Lippincott, 1947), 281.

15 Judd, *With the American Ambulance*, 49–50.

16 There are numerous claims to this effect. For two, see W. Y. Zhang and G. G. Hallock, "Gillies and Dunedin: The Birthplace of Modern Plastic Surgery," *J Plast Reconstr Aesthet Surg* 73 (2020): 1012–1017; and J. A. Chambers and P. D. Ray, "Achieving Growth and Excellence in Medicine," *Ann Plast Surg* 63 (2009): 473–78.

17   Saying attributed to Heraclitus, "Testimonia," in *Early Greek Philosophy*, vol. 3, trans. André Laks and Glenn W. Most (Cambridge: Loeb Classic Library, 2016), 168.

18   A. Roland, "Science and War," *Osiris* 1 (1985): 247–72.

19   John Jones, *Plain Concise Practical Remarks on the Treatment of Wounds and Fractures* (New York: John Holt, 1775), Preface.

20   V. Z. Cope, "The Medical Balance-Sheet of War," in *Some Famous General Practitioners and other Medical Historical Essays*, ed. V. Z. Cope (London: Pitman Medical Publishing, 1961), 169–183. War of course can be devastating in its toll of human suffering but can simultaneously stimulate groundbreaking medical research. See also Ann Westmore and Cecily Hunter, "Introduction," in *Health and History*, Special Issue: World War II and Medical Research in Australia 15 (2013): 1–10.

21   From an article in the *New York Times*, December 29, 1918, 36, contained in P. Selcer, "Standardizing Wounds: Alexis Carrel and the Scientific Management of Life in the First World War," *Brit J Hist Sci* 44 (2008): 73–107.

22   W. W. Keen, "Military Surgery in 1861 and 1918," *Ann Am Acad Pol Soc Sci* 80 (1918): 11–22.

23   George Crile, *An Autobiography*, Volumes 1 and 2 (Philadelphia: J. B. Lippincott Company, 1947), 2: 359.

24   G. H. Makins, "Introductory," *Br J Surg* 6 (1918): 1–11.

CHAPTER TWO

1   I am grateful for the eulogy to Alfred Mignon contained in *the Revue du Service de Santé Militaire* from 1936, housed in the Bibliothèque centrale du Service de santé des armées, École du Val-de-Grâce, Paris, France, and to Victor Gabella and Muriel Bret-Carlier for their help in procuring these relevant documents on Alfred Mignon.

2   Edmond Delorme, "Blessures de Guerre, Conseils aux Chirurgiens," *Comptes Rendus, Des Séances d'Académie des Sciences*, meeting August 10, 1914, 394–99.

3   Observations presented by Dr. Doyen July 7, 1915, at *la Commission de l'Armée du Sénat (Service de Santé) et à la Commission d'Hygiène de la Chambre des Députés*.

4   The editorials appeared in *L'Homme libre* and *Le Temps* in September 1914 and in *L'Homme enchainé* on October 8, 1914.

5   Vincent Viet, *La Santé en Guerre 1914–1918 : Une Politique Pionnière en Univers Uncertain* (Paris: SciencesPo, 2015), 30.

6   In this paper, the French term *ambulance* will refer to a temporary or field hospital, either mobile or "immobile," that is used to receive patients from the front, evaluate them, treat them, and prepare for further evacuation to the rear areas. For reference, see the organizational scheme for French field armies prior to World War I in A. Troussaint, *La Direction du Service de Santé en Campagne* (Paris: Henri Charles-Lavauzelle, 1914).

7   The doctrine may have stemmed from the dismal performance of French armies
     during the Franco-Prussian War, where defensive strategy resulted in utter
     routing of French field units. See also R. Way, "1914: de l'Offense à Outrance au
     Désastre Sanitaire," *Médecine et Armées* 44 (2016): 11–16.

8   P. Bonnette, "Organisation des Ambulances de Guerre," *Press Med*, August 12,
     1914 (originally published in 1912).

9   Edmond Delorme, "Blessures de guerre, Conseils aux chirurgiens" *Comptes
     Rendus, Des Séances de Académie des Sciences*, August 10, 1914, 394–99. The Société
     nationale de chirurgie, established in 1843, was an outgrowth of the Académie
     royale de chirurgie, founded in 1731, the expressed purpose of which was "per-
     fecting the practice of surgery, through experience and observation," effectively
     becoming the gatekeeper of Parisian—and eventually French—surgical practice
     and training. For a detailed history, see C. Chatelain, "Histoire de l'Académie
     Nationale de Chirurgie," *e-mémoires de l'Académie Nationale de Chirurgie* 5 (2006):
     18–23. .

10   L. Ferraton, "La Chirurgie de Guerre de Premiere Ligne au XIV Corps
     d'Armee" *Lyon Chir* 12 (1915): 565–601.

11   Master surgeon Theodor Billroth bragged that Germany was the new Paris. "I
     will add that it is now at a level which is completely equal to that of the rest of the
     world, if not more important than France at present," he crowed in 1863. The-
     odor Billroth, *Die Allgemeine Chirurgische Pathologie und Therapie* (Berlin: Georg
     Reimer, 1863), 14.

12   C. Schimmelbusch, *Anleitung zur Aseptischen Wundbehandlung* (Berlin: August
     Hirschwald, 1893), 170–175.

13   C. Langenbuch, *Ueber die Principien des Zeitgemässen Kriegswundverbandes*
     (Berlin: August Hirschwald, 1887), 9.

14   Paul Von Bruns, "Zur Wundbehandlung im Kriege," *Beitrage zur Klinischen
     Chirurgie* 10 (1916): 1–17. I am indebted to Derek Linton and his excellent sum-
     mation of German wound care contained in his publication "The Obscure Object
     of Knowledge: German Military Medicine Confronts Gas Gangrene during
     World War I," *Bull Hist Med* 74 (2000): 291–316.

15   "The surgical vehicle."

16   Frédéric Dabouis, "Le Groupe Angevin de l'Union Française pour le Suffrage des
     Femmes," in Archives de Cécile Brunschvicg (1914–1935), *Les Cahiers du CESA/
     Cercle d'Etudes Sociales Angevin*, no. 8 (November 2014); Duchesse d'Uzès, *Souve-
     nirs 1847–1933* (Paris: Editions Lacurne, 1939), 56.

17   D'Uzès, *Souvenirs 1847–1933*, 69.

18   D'Uzès, *Souvenirs 1847–1933*, 113.

19   Article found in *Le Figaro*, July 5, 1898.

20   Maurice Marcille, "Lymphatiques et ganglions ilio-pelviens par Maurice Mar-
     cille," (MD thesis, Masson et Cie Paris, 1902).

21   "Our Foreign Exchanges" (no author) *The Horseless Age*, 10 (1902): 730; also
     reported in *Le Petit Parisien*, July 29, 1904, and Georges Duhamel, *La Pesée des
     Ames, 1914–1919* (Paris: Mercure de France, 1949), 51.

22   *Chirurgien des Hôpitaux de Paris* would now mean a member of the Assistance
     publique—Hôpitaux de Paris, the public hospital system of Paris, who are ordi-
     narily high-quality surgeons, carefully selected, and often members of the Faculté
     de médecine de Paris. .

23   Marcille, M. "Pneumatic Tire" *The Motor World,* 21 (1909): 278.

24   Duhamel, *La Pesée des Ames,* 52.

25   F. Goursolas, "Chirurgie et Chirurgiens d'une Ambulance Françaises en 1915,"
     Communication presented at a meeting of the *Histoire de la Médecine* of the
     Société française, May 26, 1990.

26   "Voiture Chirurgicale Automobile Systeme Boulant," *Le Genie Civil* 61 (1912):
     222–24.

27   D. Renaud, "Voiture Chirurgicale Automobile Boulant," *La Nature* 2045 (1912):
     145–47.

28   Jean Cocteau, *Thomas l'imposteur* (Paris: Editions de la Nouvelle Revue Française,
     1923), 7.

29   André Chevrillon, ed., *Lettres d'un soldat* (Paris: Librairie Chapelot, 1916; new
     edition, Paris: Bernard Giovangeli, 2005), 143–44.

30   *Marmites* were the cast iron pots used in nearly every French household. The
     black puffs of artillery shells, igniting just above the ground, reminded troops
     of those black pots. Quotation from Fernand Engerand, *Le Secret de la Frontière,
     1815—1871—1914; Charleroi* (Paris: Brossard, 1918), 537.

31   Figures from David Stevenson, *1914–1918: The History of the First World War*
     (New York: Penguin Books, 2005), 54.

32   M. Tuffier, "Contribution à l'Etude de la Chirurgie de Guerre," session of
     October 13, 1914, *Bulletin l'Académie de Médecine* 72 (1914): 150–56.

33   Léon Werth, *Clavel chez les Majors,* (Paris: Viviane Hanny, 2006), 61.

34   Mary Borden, *The Forbidden Zone* (London: Hesperus Press Ltd, 1929, reprinted
     2008), 44.

35   Alfred Mignon, *Le Service de Santé Pendant la Guerre 1914–1918*, vol. 1 (Paris:
     Masson & Cie, Editeurs, 1926), 159.

36   O. Forcade, "Censure, Secret et Opinion en France de 1914 à 1919," *Matériaux
     pour l'histoire de notre temps* 58 (2000): 45–53.

37   Maurice Barrès, "Les Blessés sont faits pour être Guéris," *L'Echo*, September 23, 1914.

38   C. Debue-Barazer, "La Gangrène Gazeuse pendant la Première Guerre Mon-
     diale," *Annales de Démographie Historique* 103 (2002): 51–70.

39   V. Pauchet and P. Sourdat "L'amputation en 'Saucisson'" *Bulletins et Memoires de
     la Société de Chirurgie,* 40 (1914): 1216–19.

40   Viet, *La Santé en Guerre,* 77.

41   Believe it or not, in those early days of the war, horse-drawn wagons were used
     for much of the resupply effort and to transport casualties to hospitals. Their reli-
     ability in rutted, muddy roads and through farm fields was considered superior to
     the new, flimsy automobile.

42   G. Vitoux, "Les Formations Sanitaires Automobiles," *Revue d'Hygiène et de Police*
     37 (1915): 958–76.

43   A. Troussaint, "Circulaire No. 12 802 C/7," October 29, 1914, referenced in
      F. Olier, "Les Autochirs (1914–1918): Genèse d'une Epopée," *Médecine et armées*
      30 (2002): 299–320.

44   H. Hallopeau, "Fonctionnement Complet d'un Service Chirurgical Transport-
      able et Déplaçable: Destiné à Opérer, à Panser les Blessés du Front," *Press Med* 23
      (1915): 43–48.

45   Duhamel, *La Pesée des Ames*, 57–69.

46   P. Chavasse, "Circular No. 1238/S," December 25, 1914, Archives du Musée,
      Service de santé des armées, Val-de-Grâce, Paris.

47   P. Chavasse, "Circular No. 4133-c/7," February 4, 1915, Archives du Musée, Ser-
      vice de santé des armées, Val-de-Grâce, Paris.

48   J. Reinach, "Rapport Présenté au Nom de la Commission Supérieure Consulta-
      tive du Service de Santé," *Journaux Officiels*, Paris, 1915.

49   Observations presented by Dr. Doyen, July 7, 1915, before the Commission
      de l'Armée du Sénat (Service de Santé) et à la Commission d'Hygiène de la
      Chambre des Députés.

50   General Joffre, at the suggestion of Édouard de Castelnau, commander of the
      Central Army Group, had appointed General Pétain as commander of the
      defense of Verdun at the beginning of 1916.

51   Mignon, *Le Service de Santé*, 1:15.

52   *Ibid.*, 1:25; Viet also alludes to this disconnection of military and medical plan-
      ning in the Service de santé (*La Santé en Guerre*, 66).

53   Troussaint, *La Direction du Service de Santé en Campagne*, 257. French field
      ambulances were a combination of physician staff, their equipment, and hospital
      sections taken from larger units, such as so-called evacuation hospitals (*hôpitaux
      d'évacuation*) located in the *zone des étapes*.

54   Mignon, *Le Service de Santé*, 1:317–18.

55   A. Gosset, "Discussion sur les Plaies Pénétrantes de l'Abdomen," *Bulletin et
      Mémoires de la Société de Chirurgie de Paris*, meeting March 24, 1915, 759.

56   Forty-nine "*auto-chirs*" would be developed and deployed, including Marcille's
      three units donated by the Russians. Further modifications would result in almost
      unique configurations for each unit after Gosset's twenty-three ambulances had
      been completed.

57   Duhamel, *Les Pesée des Ames*, 71. Duhamel claimed, after he had reported Mar-
      cille's bizarre behavior at Lignereuil to *médecin-chef* Potherat, that Marcille pulled
      a pistol and threatened to shoot him (61). Gosset would continue to lavish praise
      on Marcille for his role in conceptualizing the mobile surgical service.

58   "Encore un Don Superb de la Russie à Nos Armées," *Le Petit Parisien*, Sep-
      tember 6, 1915; François Olier describes a circular issued by Troussaint that
      confirmed five or six mobile units of Marcille's had been donated by the
      Russians, funded, in large part, no doubt by the Duchesse (Olier, "Les Auto-
      chirs," 299–320). Previously, in March, the Formations chirurgicales franco-
      russes had donated thirty-five new, rugged ambulance transport vehicles, as
      reported in *Le Figaro*.

59   Johann Wolfgang von Goethe, *Campaign in France in the Year 1792*, translated by
      Robert Farie, (London: Chapman and Hall, 1849), 31–32.

60   Maurice Barrès, "La bataille de Verdun," *L'Echo de Paris*, September 26, 1916.

61   Jacques Péricard, *Verdun, 1914–1918* (Paris: Librairie de France, 1934), 80.

62   Maurice Barrès, *L'Ame Française et la Guerre Pendant la Bataille de Verdun* (Paris:
      Emile-Paul Frères, 1919), 175.

63   J. Horne, "Entre Expérience et Mémoire: Les Soldats Français de la Grande
      Guerre," *Annales Histoire, Sciences Sociales* 5 (2005): 903–19.

64   Mignon, *Le Service de Santé*, 2:467.

65   E. Klekowski and L. Klekowski, *Eyewitness to the Great War: American Writers,
      Reporters, Volunteers and Soldiers in France* (Jefferson: McFarland, 2012), 61.

66   Barrès, *L'Ame*, 43.

67   Mignon, *Le Service de Santé*, 2:125.

68   J. Fiolle, "Les 'Auto-Chir' et les Progrès de la Chirurgie de Guerre," *Revue de
      Paris* 6 (1917): 86–105.

69   Mignon, *Le Service de Santé*, 4:807.

70   Alfred Mignon, *La Pratique Chirurgicale Dans La Zone de L'Avant* (Paris: J.-B.
      Bailliere, 1917).

71   Mignon, *Le Service de Santé*, 2: 203.

72   Georges Duhamel, *The New Book of Martyrs* (New York: George H. Doran Com-
      pany, 1918), 112–119.

73   Viet, *La Santé en Guerre*, 236.

74   This four-volume set was published under the title of *Le Service de santé pendant la
      guerre 1914–1918* and remains a landmark study of France's Health Service efforts
      during World War I. .

75   "Alfred Mignon" *Revue du Service de Santé Militaire* 105 (1936) : 253–267.

76   American surgeon general Merritte Ireland seemed enamored of them, equip-
      ping and staffing a number of mobile hospitals (modeled after the *auto-chirs*) and
      the mobile surgical groups modeled after the *groupe complémentaire*. See Charles
      Lynch, Joseph H. Ford, and Frank W. Weed, "Evacuation Hospitals, Mobile
      Hospitals, Mobile Surgical Units, Professional Teams, Convalescent Depots,
      Evacuation Ambulance Companies, Mobile Laboratories," in *The Medical
      Department of the United States Army in the World War* Vol. VIII, ed.
      M. W. Irleland, chap. 5 (Washington, DC: Government Printing Office, 1925),
      184–201.

77   Gilbert W. Beebe and Michael E. DeBakey, *Battle Casualties: Incidence, Mortality,
      and Logistic Considerations* (Springfield, Ill.: Charles C. Thomas Publisher, 1952),
      96. See also T. S. Helling and W. S. Marble, "Surgeons to the Front: Twentieth-
      Century Warfare and the Metamorphosis of Battlefield Surgery," in *The Last 100
      Yards: The Crucible of Close Combat in Large-Scale Combat Operations*, ed. Paul E.
      Berg (Fort Leavenworth, Kan.: Army University Press, 2019), 191–210.

78   "Nécrologie: Décès de M. Maurice Marcille, Member Titulaire," *Mem Acad de
      Chir* (France) 67 (1941): 646–47.

CHAPTER THREE

1   W. B. Cannon, "The Course of Events in Secondary Wound Shock," *JAMA* 73 (1919): 174–81.

2   Homer, *Iliad* (Cambridge, Mass.: Harvard University Press, 1925), 11.812–13; 13.655–56; translations mine.

3   In antiquity most wounded on the battlefield were soon dispatched by blood-thirsty victors intent on wiping out the vanquished (or simply unwilling to care for the stricken).

4   Henri-François Le Dran, *Traité ou Réflexions Tirées de la Pratique sur les Playes d'Armes à Feu* (Paris: Charles Osmont, 1738), 68.

5   Henry-Francis Le Dran, *Observations in Surgery*, trans. J. S. Surgeon (John Sparrow) (London: James Hodges, 1740), 351. It is not entirely clear who J. S. Surgeon (John Sparrow) really was. In examining other works of medicine that he translated, it is most probable he was, in fact, a surgeon and apparent student of Claudius Amyand (1660–1740), the French surgeon who performed the first successful appendectomy and who was "Serjeant Surgeon" [sic] to the king. John Sparrow's other translations include works in syphilis and midwifery.

6   G. J. Guthrie, *Observations on Gun-Shot Wounds and on Injuries of Nerves* (London: Burgess and Hill, 1820), 10–11, 15, 27. In a later publication Guthrie seemed intrigued that the nervous system somehow played a role as he comments that a powerful blow, such as from cannon-shot that disrupts the femoral artery, often is fatal, attributed to the "double effect on the nervous and sanguiferous [sic] systems" (G. J. Guthrie, *Treatise on Gun-Shot Wounds* [London: Charles Woods, 1827], 245–46).

7   Astley Cooper, *The Lectures: Principles and Practice of Surgery*, vol. 1 (Boston: Wells and Lilly, 1825), 9–10, 12, 24. Cooper mused about the shock syndrome: how a modest loss of blood could still be lethal and whether, indeed, the nervous system could prove the culprit.

8   Samuel David Gross, *A System of Surgery: Pathological, Diagnostic, Therapeutic, and Operative*, vol. 1 (Philadelphia: Henry C. Lea's Sons & Company, 1882), 411, 414. Gross speculated that at least some of the manifestations of shock were due to a "diminution of blood."

9   John Collins Warren Jr., *Surgical Pathology and Therapeutics* (Philadelphia: W. B. Saunders, 1895), 279. John Collins Warren Jr. was from probably the most famous medical family in the United States. His great-grandfather was a founder of Harvard Medical School and his grandfather the facilitator of general anesthesia at the same medical institution. Warren Jr. was a distinguished surgeon in his own right, member of the Harvard faculty, and president of the prestigious American Surgical Association.

10   Claude Bernard, *Leçons sur les Phénomènes de la Vie, Communs aux Animaux et aux Végétaux* (Paris: J.-B. Baillière et fils, 1885), 242.

11   W. S. Savory, "Collapse," in *A System of Surgery*, ed. T. Holmes (London: Long-mans, Green, and Co., 1870), 746–65, 772.

12   H. Fischer, "Ueber den Shok," *Sammlung klinischer Vortage* 10 (1870): 69–82.
      Fischer was of the opinion, like others, that shock was caused by reflex flaring of
      the "vascular nerves," especially in the abdomen.

13   C. W. Mansell-Moullin, *On the Pathology of Shock* (London: H.G. Saunders,
      1880), 23.

14   H. Cushing, "On the Avoidance of Shock in Major Amputations by Cocainiza-
      tion of Large Nerve-Trunks Preliminary to their Division. With Observations on
      Blood-Pressure Changes in Surgical Cases," *Ann Surg* 36 (1902): 321–45. Others
      were not so eager to agree. Henry Janeway of New York had shown experimen-
      tally that trauma to the peripheral somatic nerves did not result in a reflex fall in
      blood pressure as Cushing claimied, and blocking of afferent (sensory) nerves did
      not protect against fatigue of the nerve centers as Crile maintained (see H. H.
      Janeway and E. M. Ewing, "The Nature of Shock. Its Relation to Acapnia and
      to Changes in the Circulation of the Blood and to Exhaustion of the Nerve Cen-
      tres," *Ann Surg* 59 (1914): 158–75).

15   Sphygmomanometry is the science of measurement of the pulse, from the
      Greek σφυγμός, meaning "pulse." Karl Vierordt explained his sphygmoma-
      nometer in an extensive treatise published in 1855 entitled *Die Lehre vom
      Arterienpuls in Gesunden und Kranken Zuständen* (Braunschweig: Friedrich
      Vieweg und Sohn, 1855). Karl von Basch published his more portable (but still
      cumbersome) sphygmomanometer in "Ueber die Messung des Blutdrucks am
      Menschen," *Zeitschrift für Klinische Medizin* 2 (1880): 79–96, and promoted
      his method as more accurate than Vierordt's, but refrained from applying any
      clinical significance to his blood pressure findings in humans. See also J. Booth,
      "A Short History of Blood Pressure Measurement," *Proc R Soc Med* 70 (1977):
      793–99.

16   S. Riva-Rocci, "Un Nuovo Sfigmomanometro," *Gazzetta Medica di Torino* 47
      (1896): 1001–17.

17   L. Hill and H. Barnard, "A Simple and Accurate Form of Sphygmomanometer
      or Arterial Pressure Gauge Contrived for Clinical Use," *Brit Med J* 2 (1897): 904.
      The diastolic blood pressure represents, then, the baseline arterial "tension" of the
      arteries and reflects the resistance against which the heart must work.

18   Information from R. E. Hermann, "George Washington Crile (1864–1943)," *J
      Med Bio* 2 (1994): 78–83.

19   George Crile, *An Autobiography*, Volumes 1 and 2 (Philadelphia: J. B. Lippincott
      Company, 1947), I: 22–30. The work was compiled by his widow, Grace, and
      consisted of selected letters and memoirs, and his personal recollections. His
      patient had suffered crush injuries to both legs and had undergone bilateral leg
      amputations from which he never recovered. As with most physicians, the image
      and name of this young man stayed with Crile the rest of his life.

20   Quotes mine. Personally, those nagging questions have so often pestered me and,
      in my conversations with colleagues, them, too.

21   George W. Crile and William E. Lower, *Anoci-Association* (Philadelphia:
      W. B. Saunders Company, 1914), 31. Crile and Lower felt the liver, suprarenal

glands (adrenal glands), and brain were the primary sites of energy storage. Physical trauma was only one means for producing shock and exhaustion, the authors theorized; fear, worry, starvation, excessive muscular activity, and insomnia were others.

22   In those times, blood pressure during operations, of course, was not measured. Circulation was assessed by the strength of the pulse and the beating of the heart.

23   George W. Crile, *Blood-Pressure in Surgery: An Experimental and Clinical Research* (Philadelphia: J. B. Lippincott Company, 1903), 401, 412.

24   E. W. Archibald, "Observations upon Shock, with Particular Reference to the Condition as Seen in War Surgery," *Ann Surg* 66 (1917): 280–86. Archibald, on the faculty of McGill University before the war, served for two years in France, some of that time at the Canadian No. 1 Casualty Clearing Station in the Ypres sector.

25   As an example of prevailing opinion, see Cuthbert Wallace and John Fraser, *Surgery at a Casualty Clearing Station* (London: A. & C. Black, 1918), especially "Surgical Shock," 7–22.

26   See Robert Toombs, *The War Against Paris, 1871* (Cambridge: Cambridge University Press, 1981).

27   Ross King, *The Judgment of Paris* (New York: Walker and Company, 2006), 307–09.

28   Thomas W. Evans, *History of the American Ambulance Established in Paris during the Siege of 1870–71* (London: Chiswick Press, 1873), xi.

29   Crile, *An Autobiography*, 1: 248.

30   *Ibid.*, 1: 253–55.

31   From a report Crile published in July 1915 shortly after his return from the Ambulance Américaine at Neuilly-sur-Seine: Crile, G. W., "Notes on Military Surgery," *Ann Surg* 62 (1915): 1–10.

32   Crile, *An Autobiography*, 1: 264. His anecdotal observations in France impressed upon him the possibility that pain and exhaustion alone could prove fatal. Three decades later a French surgeon by the name of Henri Laborit would use ganglionic blocking agents as an adjunct in shock to interrupt sensory input using phenothiazine derivatives and, together with cooling, called it "artificial hibernation." See H. Laborit and P. Huguenard, "L'Hibernation Artificielle par Moyens Pharmacodynamiques et Physiques," *Press Med* 59 (1951): 1329.

33   So stated surgeon Robert Greenough to the Boston Medical and Surgical Journal in 1915 (R. B. Greenough, "The American Hospital of Paris" *Bost Med Surg J* 172 [1915]: 954–55).

34   George W. Crile, *An Experimental Research into Surgical Shock* (Philadelphia: J. B. Lippincott Company, 1899), 149.

35   R. Lower, "An Account of the Experiment of Transfusion Practiced upon a Man in London," *Philos Trans R Soc* 30 (1667): 557–59.

36   See Blundell's classic paper: J. Blundell, "Experiments on the Transfusion of Blood by the Syringe," *Med Chir Trans* 9 (1818): 56–92.

37   Crile even decapitated anesthetized dogs and kept them alive with transfusions
      alone for up to eleven hours.

38   Crile, *An Autobiography*, 1: 166. Alexis Carrel had perfected the technique
      of anastomosing blood vessels together for unimpeded flow of blood. As for
      Crile's poor donor, he remarked that the fellow "seemed to have shrunk to
      half his size."

39   George W. Crile, *Hemorrhage and Transfusion: An Experimental and Clinical
      Research* (New York: D. Appleton and Company, 1909). Pay particular attention
      to 283–99 and 407–99; quote from 533.

40   "The Transfusion of Blood," *Brit Med J* 2 (1907): 1006–07. Reference was made
      to G. W. Crile, "On the Direct Transfusion of Blood—An Experimental and
      Clinical Research," *Canada Lancet* 60 (1907): 1057–68.

41   E. Lindeman, "Simple Syringe Transfusion with Special Cannulas," *Am J Dis
      Children* 6 (1913): 28–32.

42   J.-P. Aymard and P. Renaudier, "La Transfusion Sanguine Pendant la Grande
      Guerre (1914–1918)," *Hist Sci Med* 50 (2016): 353–66. The soldier, Henri
      Legrain, recovered and lived to be ninety-seven. Jeanbrau favored the Kimpton-
      Brown tube that allowed rapid, gravity-driven, and measured blood transfusions,
      all done speedily before blood clotted. See A. R. Kimpton and J. H. Brown, "A
      New and Simple Method of Transfusion," *JAMA* 61 (1913): 117–18. In his *An
      Autobiography*, 2:337, George Crile claimed the first transfusion was done by his
      Lakeside unit at the Ambulance Américaine in 1914 (they did not even arrive
      until January 1915), but that does not seem to be the case.

43   Crile, *An Autobiography*, 1: 262.

44   See B. Vincent, "Blood Transfusion: Indications, Methods, and Results," *Boston
      Med Surg J* 147 (1912): 239–42. Vincent wisely felt that blood transfusion was a
      perfect substitute for acute hemorrhagic blood loss, restored the cellular elements,
      and contributed to hemostasis.

45   Elliot Carr Cutler, *A Journal of the Harvard Medical School Unit to the American
      Ambulance Hospital in Paris: Spring of 1915* (New York: Evening Post Job Printing
      Office, 1915), 30, 49.

46   Following his time at Bellevue, Robertson returned to Toronto where it is
      reported that he performed the first blood transfusion there. See L. B. Robertson
      and A. Brown, "Blood Transfusion in Infants and Young Children," *Can Med
      Assoc J* 5 (1915): 298–305.

47   The No. 2 Canadian Casualty Clearing Station was organized in Toronto in Feb-
      ruary 1915 and commanded by Lieutenant Colonel G. S. Rennie (Library and
      Archives Canada).

48   Information from the rather detailed obituary published by C. L. Starr, "Law-
      rence Bruce Robertson, B.A., M.B.," *Can Med Assoc J* 13 (1923): 216–17.

49   L. B. Robertson, "The Transfusion of Whole Blood: A Suggestion for Its More
      Frequent Employment in War Surgery," *Brit Med J* 2 (1916): 38–40.

50   L. B. Robertson and C. G. Watson, "Further Observations on the Results of
      Blood Transfusions in War Surgery, with Special Reference to the Results in

Primary Haemorrhage," *Br Med J* 2 (1917): 679–83. Statistics from War Diaries—2nd Canadian Casualty Clearing Station, 1915–1919; War Diaries of the First World War, Library and Archives Canada.

51   Letter from Mr. James Kerr-Lawson to Mrs. Bruce Robertson, 1923, Archives of Ontario. For example, on one day, July 31, 1917, No. 2 Casualty Clearing Station admitted 5,092 patients. This hospital apparently handled the most wounded of any hospital in the Remy Siding (War Diaries—2nd Canadian Casualty Clearing Station, RG9-III-D-3, Archives of Ontario).

52   A. Primrose and E. S. Ryerson, "The Direct Transfusion of Blood: Its Value in Haemorrhage and Shock in the Treatment of the Wounded in War," *Br Med J* 2 (1916): 384–86.

53   G. H. Makins, "The Development of British Surgery in the Hospitals on the Lines of Communication in France," *Br Med J* 1 (1917): 789–806. Makin referred to the use of transfusions in British general hospitals and not nearer the front in casualty clearing stations. In fact, an article two weeks earlier in the *British Medical Journal* by Anthony Bowlby and Cuthbert Wallace on surgery at the front specifically did not reference use of blood in resuscitation of casualties in shock or prior to operation in casualty clearing stations (see A. Bowlby and C. Wallace, "The Development of British Surgery at the Front," *Br Med J* 1 (1917): 705–21).

54   See N. Guiou,"Blood Transfusion in a Field Ambulance," *Br Med J* 1 (1918): 695–96.

55   For characterization of the surgeon and the man, see his very informative obituary written by Jonathan Meakins, "Edward William Archibald, B.A., M.D.," *CMAJ* 54 (1946): 194–98.

56   Archibald, E., "A Note Upon the Employment of Blood Transfusion in War Surgery," *Lancet* 2 (1916): 429–31.

57   *Ibid.*

58   Duhamel, *Vie Des Martyrs*, 111, 113.

59   T. Howard Somervell, *After Everest* (London: Hodder and Stoughton, 1936), 27.

60   John Keegan, *The Face of Battle* (New York: Penguin Books, 1976), 272.

61   One must remember that in 1916 "shock" was not a reportable diagnosis and there were few agreed upon criteria to label clinical findings as such. It is hard, therefore, to know exactly how many of the cases in the "moribund ward" were truly in shock. No doubt a good many were, at some point or other, suffering from it. In some shock was due to uncontrollable hemorrhage; in others sepsis and the effects of progressing infections; in still others, shock produced that indefinable syndrome of dwindling vital signs and consciousness.

62   See his detailed studies and theories outlined in E. W. Archibald and W. S. McLean, "Observations Upon Shock" *Ann Surg* 66 (1917): 280–286.

63   Read his experimental and human trial in A. Hustin, "Note sur une Nouvelle Méthode de Transfusion," *Ann Bull Soc Méd et Nat Bruxelles* 72 (1914): 104–11. For a more complete discussion of citrate in blood see P. I. Mollison, "The Introduction of Citrate as an Anticoagulant for Transfusion and of Glucose as a Red Cell Preservative," *Brit J Haematology* 108 (2000): 13–18.

64   P. Rous and J. P. Turner, "The Preservation of Living Red Blood Cells in Vitro: I. Methods of Preservation," *J Exp Med* 23 (1916): 219–37.

65   E. A. Archibald, "A Brief Survey of Some Experiences in the Surgery of the Present War," *Can Med Assoc J* 6 (1916): 793. Most his patients, he admitted, "were in very desperate condition, indeed practically moribund" at the time he administered his transfusions.

66   *Ibid.*

67   See a rich discussion of the role of the Canadian Army Medical Corps in blood transfusions in K. Pelis, "Taking Credit: The Canadian Army Medical Corps and the British Conversion to Blood Transfusion in WWI," *J Hist Med Allied Sci* 56 (2001): 238–77.

68   In Greek mythology, Sirens were devilish creatures who lured naïve seamen by their sweet songs to shipwreck on rocky coasts. Hardly were blood transfusions worthy of such catastrophes, but, during the Great War, still filled with potential dangers.

69   Of course, grouping of blood into three and then four types (A, B, C [O], AB) had already been defined by the Karl Landsteiner in 1900. See K. Landsteiner, "Zur Kenntnis der Antifermentativen, Lytischen und Agglutinierenden Wirkungen des Blutserums und der Lymphe," *Centralblatt für Bakteriologie, Parasitenkunde* 27 (1900): 357–62.

70   See R. I. Lee, "A Simple and Rapid Method for the Selection of Suitable Donors for Transfusion by the Determination of Blood Groups," *Br Med J* 2 (1917): 684–85.

71   O. H. Robertson, "Transfusion with Preserved Red Blood Cells," *Brit Med J* 1 (1918): 691–95.

72   Memorandum Peyton Rous to Franklin McLean (University of Chicago), Rockefeller Institute for Medical Research, November 23, 1949.

73   Crile, *An Autobiography*, 1: 287.

74   For example, by May 1917 No. 2 Canadian Casualty Clearing Station had officially designated the resuscitation ward as a place to move moribund and "collapsed" cases (no doubt those thought to be in shock). War Diaries—2nd Canadian Casualty Clearing Station, RG9-III-D-3, Archives of Ontario.

75   Crile, *An Autobiography*, 1: 281, 337.

76   The Medical Research Committee, "Memorandum upon Surgical Shock and Some Allied Conditions," *Br Med J* 1 (1917): 381–83.

77   Saul Benison, A. Clifford Barger, and Elin L. Wolfe, *Walter B. Cannon: the Life and Times of a Young Scientist* (Cambridge, Mass.: Harvard University Press, 1987), 71.

78   *Ibid.*, 384.

79   *Ibid.*, 391–92.

80   Walter Bradford Cannon, *The Way of an Investigator* (New York: W. W. Norton & Company, 1945), 133.

81   Quotes taken from Walter Cannon's letters home, reproduced in S. Benison, A. C. Barger, and E. L. Wolfe, "Walter B. Cannon and the Mystery of Shock:

A Study of Anglo-American Co-operation in World War I," *Med Hist* 35 (1991): 217–49.

82   William Townsend Porter, *Shock at the Front* (Boston: Atlantic Monthly Press, 1918), 44, 54–55. There was no love lost between Porter and Walter Cannon. Cannon had replaced him as chairman of physiology at Harvard in 1906, a move that rankled Porter in that he had recruited Cannon to Harvard some years earlier.

83   For a lengthier explanation of this theory see E. Cowell, "The Pathology and Treatment of Traumatic (Wound) Shock," *Proc Royal Soc Med* 21 (1928): 1611–18. See also E. M. Cowell, "Memorandum: The Initiation of Wound Shock, with Suggestions for its Early Treatment," November 7, 1917, RAMC/466/5 Wellcome Library, London. Some cases of low blood pressure immediately after wounding have been ascribed by others to syncope, more psychosomatic than a strictly physiologic hemorrhagic depletion of blood.

84   Cannon, "Secondary Wound Shock." The report of the Medical Research Committee on February 27, 1917, indicated that the acidosis observed in "circulatory failure" (the overriding explanation of shock at the time) should be treated with sodium bicarbonate not only to ease symptoms but also to improve the viscosity of a reduced blood volume following hemorrhage, particularly in the all-important capillary bed where critical exchange of oxygen must occur. See The Medical Research Committee "Acidosis and Shock, Reports of the Special Investigation Committee on Surgical Shock and Allied Conditions. No. 7," London, 1918.

85   Gum arabic is a mixture of the complex sugars arabinose and galactose in an inert formula that seems well tolerated by subjects and is eventually metabolized. It was the first of a long series of "colloid" solutions to be used to treat shock, the value of which is still disputed to this day. See W. M. Bayliss, *Intravenous Injection in Wound Shock* (London: Longmans, Green, and Co., 1918), 80–93.

86   For an extended summary of wound shock, both concepts of origin and treatment, as it developed during World War I see W. G. Macpherson, *Medical Services: Surgery of the War* (London: His Majesty's Stationery Office, 1922), chapters 4 and 5, 58–107.

CHAPTER FOUR

1   Saying attributed to Guilhelmus Fabricus Hildanus, *De Gangraena et Sphacelo* (Oppenheimii: Typis Hieronymus Gallerus, 1617), 7.

2   *Emphysema* comes from the Greek ἐμφυσᾶν, meaning to inflate or "puff up." In this context it signifies air (gas) in the tissues below the skin—subcutaneous fat and, below that, muscle. Unless introduced through the skin in the process of wounding with penetrating-type trauma, the gas originates from the metabolism of microorganisms. Such findings are harbingers of dread.

3   *Gangrene* is a term that probably originated from the Greek γάγγραινα, meaning putrefaction of tissues. The 17th-century physician Guilhelmus Hildanus characterized gangrene as "a disease that eats away the flesh" and represents "the

principle of mortification, following the greatest inflammation and corruption of the soft parts of the human body, that is, the skin, muscles, veins, arteries, and nerves" (Hildanus, *De Gangraena et Sphacelo*, 36).

4   M. Maisonneuve, "De la Gangrène Foudroyante, avec Développement et Circu-lation de Gaz Putrides dans les Veines (pneumo-hémie putride)," *Comptes rendus l'Académie des Sciences* 37 (1853): 425–27. Maisonneuve was a surgeon of some renown in Paris in the mid–19th century, serving with distinction in a number of Parisian hospitals such as the Hôtel-Dieu, Charité, and Pitié. His interests were eclectic, ranging from maxillo-facial disorders to orthopedic injuries to dis-eases of the viscera and ovaries. It was Maisonneuve who introduced the cautery, allowing surgeons bloodless access to all depths of an affected part (from M. W. Duckett, ed., *Dictionnaire de la Conversation et de la Lecture*, vol. 4 [Paris: Dirmin-Didot et Cie, 1876], 561–62).

5   A. Velpeau, *Nouveaux Éléments de Médecine Opératoire*, vol. 1 (Paris: J.-B. Bail-lière, 1832), 270.

6   D. J. Larrey, *Clinique Chirurgical* (Paris: Gabon, 1829), 538–42.

7   M. Salleron, *Compte-Rendu des Amputations Primitives et des Amputations Con-sécutives* (Paris: Henri et Charles Noblet, 1858), 41–46. Almost three quarters of amputations prompted by this gangrene were found in the leg, thigh, or shoulder areas—large muscle mass groups (43).

8   *Ibid.*, 50, 61.

9   *Ibid.*, 66.

10   Hospital gangrene is discussed in some detail by medical chroniclers of the Civil War. The deep muscle involvement frequently led to rivulets of liquid pus and tissue destruction that seemed to follow fascial planes and eventually pro-duced systemic symptoms of inanition, fever, and prostration. Fatality rates were impressive, sometimes exceeding 50 percent in extremity cases. This disorder is probably analogous to "necrotizing fasciitis" that is seen today, an infection caused by any number of bacteria that spreads much like hospital gangrene did in Civil War times. See Joseph K. Barnes, *The Medical and Surgical History of the War of the Rebellion*, vol. 2 (Washington, DC: Government Printing Office, 1883), 823–51. Nor does the subject of emphysematous gangrene come up in reviews of wound problems as discussed by L. A. Dugas, "A Lecture on Suppuration," *South Med Surg J* 21 (1867): 36–55, or in a case of ligation of the subclavian artery resulting in gangrene and death (W. H. Doughty, "Report of Two Cases of Liga-tion of the Subclavian Artery," *South Med Surg J* 21 [1867]: 30–36).

11   Joseph Jones, *Surgical Memoirs of the War of the Rebellion: II: The Nature, Causes, and Treatment of Hospital Gangrene, as it Prevailed in The Confederate Armies 1861–1865* (Cambridge: Hurd and Hougton, 1871), 148.

12   J. Julian Chisolm, *Manual of Military Surgery* (Columbia, S.C.: Evans and Cog-swell, 1864), 2.

13   For an in-depth study of Pasteur's work in anaerobic organisms see M. Sebald and D. Hauser, "Pasteur, Oxygen and the Anaerobes Revisited," *Anaerobe* 1 (1995): 11–16.

14   Leeuwenhoek named the tiny organisms he viewed through his microscope *dier-kens*, which translated to English as *animalcules* (tiny animals). See N. Lane, "The Unseen World: Reflections on Leeuwenhoek (1677) 'Concerning Little Animals,'" *Phil Trans R Soc B* 370 (2015): 1–10.

15   See Filippo Pacini, "Osservazioni Microscopiche e Deduzioni Patologiche sul Cholera Asiatico," *Gazzetta Medica Italiana* 4 (1854): 397–401.

16   "Cursed fields" taken from Émile Duclaux, *Pasteur: The History of a Mind* (Philadelphia: W. B. Saunders Company, 1920), 236.

17   Actually, Casimir Davaine (1812–82), in 1863, was the first to uncover the etiologic agent of anthrax as stick-shaped corpuscles (named by him *bacteridia*) that, when injected into laboratory animals, soon produced death. However, clear transmissibility eluded him because he could not identify the resilient spore of the germ (that Pasteur later did). He defined his septicemia as a "putrefaction which takes place in the blood of a living animal." (From J. Théodoridès, "Casimir Davaine [1812–1882]: A Precursor of Pasteur" *Med Hist* 10 (1966): 155–65). For unraveling of the anthrax mystery see Patrice Debré, *Louis Pasteur* (Baltimore: Johns Hopkins University Press, 1994), especially 314–18.

18   L. Pasteur, "Étude sur la Maladie Charbonneuse," in *Oeuvres de Pasteur* vol. 6, ed. P. Vallery-Radot (Paris: Masson et Cie, 1933), 164–71. This work was originally presented before the Société du biologie in April 1877 and can be found in *Comptes Rendus de Séances et Mémoires des Société du Biologie* 84 (1877): 900–06.

19   Debré, *Pasteur*, 408–09.

20   R. Koch, "Die Ätiologie der Milzbrand-Krankheit, begründet auf die Entwicklungsgeschichte des Bacillus Anthracis," *Beiträge zur Biologie der Pflanzen* 2 (1877): 277–310. For an extended discussion of this bitter rivalry, see K. C. Carter, "The Koch-Pasteur Dispute on Establishing the Cause of Anthrax," *Bull Hist Med* 62 (1988): 42–57.

21   See L. P. Elliott, "William Henry Welch: Pioneer American Microbiologist and Physician," *Bios* 50 (1979): 73–77. William Welch was of such renown that he was known as one of the "Big Four" founding faculty of Johns Hopkins Hospital, the other three being William Osler, William Halsted, and Howard Kelly.

22   W. H. Welch, and G.H.F. Nuttall, "A Gas-Producing Bacillus (Bacillus Aerogenes Capsulatus, Nov. Spec.) Capable of Rapid Development in the Blood-Vessels After Death," *Bull Johns Hopkins Hosp* 3 (1892): 81–91.

23   *Phlegmon* is a term meaning "inflammation of the tissues under the skin (subcutaneous)" and comes from the Greek φλεγμονή, meaning, of course, "inflammation."

24   E. Fraenkel, "Ueber die Aetiologie der Gasphlegmonen (Phlegmone Emphysematosa)," *Centralbl für Bakteriol u Parasitenk* 13 (1893): 13–16, including preceding quote. Malignant edema and blackleg were two conditions sometimes seen in herbivorous farm animals (cattle, sheep, hogs) with similar necrotizing changes and an often fatal course. The causative agents seemed to be some variant

of anaerobic organisms, but differentiation by species had been a matter of some dispute among bacteriologists of the day. For a fuller compilation of the confusion that reigned in the early 20th century about this, see H. H. Heller, "Etiology of Acute Gangrenous Infections of Animals: A Discussion of Blackleg, Braxy, Malignant Edema and Whale Septicemia: Studies on Pathogenic Anaerobes I," *J Infect Dis* 27 (1920): 385–451.

25   Eugen Fraenkel, *Üeber Gasphlegmonen* (Hamburg und Leipzig: Leopold Voss, 1893), 16–17; W. H. Welch, "Morbid Conditions Caused by Bacillus Aerogenes Capsulatus," *Bull Johns Hopkins Hosp* 11 (1900): 185–204.

26   W. C. Cramp, "A Consideration of Gas Bacillus Infection with Special Reference to Treatment," *Ann Surg* 56 (1912): 544–64.

27   *Ibid.*

28   The Danish physician Hans Christian Gram (1853–1938) had developed a stain that separated known bacteria into two groups: those that took up his stain and those that did not. See H. C. Gram, "Über die isolierte Färbung der Schizomyceten in Schnitt- und Trockenpräparaten," *Fortschritte der Medizin* 2 (1884): 185–89.

29   See Franz Hutyra and Josef Marek, *Spezielle Pathologie und Therapy der Haustiere* (Jena: Gustav Fischer, 1913), 34–41, 41–60.

30   Chief among these would be microbiologists Conradi and Bieling, who radically claimed one polymorphic species of anaerobes—the bacillus of Fraenkel—was implicated in all gas gangrene cases. See H. Conradi and R. Bieling, "Zur Aetiologie und Pathogenese des Gasbrands," *Münchener Med Wochenschrift* 63 (1916): 133–178, 1023–68, 1561–1608. One must remember that purification of bacteria in wartime was notoriously unreliable, as Hilda Heller pointed out in her article "Classification of the Anaerobic Bacteria," *Bot Gazette* 73 (1922): 70–79.

31   Ernst Bergmann, *Die Behandlung der Schusswunden des Kniegelenks im Kriege* (Stuttgart: Ferdinand Enke, 1878), 8. Bergmann's approach to wound care is also discussed in Arend Buchholtz's comprehensive biography *Ernst von Bergmann* (Leipzig: C. W. Vogel, 1913). Iodine preparations were widely believed to be potent antiseptics.

32   August Hildebrandt, *Die Verwundungen durch die modernen Kriegsfeuerwaffen ihre Prognose und Therapie im Felde* (Berlin: August Hirschwald, 1905), 125–26; this book received acclaim as a detailed portrayal of firearm ballistics and wounding, so much so that "probably in no other work of a similar kind is so much accurate and valuable information to be found" as one reviewer wrote (W. G. M., *J R Army Med Corps*, 11 [1908]: 103).

33   The Société nationale de chirurgie, established in 1843, was an outgrowth of the Académie royale de chirurgie, founded in 1731, the express purpose of which was "perfecting the practice of surgery, through experience and observation," effectively becoming the gatekeeper of Parisian—and eventually French—surgical practice and training. For a detailed history, see C. Chatelain, "Histoire de l'Académie Nationale de Chirurgie," e-mémoires de l'Académie Nationale de Chirurgie 5 (2006): 18–23. For the 1914 regulations on wound care, see Delorme "Blessures de guerre," 394–399.

34   Military planners did not appreciate the destructive power of rapid-fire machine guns like the German Maxim and French Saint Étienne, which, in covered emplacements, were almost impervious to prepping artillery fire and loosed their terrible energy within minutes of the appearance of an approaching enemy.

35   Fernand Engerand, *Le Secret de la Frontière 1815—1871—1914, Charleroi* (Paris: Éditions Bossard, 1918), 504.

36   Millicent Leveson-Gower, Duchess of Sutherland, *Six Weeks at the War* (London: The Times, 1914), 27–28.

37   David Stevenson, *1914–1918: The History of the First World War* (New York: Penguin Books, 2005), 54.

38   Holger H. Herwig, *The Marne, 1914: The Opening of World War I and the Battle that Changed the World* (New York: Random House, 2011), 315.

39   E. Delorme, "Considérations Générales sur le Traitement des Blessures de Guerre," *Comptes rendus de l'Académie des Sciences*, 159 (1914): 543–55.

40   Harvey Cushing, *From a Surgeon's Journal* (Boston: Little, Brown, and Company, 1936), 44. *Blessés* is a French term for wounded. Cushing was serving with the Harvard University volunteer unit in France.

41   M. Weinberg, "Bacteriological and Experimental Researches on Gas Gangrene," *Proc Royal Soc Med* 9 (1916): 119–44.

42   Figure cited by Dr. Franz in "Anaerobe Wundinfektion (Absegehen von Wundstarrkrampf)," *Beiträge zur Klinischen Chirurgie* 101 (1916): 331–32.

43   Woods Hutchinson, *The Doctor in War* (Boston: Houghton Mifflin Company, 1918), 135–36.

44   W. G. Macpherson, *Medical Services: Surgery of the War* (London: His Majesty's Stationery Office, 1922), 134.

45   Kate John Finzi, *Eighteen Months in the War Zone* (London: Cassell and Company, 1916), 43.

46   G. W. Crile, "Notes on Military Surgery," *Ann Surg* 62 (1915): 1–10.

47   The Pasteur Institute was founded on June 4, 1887, by Louis Pasteur and would come to house the preeminent laboratories for the study of infectious diseases.

48   M. Weinberg, "Recherches Bactériologiques sur la Gangrène Gazeuse," *Compte rendus Société Biologie* 77 (1914): 506–08. During his medical school education the young Fleming had become associated with the bacteriologist Almroth Wright at Saint Mary's Hospital, London, initially for his prowess on the rifle team rather than his interest in bacteria. In 1928 Fleming went on to discover the bactericidal properties of a mold he labeled *penicillin* (see L. Colebrook, "Alexander Fleming 1881–1955," *Bio Mem Royal Soc* 2 [1956]: 117–26).

49   A. Fleming, "On the Bacteriology of Septic Wounds," *Lancet* 2 (1915): 638–43.

50   B. Moynihan, "The Treatment of Gunshot Wounds." *Brit Med J* 2879 (1916): 333–37.

51   Wolfgang U. Eckart, Christoph Gradmann, *Die Medizin und der Erste Weltkrieg* (Herbolzheim: Springer-Verlag, 2017), 299.

52   A. Von Rothe, "Chirurgie im Kriegslazarette," *Beiträge zur Klinischen Chirurgie* 96 (1915): 204.

53 W. Kausch, "Ueber die Gasphlegmone," *Beiträge zur Klinischen Chirurgie* 2 (1915): 7–31.

54 H. Kümmell, "Wundinfektion insbesondere Wundstarrkrampf und Gasbrand," *Beiträge zur Klinischen Chirurgie* 1 (1915): 421–39. There were actually three Congresses of Surgeons held by the Germans during the War, the first April 7, 1915, in Brussels, the second in Berlin, April 26–27, 1916, and the third in Brussels, February 11–12, 1918. I am indebted to Derek S. Linton and his superb article "The Obscure Object of Knowledge: German Military Medicine Confronts Gas Gangrene during World War I," *Bull Hist Med* 74 (2000): 291–316, for guiding me to pertinent German literature on this subject.

55 H. Coenen, "Ein Rückblick auf 20 Monate Feld Ärztlicher Tätigkeit, mit Besonderer Berflicksichtigung der Gasphlegmone," *Beiträge zur Klinischen Chirurgie*. 6 (1916): 397–464.

56 E. Payr, "Ueber Gasphlegmonen im Kriege," *Deutsche Med Wochensch* 2 (1915): 57–58.

57 E. Fraenkel, "Ueber Gasbrand," *Deutsche Med Wochensch* 42 (1916): 1533–535.

58 L. Aschoff, "Zur Frage der Aetiologie und Prophylaxe der Gasödeme," *Deutsche Med Wochensch* 42 (1916): 469–71. Simond had examined bacteria in terms of their ability to ferment butyric acid (Aschoff would call them *Buttersäurebazillen*). These were basically, anaerobes. Simonds then classified these into firstly, nonmotile types (*Bacillus aerogenes capsulatus* [Welch's bacillus], *Bacillus phlegmones emphysematose* [Fraenkel's bacillus], *Bacillus enteritidis sporogenes*, *Bacillus perfringens* [Weinberg's bacillus]); secondly, motile types; and thirdly, the putrifying bacilli that included the anthrax bacillus, the bacillus of the malignant edema, and the *Bacillus putrificus*. For an in-depth discussion of the anaerobic fermenters see J. P. Simonds, "Studies in Bacillus Welchii with Special Reference to Classification and to its Relation to Diarrhea," *Rockefeller Institute Monograph* 5 (1915): 1–130.

59 H. Tissier, "Recherches sur la Flore Bactérienne des Plaies de Guerre," *Ann d'Institut Pasteur* 30 (1916): 681–90.

60 A. Chalier and R. Glenard, "Les Grandes Blessures de Guerre," *Revue de Chirurgie* 51 (1916): 210–73; *"gazeuse gangrène,"* 239–44 (including quotes). Once again the authors documented that 42 percent of the 1,500 wounds studied were a result of artillery, which is a lower figure than others had reported.

61 *Ibid.*

62 C. Ritter, "Ueber Gasbrand," *Beiträge zur Klinischen Chirurgie* 3 (1916): 47–72.

63 Edmond Delorme, *Les Enseignements Chirurgicaux de la Grande Guerre (Front Occidental)* (Paris: A Maloine et Fils, 1919), 397.

64 J. W. McNee and J. S. Dunn, "The Method of Spread of Gas Gangrene into Living Muscle," *Lancet* 1 (1917): 727–29. The authors documented that, even when organisms were filtered out, injection of the liquid broth produced muscle necrosis, indicating a potent exotoxin secreted by the bacillus.

65 Ellen N. La Motte, *The Backwash of War* (New York: The Knickerbocker Press, 1916), 49.

66 D. S. Edwards, E. R. Mayhew, and A.S.C. Rice, "'Doomed to go in Company with Miserable Pain': Surgical Recognition and Treatment of

Amputation-Related Pain on the Western Front during World War 1," *Lancet* 384 (2014): 1715–19.

67   Georges Duhamel, *Vie des Martyrs 1914–1916* (Paris: Mercure de France, 1917), 126.

68   His innovative publication appeared in *Lyon Médical* in June 1902 (A. Carrel, "La Technique Opératoire des Anastomoses Vasculaires et la Transplantation des Viscères," *Lyon Médical* 98 [1902]: 859–64).

69   R. M. Sade, "Transplantation at 100 Years: Alexis Carrel, Pioneer Surgeon," *Ann Thorac Surg* 80 (2015): 2415–18.

70   "Une Guerison Miraculeuse à Lourdes," *Le Nouvelliste de Lyon*, June 10, 1902.

71   For Alexis Carrel's experiences at Lourdes, see his fictionalized account, published six years after his death, in Alexis Carrel and Virgilia Peterson, *The Voyage to Lourdes* (New York: Harper & Brothers, 1950), 61. See also A. Hartmann, "Cicatrization of Wounds. I. The Relation Between the Size of a Wound and the Rate of its Cicatrization," *J Exp Med* 24 (1916): 429–50. For his involvement at Lourdes, see B. François, G. Sternberg, and E. Fee, "The Lourdes Medical Cures Revisited," *J Hist Med Allied Sci* 69 (2014): 135–62. His turmoils after his Lourdes experience are discussed superbly in Andrés Horacio Reggiani, *God's Eugenicist: Alexis Carrel and the Sociobiology of Decline* (New York: Berghahn Books, 2007), 18–19; and David Hamilton, *The First Transplant Surgeon: The Flawed Genius of Nobel Prize Winner, Alexis Carrel* (Singapore: World Scientific Publishing, 2017), 25–28.

72   From Alexis Carrel, *Man the Unknown* (New York: Harper & Brothers, 1935, 1939), quotes 148–149.

73   L. Baguenier-Desormeaux, "Henry Drysdale Dakin à Compiègne en 1915," *Revue d'histoire de la pharmacie* 249 (1981): 79–88.

74   A. Carrel, "Science has Perfected the Art of Killing—Why not of Saving?," *Surg Gynecol Obstet* 20 (1915): 710–11.

75   P. Selcer, "Standardizing Wounds: Alexis Carrel and the Scientific Management of Life in the First World War," *Brit J Hist Sci* 41 (2008): 73–107.

76   H. D. Dakin, "On the Use of Certain Antiseptic Substances in the Treatment of Infected Wounds," *Br Med J* 2 (1915): 318–20. Sodium hypochlorite was actually "discovered" by the French chemist Claude Louis Berthollet in 1788 and used intermittently throughout the 19th century. Dakin humbly deflected the enormous praise heaped on him as a result of his initial 1915 paper, pointing out that his antiseptic solution was nothing novel (for further discussion, see H. D. Dakin, "The Antiseptic Action of Hypochlorites: The Ancient History of the 'New Antiseptic,'" *Br Med J* 2 [1915]: 809–19).

77   Richard Jay Hutto, *Their Gilded Cage: The Jekyll Island Club Members* (Macon, Ga.: Henchard Press, 2006), 75. Christian Herter was a founding member of the Rockefeller Institute for Medical Research and served on its original board of directors (see George W. Corner, *A History of the Rockefeller Institute: 1901–1953, Origins and Growth* [New York: The Rockefeller Institute Press, 1964], 32–33). In fact microbiologist William Welch was also approached to work but declined the offer.

78   Their seminal work on pulmonary artery valvuloplasty was published as:
      T. Tuffier and A. Carrel, "Patching and Section of the Pulmonary Orifice of
      the Heart," *J Exp Med* 20 (1914): 3–8. Carrel had received the Nobel Prize
      in Physiology or Medicine in 1912 for his work on vascular suturing and
      anastomoses.

79   Carrel seemed extremely attached to this magnanimous French surgeon who
      died in 1929. In 1932, in the journal *Revue de Paris*, Carrel provided a glowing
      tribute to the great Tuffier, who was instrumental in organizing a collaborative
      effort among the Allies in wound care. "Neither distance, nor time, nor fatigue
      exists for him when he knows that, by his training, he can help one who suf-
      fers," Carrel wrote of his dear friend and mentor (A. Carrel, "Tuffier," *Revue de
      Paris* 39 [1932]: 347–59). See also comments regarding the two from Carrel's
      biographer Robert Soupault in *Alexis Carrel 1873–1944* (Paris: Librairie Plon,
      1952), 107–42.

80   Cushing, *From a Surgeon's Journal*, 31.

81   Corner, *A History of the Rockefeller Institute*, 136. For a discussion of Alexis Car-
      rel's trials and achievements with wound care during World War I see Hamilton,
      The First Transplant Surgeon, 196–204.

82   Carrel had requested these quality nurses on the advice of his friend and col-
      league, the distinguished Swiss surgeon Theodor Kocher, who himself had used
      these nurses since 1908. The École d'Infirmières de la Source was founded in
      1859 by Countess Valérie de Gasparin and her husband, the Count Agénor de
      Gasparin, and was the first secular school for nursing in the world.

83   Carrel's rather detailed description of combined surgical, medical, and bacte-
      riological interrogation of the recently wounded is contained in his presenta-
      tion before l'Académie de médecine in October 1915 and can be reviewed in
      A. Carrel, H. Dakin, M. Daufresne, et al., "Traitement Abortif de l'Infection
      des Plaies," *Bull l' Académie Natl Med* 74 (1915): 361–68. The paper was actually
      presented by longtime Carrel admirer Samuel Pozzi, who claimed that Théodore
      Tuffier ascribed eight hundred of the one thousand amputations he witnessed to
      infectious complications and not the degree of trauma.

84   For a rather lively and not always gentlemanly discussion of the topic, see
      P. Delbert, "Actions de Certains Antiseptiques sur le Pus," *Bull et Mem Société
      Chir* 42 (1916): 92–110, from which this quote was taken.

85   Alexis Carrel and Georges Dehelly, *The Treatment of Infected Wounds* (Toronto:
      The Macmillan Company, 1917), 10–12. Alexis Carrel had a fiery temper and
      held his tongue almost never. In a chance encounter, he had once called Madame
      Marie Curie "a most conceited and ugly old woman" (see N. Whitfield, "Surgical
      Skills Beyond Scientific Management," *Med Hist* 59 [2015]: 421–42).

86   Read his complete address in A. Depage, "War Surgery," *Ann Surg* 60 (1914):
      137–42.

87   A. Depage and G. Maloens, "L'Ambulance de l'Océan à La Panne Aperçu Cli-
      nique sur les Effets Comparés de Divers Traitements des Plaies de Guerre," *Trans
      Ambul Océan La Panne* 2 (1917): 1–19. For a study of Depage's interactions with

the Belgian royal family see R. Van Hee, "Antoine Depage's Relationship with Queen Elisabeth of Belgium," *Acta Chir Belg* 112 (2012): 170–81. The term *exérèse* (excision) was used to indicate the actual parring or removal of dead or contused tissue. *Débridement* referred to the incision into skin, subcutaneous tissue, fascia, and on into muscle compartments to explore and visualize. Now *débridement* is used to indicate both techniques. For further review see T. S. Helling and E. Daon, "In Flanders Fields: The Great War, Antoine Depage, and the Resurgence of Débridement," *Ann Surg* 228 (1998): 173–81.

88 G. Ahreiner, "Ueber Behandlung der Schußwunden und den Wert der Dakin'schen Lösung," *Beiträge zur Klinischen Chirurgie* 107 (1917): 286–96.

89 Bier wrote a rather lengthy treatise on the subject: Auguste Bier, *Hyperämie als Heilmittel* (Leipzig: F. C. W. Vogel, 1903).

90 A. Bier, "Anaerobe Wundinfektion (Abgesehen von Wundstarrkrampf)," *Beiträge zur Klinischen Chirurgie* 101 (1916): 271–335.

91 A. Thies, "Ueber Zwei Hauptformen der Gasinfektion," *Beiträge zur Klinischen Chirurgie* 109 (1918): 157–93.

92 Thies detailed his method in a 1917 publication, even providing a number of anecdotal cases and pictures, in A. Thies, "Die Behandlung der Gasphlegmone mit der Rhythmischen Stauung," *Beiträge zur Klinischen Chirurgie* 105 (1917): 595–636.

93 E. Behring and S. Kitasato, "Ueber das Zustandekommen der Diphtherie-Immunität und der Tetanus-Immunität bei Thieren," *Dtsch Med Wochenschr* 16 (1890): 1113–14. Behring and Kitasato actually used rabbit sera in their animal experiments. See P. Ehrlich, "Experimentelle Untersuchungen über Immunität," *Dtsch Med Wochenschr* 17 (1891): 1218–19. "In the blood there is a body [*Körper*]," Ehrlich wrote, which "paralyzes" offensive agents. He ascribed *antikörperbedingen* (antibody-related) properties to it. Regarding the conquest of tetany, see P. Wever and L. van Bergen, "Prevention of Tetanus During the First World War," *Med Humanit* 38 (2012): 78–82. Mortality figures are cited in this article.

94 F. Klose, "Ueber Toxin- und Antitoxinversuche mit dem Fränkelschen Gas-brandbazillus," *Feldarztliche Beilage zur Münch. Med. Wochenschrift* 63 (1916): 723–26.

95 Read the field directive in: Sanitäts-Department des Königlich Preussischen Kriegsministeriums, *Veröffentlichungen aus dem Gebiete des Militär-Sanitätswesens* (Berlin: Springer-Verlag, 1918), 1–20.

96 F. Klose, "Gasödemschutz und–Bekämpfung," *Beiträge zur Klinischen Chirurgie*, 113 (1918): 76–98 (Klose 87–98). Later testing of the German antisera after War's end showed primary activity against *B. sporogenes* (probably *B. oedematiens*) and *V. septique*, and almost no activity against *B. perfringens*, very similar to the Entente vaccine; see H. Henry, "On the Antitoxin Content of some Gas Gangrene Sera used in the Later Stages of the War," *J Path* 23 (1920): 270–72.

97 M. Weinberg, "Bacteriological and Experimental Researches ion Gas Gangrene," *Proc Roy Soc Med* 9 (1916): 119–44.

98 C. Franz, "Die Wundinfektionskrankheiten," in *Kriegschirurgie*, ed. Carl Franz (Leipzig: Werner Klinkhardt, 1920) 65. Franz admits that the true frequency is hard to come by. Some doctors overreported, some underreported. Nevertheless, despite its voracity it was an uncommon occurrence. "A final verdict on the number [of gas gangrene cases] is still hard to come by. What is certain is that among rank and file doctors many cases have been incorrectly subsumed under this disease." (Franz, "Die Wundinfektionskrankheiten," 66).

99 Information from "Statistiques de la guerre 14–18", *Centre de documentation de Val-de-Grâce, Archives du Service de Santé des Armées*, Paris.

100 G. D. Shanks, "How World War 1 Changed Global Attitudes to War and Infectious Diseases," *Lancet* 384 (2014): 1699–1707.

101 L. S. Pilcher, "The Influence of War Surgery upon Civil Practice," *Ann Surg* 69 (1919): 565–74.

CHAPTER FIVE

1 John. J. Pershing, *Final Report* (Washington, DC: Government Printing Office, 1919).

2 See also Augustin M. Prentiss, *Chemicals in War: A Treatise on Chemical Warfare* (New York: McGraw-Hill Book Company, 1936).

3 See Dietrich Schindler and Jiri Toman, *The Laws of Armed Conflicts* (Leiden: Martinus Nijhoff Publishers, 1988), 22–34. See also, T. L. Dowdeswell, "The Brussels Peace Conference of 1874 and the Modern Laws of Belligerent Qualification," *Osgoode Hall Law Journal* 54 (2017): 805–50.

4 James Brown Scott, Director, *The Proceedings of the Hague Peace Conferences: The Conference of 1899* (New York: Oxford University Press, 1920), 266–68. For an in-depth discussion of this topic, see S. Barcroft, "The Hague Peace Conference of 1899," *Irish Studies in International Affairs* 3 (1989): 55–68.

5 Account related in *Der Weltkrieg 1914 bis 1918: Die Operationen des Jahres 1915*, Reicharchiv (Berlin: E. S. Mittler & Sohn, 1932), 39–41; and C. E. Heller, "The Introduction of Gas Warfare in World War I," in *Chemical Warfare in World War I: The American Experience, 1917–1918*, ed. Charles E. Heller (Fort Leavenworth, Kan.: Combat Studies Institute, 1984), 3–34.

6 Harry L. Gilchrist, *A Comparative Study of World War Casualties from Gas and Other Weapons* (Edgewood, Md.: Chemical Warfare School, 1928), 9.

7 From the journal of Willi Siebert, a German soldier who witnessed the first gas attack, courtesy of In Flanders Fields Museum, Ypres, Belgium. https://www.inflandersfields.be/nl/in-flanders-fields-museum/mensen, accessed 9/10/2021.

8 Will Irwin, "The German Army Dispersed Chlorine Gas Over Allied Lines at Ypres on 22 April 1915," *New York Tribune*, April 27, 1915.

9 "Germany Forswore Gas," *New York Times*, May 26, 1916, 1, from which quotes were taken.

10   For example, see the report in the periodical *Current Opinion*, a quasi-scientific review at the time: "Nature and Effect of Asphyxiating Gases in the Trenches," *Current Opinion* 59 (July 1915): 36–37.

11   Allies and Entente were interchangeable terms designating the coalition of Western powers opposed to Germany, primary of which were England, France, Belgium, and Italy.

12   Cables were dredged up and severed on August 5, 1914, after the British ultimatum to Berlin had expired. See P. M. Kennedy, "Imperial Cable Communication and Strategy, 1870–1914," *English Historical Review* 86 (1971): 728–52.

13   "Berlin Statement Cites Alleged French War Ministry Note—Calls Gas Humane Weapon," *New York Times*, June 26, 1915, 2.

14   Harvey Cushing, *From a Surgeon's Journal* (Boston: Little, Brown, and Company, 1936), 69.

15   The vivid descriptions of men affected by chlorine gas can be found in J. R. Bradford and T. R. Elliott, "Cases of Gas Poisoning among the British Troops in Flanders," *Br J Surg* 3 (1915): 234–46. Chlorine gas is a respiratory irritant that can affect the entire tracheobronchial tree and lung tissue itself. Acute lung injury can result in massive pulmonary edema, a condition known as adult respiratory distress syndrome (ARDS).

16   Information from No. 8 Casualty Clearing Station: J. E. Black, T. G. Glenny, and J. W. McNee, "Observations on Six Hundred and Eighty-five Cases of Poisoning by Noxious Gases Used by the Enemy," *Br Med J* 24 (1915): 509–18.

17   Fritz Haber, *Fünf Vorträge aus den Jahren 1920–1923* (Berlin: Julius Springer, 1924), 36.

18   E. Jones, "Terror Weapons: The British Experience of Gas and its Treatment in the First World War," *War Hist* 21 (2014): 355–75.

19   "Comment Bonnot Fut Pris et Tué," *Le Petit Parisien*, April 29, 1912.

20   Ministère de la Guerre, "Notice sur les Engins Suffocants, 21 févier 1915," Service Historique de la Défense, Vincennes. This circular apparently fell into German hands and may have contributed to their decision to employ chemical weapons that spring. See U. Trumpener, "The Road to Ypres: The Beginning of Gas Warfare in World War I," *J Modern Hist* 47 (1975): 460–80.

21   P.-L. Weiss, "Rapport sur l'Organisation d'une Commission Permanente auprès de la Commission des Etudes Chimiques de Guerre," Service Historique de la Défense (Vincennes), Paris, August 17, 1915, 16n826.

22   Justification for the German decision to use chemical weapons at Ypres can be found in W. Volkart, "Der Giftgaskrieg und seine Entstehung" *Allgemeine schweizerische Militärzeitung* 72 (1926): 69–78.

23   Apparently, one way chlorine was detected was by the observation that it had discolored brass buttons on dead soldiers' uniforms.

24   Thiosulfate reduces the chlorine molecule to its harmless anion. See also O. Lepick, "France's Political and Military Reaction in the Aftermath of the First German Chemical Offensive in April 1915: The Road to Retaliation in Kind," in *One Hundred Years of Chemical Warfare: Research, Deployment,*

Consequences, eds. B. Friedrich et al. (Berlin: Springer, 2017), 69–76. France's response to the German chemical attack is difficult to extract from the historiography. The best source, written after the war, is probably Charles Moureu, *La Chimie et la Guerre: Science et Avenir* (Paris: Masson, 1920), although even there, the time sequences for development of protective devices are a bit confusing.

25   Weiss, *"Rapport."*

26   For an in-depth description of the French chemical weapons program, see E. Vinet, "La Guerre des Gaz et les Travaux des Services Chimiques Français," *Chimie & Industrie* 2 (1919): 1377–1415.

27   M. D'Aubigny, "Rapport sur les Armements," *Les Archives de la Grande Guerre* 8 (1921): 487–538.

28   See Denis Varaschin and Lodovic Laloux, *10 Mars 1906, Courrières, aux Risques de l'Histoire* (Paris: Éditions GRHEN, 2006). So impressive were the respirators that mine rescue workers in the United States were known as Drägermen.

29   See Dietrich Stoltzenberg, *Fritz Haber: Chemist, Nobel Laureate, German, Jew* (Philadelphia: Chemical Heritage Press, 2004), 14–243.

30   Moureu, *Le Chimie et Guerre*, 60.

31   War Office (Chemical Warfare Department), National Archives, London, UK, WO 142/183. See also Simon Jones, *World War I Gas Warfare Tactics and Equipment* (Oxford: Osprey Publishing, 2007), 16–21.

32   Arthur Alan Hansbury-Sparrow, *The Land-Locked Lake* (London: Arthur Barker, 1932), 309.

33   B. Evans, "A Doctor in the Great War—An Interview with Sir Geoffrey Marshall," *Brit Med J* 285 (1982): 1783.

34   Marion Leslie Girard, *A Strange and Formidable Weapon* (Lincoln: University of Nebraska Press, 2008), 76–101.

35   Georges Duhamel, *Vie des Martyrs 1914–1916* (Paris: Mercure de France, 1917), 128.

36   Figures and description of this tragic attack can be found in Alan Clark, *The Donkeys* (London: Pimlico, 1961), 173.

37   T. C. Nicholson-Roberts, "Phosgene Uses in World War 1 and Early Evaluations of Pathophysiology," *J R Army Med Corps* 165 (2019): 183–87.

38   Woods Hutchinson, *The Doctor in War* (Boston: Houghton Mifflin Company, 1918), 181.

39   W. G. Macpherson, "Development of Gas Warfare" in W. G. Macpherson [Ed] *Medical Services, Diseases of the War*, Vol II (London: His Majesty's Stationery Office, 1923), 271–323.

40   *Le Filon*, March 20, 1917, in Stéphane Audoin-Rouzeau, *Men At War 1914–1918* (Oxford: Berg, 1992), 72. Trench newspapers were literally composed and produced in the trenches by soldiers under fire on the western front. Most publications described conditions and events as they actually occurred without the whitewashing of the government.

41   See J. Krause, "The Origins of Chemical Warfare in the French Army," *War in History* 20 (2013): 545–56; and Heller, "The Introduction of Gas Warfare," 18.

42   See H. S. Hulbert, "Gas Neurosis Syndrome," *Am J Insanity* 77 (1920): 213–16.

43   Robert Graves, *Good-bye To All That* (New York: Doubleday, 1929), 154–55.

44   Prentiss, *Chemicals in War*, 658–60.

45   The Yellow Cross (*Gelbkreuz*) shell was so named because a yellow cross was painted on the shaft of the canister to indicate a vesicant agent. For further information on mustard gas, see also Amos A. Fries and Clarence J. West, *Chemical Warfare* (New York: McGraw-Hill Book Company, 1921), 150.

46   A. S. Warthin and C. V. Weller, "The Lesions of the Respiratory and Gastrointestinal Tracts Produced by Mustard Gas (Dichlorethylsulfide)," *J Lab Clin Med* 4 (1919): 229–64.

47   Prentiss, *Chemicals in War*, 180. These figures are at odds with those tallied by Macpherson, *Development of Gas Warfare*, 292–93. He recorded 2,143 gas admissions and 86 deaths to 4 casualty clearing stations in that sector.

48   L. F. Haber, *The Poisonous Cloud* (Oxford: Clarendon Press, 1986), 218. See also Roy MacLeod and Jeffrey A. Johnson, *Frontline and Factory: Comparative Perspectives on the Chemical Industry at War, 1914–1924* (Berlin: Springer Science, 2007), 209–10.

49   Moureu, *Le Chimie et Guerre*, 79, 85.

50   Figures from James E. Edmonds, *Military Operations France and Belgium 1918* (London: Macmillan and Co., 1935), 153, 158. Haber also mentioned the same distribution of gas to high explosive rounds (Haber, *Poisonous Cloud*, 214).

51   Like Yellow Cross shells, Green Cross (*Grünkreuz*) shells had the fuse tip painted green and a green cross at the bottom of the cartridge to indicate a pulmonary agent. Similarly, Blue Cross (*Blaukreuz*) shells had the canister shaft colored blue to indicate an upper-respiratory agent. The larger caliber howitzers could fire an enormous amount of the mustard. The German 8.3-inch howitzer tossed shells containing almost three gallons of the liquid for a distance of six miles. See S.J.M. Auld, *Gas and Flame in Modern Warfare* (New York: George H. Doran Company, 1918), 173.

52   Prentiss, *Chemicals in War*, 190.

53   See commentary by Fries, *Chemical Warfare*, 177–78.

54   *Reports of the Secretary of War and Surgeon General, War Department Annual Reports, 1917* (Washington, DC: Government Printing Office, 1918), 52–53 and 335–789.

55   See Fries, *Chemical Warfare*, 32–34. Soon work outstripped the facilities in Washington, DC, and other laboratories in Pittsburgh, Cleveland, and Madison, Wisconsin were recruited.

56   War Department, *Annual Report 1918, Director Chemical War Service* (Washington, DC: Government Printing Office, 1919), 1399–1403.

57   War College, *Memorandum on Gas Poisoning in Warfare* (Washington, DC: Government Printing Office, 1917).

58   Leo P. Brophy, Wyndham D. Miles, and Rexmond C. Cochrane, *The Chemical Warfare Service: From Laboratory to Field* (Washington, DC: Office of Military History, 1959), 7–8.

59   See L. P. Brophy, "Origins of the Chemical Corps," *Military Affairs* 20 (1956):
     217–26; and W. D. Bancroft, et al., "Medical Aspects of Gas Warfare," in *The
     Medical Department of The United States Army in the World War*, vol. 14 (Wash-
     ington, DC: Government Printing Office, 1926), 25–771.

60   Robert Lee Bullard, *Personalities and Reminiscences of the War* (New York: Dou-
     bleday, Page & Company, 1925), 159.

61   "Memorandum No. 45: Instruction and Training—Gas, Headquarters First Divi-
     sion, American Expeditionary Forces, France, December 1, 1917" (World War
     Records: First Division, A.E.F., vol. 20, 1928). Six lectures on various aspects of
     gas warfare were also developed to be given at the regimental and battalion level by
     gas officers. As a final test, the commanding general of the First Division required
     his men to play a baseball game with masks on (Bullard, *Personalities*, 159).

62   A. W. Catlin, *"With the Help of God and a Few Good Marines"* (New York: Dou-
     bleday, Page & Company, 1919), 55.

63   "Defense Against Gas," Memorandum A.E.F. No. 1433, General Headquarters,
     American Expeditionary Force, 1918, 7.

64   Rexmond C. Cochrane, *The 1st Division at Ansauville, January—April 1918*
     (Washington, DC: US Army Chemical Corps Historical Office, 1958).

65   *History of the First Division during the World War 1917–1919* (Philadelphia: John
     C. Winston Company, 1922), 52.

66   Cochrane, "The 1st Division at Ansauville," 24–25.

67   Erich Maria Remarque, *All Quiet on the Western Front* (New York: Ballantine
     Books, 1928, 1956), 130–31.

68   Harry L. Gilchrist and Philip B. Matz, *The Residual Effects of Wartime Gases*
     (Washington, DC: Government Printing Office, 1933), 44.

69   A topical paste, called SAG paste (*GAS* spelled backward), was applied to many
     victims. The paste, an ointment of zinc stearate, had some mollifying effect on
     blistered skin. It had the consistency of Vaseline. See reports in Bancroft, "Med-
     ical Aspects of Gas Warfare," 769–70.

70   By the end of the war, numbers of gassed men were so great that one in four divi-
     sional field hospitals was reserved for chemical victims.

71   See Prentiss, *Chemicals in War*, 578–85.

72   Charles Grasty, "New German Gas Causes Blindness," *New York Times*, Sep-
     tember 2, 1918, 4.

73   Quoted in Robert B. Asprey, *At Belleau Wood* (Denton: University of North Texas
     Press, 1996), 289–90.

74   H. Cale, "The American Marines at Verdun, Chateau Thierry, Bouresches, and
     Belleau Wood," *Indiana Magazine of History* 15 (1919): 179–91.

75   Rexmond C. Cochrane, *Gas Warfare at Belleau Wood, June 1918* (Washington,
     DC: US Army Chemical Corps Historical Office, 1957), 34.

76   P. Brown, "Memorandum for Colonel Gilchrist, Medical Corps, June 16, 1918,"
     quoted in Wilder D. Bancroft et al., "Medical Aspects of Gas Warfare," in *The
     Medical Department of the United States Army in the World War*, vol 14, ed. M. W.
     Ireland (Washington, DC: Government Printing Office, 1926), 70.

77 It is difficult to say where the term *Devil Dogs* originated. It certainly was the Fourth Brigade at Belleau Wood responsible for it, however. Some say the Germans, seeing the Marines advance uphill at one point, often on all fours and with gas masks on, had the appearance of unworldly beasts rather than humans.

78 Cochrane, *Gas Warfare*, 66.

79 Asprey, *At Belleau Wood*, 175.

80 A. A. Fries, "Chemical Warfare Service," *Infantry Journal* 21 (1923): 530.

81 Edward G. Lengel, *To Conquer Hell* (New York: Henry Holt and Company, 2008), 391.

82 Statistics from: A. G. Love, "Medical and Casualty Statistics," in *The Medical Department of the United States Army in the World War*, vol. 15, ed. M. W. Ireland (Washington, DC: Government Printing Office, 1925), 1019, 1021; A. G. Love, "War Casualties," *Army Medical Bulletin No. 24*, (Carlisle Barracks, Penn., 1931), 76; Gilchrist, *World War Casualties*, 10–21; and Prentiss, *Chemicals in War*, 671.

83 J. B. S. Haldane, *Callinicus: A Defence of Chemical Warfare* (New York: E.P. Dutton & Company, 1925), 52.

84 Frederick W. Holls, *The Peace Conference at The Hague* (New York: The Macmillan Company, 1900), 119.

85 Prentiss, *Chemicals in War*, 679–80.

86 Constance M. Pechura and David P. Rall, eds., *Veterans at Risk: The Health Effects of Mustard Gas and Lewisite* (Washington: National Academy Press, 1993), 8.

87 See J. A. Vilensky and P. R. Sinish, "The Dew of Death," *Bull Atomic Scientists* 60 (2004): 54–60. Apparently, German chemists were familiar with Lewis's arsenic compound but had discarded it as it was not stable in water.

88 Prentiss, *Chemicals in War*, 696.

89 See William Augerson, *A Review of the Scientific Literature as it Pertains to the Gulf War Illnesses* (Santa Monica, Calif.: RAND Corporation, 2000).

CHAPTER SIX

1 See Edward Berenson, *The Trial of Madame Caillaux* (Berkeley: University of California Press, 1992), 130.

2 See Crookes's theory developed in R. K. DeKosky, "William Crookes and the Fourth State of Matter," *Isis* 67 (1976): 36–60.

3 W. Robert Nitske, *The Life of Wilhelm Conrad Röntgen, Discoverer of the X Ray* (Tucson: University of Arizona Press, 1971), 5. This intriguing biography by Robert Nitske served as a primary reference source on Wilhelm Röntgen.

4 W. C. Röntgen, "Uber Eine Neue Art von Strahlen," *Sitzungsberichte der Physika-lische-Medizinischen Gesellschaft zu Würzburg* (1895): 137–47.

5 Otto Glasser, *Wilhelm Conrad Röntgen and the Early History of the Roentgen Rays* (Springfield, Ill.: Norman Publishing, 1993), 199. Also see Otto Glasser and Margret Boveri, *Wilhelm Conrad Röntgen und Die Geschichte der Röntgenstrahlen* (Berlin: Springer-Verlag, 2013), 147–48.

6   "Un Decouverte Sensationnelle," *Le Petit Parisien*, January 10, 1896, 1.

7   Nitske, *Wilhelm Conrad Röntgen*, 162.

8   Susan Quinn, *Marie Curie: A Life* (Boston: Da Capo Press, 1995), figures 140.

9   "Notes," *Nature* 53 (1896): 253.

10   M. Oudin and M. Barthelemy, "Communiquent une Photographie des Os de la Main Obtenue a l'aide des 'X.-Strahlen.'" *Comptes Rendus de l'Acad Sci* 122 (1896): 150–51.

11   See J. A. del Regato, "Antoine Béclère," *Int J Radiation Oncology Biol Phys* 4 (1978): 1069–79.

12   For reference, see J. D. Rolleston, "Dr. Antoine Béclère," *Nature* 143 (1939): 591.

13   Destot eventually lost a number of fingers to the harmful effects of radiation, although he still consulted in radiology during the war years. He died in 1918. See V. Baca, D. Kachlik, T. Bacova, et al., "Anatomist and the Pioneer of Radiology Étienne Destot—95th Anniversary of his Death," *Clin Anat* 27 (2014): 282–85; and N. Foray, M. Amiel, and R. Mornex, "Étienne Destot (1864–1918) ou l'Autre Père de la Radiologie Française," *Cancer/ Radiothérapie* 21 (2017): 138–47.

14   See as an example A. Buguet and A. Gascard, "Détermination à l'aide des rayons X de la profondeur où siège un corps étranger dans les tissus," *Comptes Rendus de l'Acad Sci* 122 (1896): 786–87.

15   T. Dineur, "Balle de Revolver Perdue dans la Jambe et Découverte par la Radiographie," *Arch Med Belges* 21 (1896): 330–35.

16   See G. Pallardy, "La Radiologie est Entrée Avant l' Électricité dans les Hôpitaux de Paris," *Hist Sci Med* 33 (1999): 333–42.

17   G. Alvaro, "I Vantaggi Practici della Scoperta de Röntgen in Chirurgia," *Giornale medico del Regio Esercito* 44 (1896): 385–94.

18   H. Küttner, "Ueber die Bedeutung der Röntgenstrahlen für die Kriegschirurgie: Nach Erfahrungen im Griechisch-Türkischen Krieg 1897," *Beitr Klinische Chir* 20 (1898): 167–229.

19   H. Niehues, "Ueber den Heutigen Stand der Verwendung von Röntgenstrahlen im Kriege," *Berliner Klinische Wochenschrift* 46 (1909): 2293–96.

20   W. C. Borden, *The Use of the Röntgen Ray by the Medical Department of the United States Army in the War with Spain (1898)* (Washington, DC: Government Printing Office, 1900), 11.

21   N. Senn, "Recent Experience in Military Surgery After the Battle of Santiago," *J. Mil Service Institute* 23 (1898): 309–23.

22   J. C. Battersby, "The Roentgen Rays in Military Surgery," *Brit Med J* 1 (1899): 112–14.

23   J.-J. Ferrandis and A. Segal, "L'Essor de la Radiologie Osseuse Pendant la Guerre de 1914–1918," in *Journées d'Histoire des Maladies des Os et des Articulations*, ed. B.-P. Amor, P. Bonnichon, and D. Gourevitch, *Rhumatologie Pratique* 267 (2009): 48–50.

24   Ève Curie, *Madame Curie*, trans. Vincent Sheean (London: William Heinemann, 1938), 280.

25 Shelley Emling, *Marie Curie and Her Daughters* (New York: Palgrave Macmillan, 2012), 25.

26 Quinn, *Curie*, 355.

27 *Ibid.*, 356.

28 Marie Curie, *La Radiologie et la Guerre* (Paris: Felix Alcan, 1921), 4.

29 Marie Curie, *Pierre Curie*, trans. Charlotte Kellogg and Vernon Kellogg (New York: The Macmillan Company, 1923), 210.

30 Curie, *La Radiologie et la Guerre*, 11, 115.

31 Quinn, *Curie*, 361. The French had partitioned the country into two basic zones: the *zone de l'intérieur* consisted of areas far removed from the front lines—what would be considered the rear areas—and under control of the central government; and the *zone des armées*—areas much nearer combat and under firm control by the military. At the start of the war radiology facilities were basically confined to the *zone de l'intérieur*.

32 G. Pallardy and M.-J. Pallardy, "Georges Massiot: Ingénieur-Constructeur et Manipulateur," in *1895–1995 Le Premier Siècle de la Radiologie* (l'Association Française du Personnel Paramédical d'Electroradiologie [Special Issue]) (1995): 32–38. See also J. LeVot, "La Radiologie Militaire au Cours du Premier Conflit Mondial," *Médecine et Armées* 44 (2015): 55–61. Germans were working on a portable automobile unit, too. They had in mind a two-car system with all elements for radiology services contained. Later units could store all equipment in one vehicle carrying four tons of dynamos, tubes, tables, and plates. See L. Brauer and F. Haenisch, "Eins selbständige, transportable Feldröntgenanlage fiir interne und chirurgische Untersuchungen," *Fortschritte auf dem Gebiete der Röntgenstrahlen [RöFo]* 23 (1915/1916): 38–46.

33 Read Haret's compelling argument in M. Haret, "Le Role de la Voiture Radiologique du Service de Santé aux Armées," *J de Radiol et d'Electrol* 1 (1915): 497–99.

34 Ferrandis and Ségal, "L'Essor de la Radiologie."

35 Quinn, *Curie*, 364.

36 Curie, *La Radiologie et la Guerre*, 36.

37 See G. Pallardy and J. P. Mabille, "Antoine Béclère," *J Radiol* 80 (1999): 600–03.

38 Comprising the Patronage national des blessés were members of the Parisian intelligentsia who donated time, money, and prestige to projects directed toward providing medical supplies (now including X-rays) to the front. It was directed by Ernest Lavisse, head of the École normale supérieure.

39 Ève Curie, *Madame Curie*, 287.

40 *Ibid.*, 289.

41 Marie Curie and Irène Curie, *Correspondence: Choix de Lettres, 1905–1934*, ed. Gillette Ziegler (Paris: Éditeurs français réunis, 1974), 129.

42 Curie, *Pierre Curie*, 215.

43 Curie, *Madame Curie*, 289–90.

44 Quinn, *Curie*, 366.

45 Ferrandis and Ségal, "L'Essor de la Radiologie."

46 Emling, *Marie Curie*, 26.

47   Universal conscription originated in France during the Revolution of 1798 and
      continued through the Great War, even for men up to the age of forty-five.

48   Edith Cavell was an English nurse who was executed as a spy by the Germans in
      1915. She became a rallying point for the Allies.

49   Curie, *La Radiologie et la Guerre*, 111.

50   *Ibid.*, 112.

51   For further discussion see C. M. Bourne and R. K. Chhem, "War Medicine as
      Springboard for Early Knowledge Construction in Radiology," *Med Studies* 4
      (2014): 53–70.

52   "Le Rôle de Mme Curie Pendant la Guerre," *Le Figaro*, February 14, 1922
      (reported first in *L'Echo National*).

53   In fact, Curie had moved her supply of radium to Bordeaux at the start of the
      war, fearing it would fall into German hands if Paris were occupied. It was
      returned to Paris in 1915. Marie tried to find some application of radium therapy
      for wounded soldiers but her efforts were to be of no proven benefit.

54   Hans Wehberg, *Wider den Aufruf der 93!* (Berlin: Deusche Verlagsgesellschaft für
      Politik u. Geschichte, 1920), 16.

55   See Gerd Rosenbusch and Annemarie de Knecht-van-Eekelen, *Wilhelm Conrad
      Röntgen: The Birth of Radiology* (Berlin: Springer, 2019), 139–52.

CHAPTER SEVEN

1   Harvey Cushing, *From a Surgeon's Journal* (Boston: Little, Brown, and Company,
      1936), 177.

2   Cushing, *From a Surgeon's Journal*, 47.

3   John F. Fulton, *Harvey Cushing: A Biography* (Springfield, Ill.: Charles C.
      Thomas, 1946), 205.

4   George H. B. MacLeod, *Notes on the Surgery of the War in the Crimea with
      Remarks on the Treatment of Gunshot Wounds* (Philadelphia: J. B. Lippincott &
      Co., 1862), 160.

5   *Ibid.*, 178.

6   *Ibid.*, 183.

7   A. H. Bennett and R. J. Godlee, "Case of Cerebral Tumour—The Surgical
      Treatment," *Brit Med J* 1 (1885): 988–89. See also "Alexander Hughes Ben-
      nett (1848–1901) and Rickman John Godlee (1849–1925)," *CA Cancer J Clin* 24
      (1974): 169–70.

8   H. Cushing, "The Special Field of Neurological Surgery," *Bull Johns Hopkins Hosp*
      16 (1905): 77–87.

9   Michael Bliss, *Harvey Cushing: A Life in Surgery* (Oxford: Oxford University
      Press, 2005), 171.

10   W. Macewen, "An Address of the Surgery of the Brain and Spinal Cord," *Brit
      Med J* 2 (1888): 302–09.

11   E. Bergmann, "Surgical Treatment of Diseases of the Brain," in *Wood's Medical
      and Surgical Monographs*, vol. 6, ed. W. Wood (New York: William Wood &
      Co., 1890), 768.

12   Ernst von Bergmann, *Die Lehre von den Kopfverletzun* (Stuttgart: Ferdinand
      Enke, 1880), 130.

13   *Ibid.*, 893.

14   Theodor Kocher, *Hirnerschütterung Hirndruck und Chirurgische Eingriffe bei Herz-
      krankheiten* (Wien: Alfred Hölder, 1901), 361.

15   Kocher, *Hirnerschütterung*, 441.

16   P. Coryllos, "Le Traitement des Plaies du Crane par Projectiles de Guerre," *Arch
      Chir* (Le Mans) 50 (1915): 1–49.

17   R. Bárány, "Die Offene und Geschlossene Behandlung der Schussverletzungen
      des Gehirns," *Beiträge zur Klinischen Chirurgie* 97 (1915): 397–417. Actually,
      Bárány's patients had not been subjected to the manured soil of France's farms
      and so were spared exposure to the bacilli of gas gangrene. Yet, undoubtedly,
      early operation helped.

18   W. Penfield, "Sir Percy Sargent, 1873–1933," *Arch NeurPsych* 30 (1933): 413–14. See
      also a synopsis of the life of Sir Victor Horsley by M. P. Powell, "Sir Victor Horsley
      at the Birth of Neurosurgery," *Brain* 139 (2016): 631–34. Horsley himself would
      become a victim of the war, dying of heatstroke and typhus in present-day Iraq.

19   See P. Sargent and G. Holmes, "The Treatment of the Cranial Injuries of War-
      fare," *Brit Med J* 1 (1915): 537–41.

20   Fulton, *Harvey Cushing*, 184.

21   The hemodynamic relationship of flow (F), pressure (P), and resistance (R) is
      depicted in the equation $\Delta P = F \times R$. As intracranial resistance (tissue swelling
      from trauma, as an example) increases, then either blood flow must decrease or
      pressure inside the cranium will increase.

22   See H. Cushing, "Surgery of the Head," in *Surgery: Its Principles and Practice*,
      vol. 5, ed. William Williams Keen (Philadelphia: W. B. Saunders Company,
      1908), 17–276. Of interest are the drawings depicting various surgical maneuvers
      on the brain, all surgeons working with bare hands.

23   Fulton, *Harvey Cushing*, 268.

24   *Ibid.*, 270.

25   Cushing, "Surgery of the Head," 64.

26   For details of his operative preparations for craniotomy, see H. Cushing, "Tech-
      nical Methods of Performing Certain Cranial Operations," *Surg Gynecol Obstet* 6
      (1908): 227–46.

27   Fulton, *Harvey Cushing*, 388.

28   Cushing, *From a Surgeon's Journal*, 17.

29   *Ibid.*, 46.

30   Harvey Cushing, *Tumors of the Nervus Acusticus and the Syndrome of the Cerebel-
      lopontine Angle* (Philadelphia: W. B. Saunders Company, 1917), 14. It is not clear,
      in his summation of cases, whether he had personally performed that many cases
      or whether this is a compilation of the experiences of all faculty of those institu-
      tions (Johns Hopkins Hospital and the Peter Bent Brigham Hospital).

31   Cushing gave a thorough discussion of his experiences in Paris, including
      detailed case histories and illustrative radiographs, in H. Cushing, "Concerning

Operations for the Cranio-Cerebral Wounds of Modern Warfare," *Mil Surg* 38 (1916): 601–15.

32   See A. Bowlby, "The Development of British Surgery at the Front," *Brit Med J* 1 (1917): 705–21. This article, published before Cushing's involvement in the Ypres sector, probably embodied views not necessarily representative of Cushing's phi-losophy of management at the time.

33   Cushing, *From a Surgeon's Journal*, 160, 165. While Cushing did not mention Bowlby's directive in his journal there, is mention made of Casualty Clearing Station No. 46 to be designated for head cases in Bliss, *Harvey Cushing*, 321.

34   The Battle of Passchendaele, as it has come to be called, was also named the Third Battle of Ypres. Passchendaele was a small town that lay on the last ridge east of Ypres and, if captured, would have allowed the Allies easier access to the German rear areas in Belgium. The town itself was literally wiped off the face of the earth. The British eventually captured Passchendaele ridge but found additional bands of German defenses beyond and simply gave up, all at a cost of almost 250,000 British troops.

35   David Lloyd George, *War Memoirs 1917* (Boston: Little, Brown, and Company, 1934), 320.

36   Cushing, *From a Surgeon's Journal*, 176.

37   C. W. Rand, "Doctor Cushing As I Knew Him," *Bull Los Angeles Neurological Soc* 5 (1940): 1–8.

38   Fulton, *Harvey Cushing*, 163.

39   Fulton makes this comment in his biography (Fulton, *Harvey Cushing*, 441). Cushing proclaimed his better results by virtue of his careful, uncompromising operative approach.

40   See M. Rollet, "Extraction des Balles Allemandes et des Éclats d'Obus a l'Électro-aimant Géant," *Comptes rendus Séances de l'Académie des Sciences* 159 (1914): 562–64. For an entertaining synopsis of electromagnetism and medicine see J. R. Basford, "A Historical Perspective of the Popular Use of Electric and Magnetic Therapy," *Arch Phys Med Rehab* 82 (2001): 261–69. The magnet would only work with fragments containing nickel or iron alloys.

41   This new stereotactic technique was the brainchild of a little-known Parisian scientist by the name of Gaston Contremoulins. Teaming with surgeon Charles Rémy in 1897 the two had successfully manually extracted projectiles from the heads of two patients using their new "bullet finder." See P. Bourdillon, C. Apra, and M. Lévêque, "First Clinical Use of Stereotaxy in Humans: The Key Role of X-ray Localization Discovered by Gaston Contremoulins," *J Neurosurg* 128 (2018): 932–37.

42   M. Henrard and M. Janssen, "Extraction des Projectiles Magnétique Intracéré-braux au Moyen de l'Electro-aimant et de l'Appareil Téléphonique de Hedley," *Bull et Mem Soc Chir* (Paris) 43 (1917): 1850–58. Henrard's sterotactic technique involved the three-dimensional isolation of objects within an enclosed space in order to precisely advance instruments directly to the target from *some distance away*.

43 Cushing, *From a Surgeon's Journal*, 51.

44 Charles Willems, *Manuel de Chirurgie de Guerre* (Paris: A. Maloine et fils, 1917), 119.

45 H. Cushing, "Notes on Penetrating Wounds of the Brain," *Brit Med J* 1 (1918): 221–26.

46 Cushing, *From a Surgeon's Journal*, 231.

47 Fulton, *Harvey Cushing*, 424.

48 Cushing, *From a Surgeon's Journal*, 241.

49 Cushing, "A Study of a Series of Wounds Involving the Brain and its Enveloping Structures," *Brit J Surg* 5 (1918): 558–684.

50 Casualty Clearing Stations were not infrequently bombed and shelled with occasional loss of life to patients, support staff, and medical personnel. Proven, a town in Flanders, was one of the locations for Casualty Clearing Station No. 46.

51 Fulton, *Harvey Cushing*, 439.

52 Information from Cushing, "Neurosurgery," in Charles Lynch, Frank W. Weed, Loy McAfee, *The Medical Department of the United States Army in the World War* (Washington, DC: Government Printing Office, 1927), 749–58. Cushing believed firmly in his neurosurgical teams. He claimed they were able to reduce mortality in penetrating injuries to a respectable 29 percent, compared to over 60 percent in work done by a variety of general surgeons (Cushing, "Neurosurgery," 755). Mobile hospitals of the AEF were similar to British casualty clearing stations—well-equipped and spacious surgical field hospitals.

53 See Samuel H. Greenblatt, *A History of Neurosurgery in its Scientific and Professional Contexts* (Park Ridge, Ill.: American Association of Neurological Surgeons, 1997), 311.

54 Fulton, *Harvey Cushing*, 440.

55 Cushing, *From a Surgeon's Journal*, 499.

56 See the argument for Guillain-Barrè syndrome in S. G. Reich, "Harvey Cushing's Guillain-Barrè Syndrome: An Historical Diagnosis," *Neurosurgery* 21 (1987): 135–41.

57 Ernest Sachs, *Fifty Years of Neurosurgery: A Personal Story* (New York: Vantage Press, 1958), 68.

58 Rand, "Doctor Cushing."

59 C. W. Hart, "Harvey Cushing, M.D., in His World," *J Rel Health* 53 (2014): 1923–29.

60 H. Cushing, "The Special Field of Neurological Surgery After Another Interval," *Arch Neurol Psych* 4 (1920): 603–36.

CHAPTER EIGHT

1 Ward Muir, *The Happy Hospital* (London: Simpkin, Marshall, Hamilton, Kent & Co, 1918), 143–44. Of course, one could take exception to the title "Happy" for any hospital, particularly one that contained the young, mutilated victims of war. For the disfigured, these places, without a doubt, were not happy.

2   S. A. Davidson, "Dr. Robert Tait McKenzie: A Man for all Seasons," *CMAJ* 138 (1988): 70–72.

3   R. Tait McKenzie, *Reclaiming the Maimed: A Handbook of Physical Therapy* (New York: The Macmillan Company, 1918), 117.

4   D. Le Breton, "Handicap d'Apparence: Le Regard des Autres," *Ethnologie française* 21 (1991): 323–30.

5   James R. Judd, *With the American Ambulance in France* (Honolulu: Star-Bulletin Press, 1919), 50.

6   F. X. Long, "Les Blessés de la Face Durant la Grande Guerre: Les Origines de la Chirurgie Maxillo-Faciale," *Hist Sci Med* 36 (2002): 175–83.

7   S. Delaporte, "Les Défigurés de la Grande Guerre," *Guerres Mondiales et Conflits Contemporains* 175 (1994): 103–21.

8   See V. H. Kazanjian, "Remembrance of Things Past," *Plast Reconstr Surg* 35 (1965): 5–13.

9   H. Morestin, "La Réduction Graduelle des Difformités Tégumentaires," *Bull Mem Soc Chir de Paris* 41 (1915): 1233–53. For sources on Morestin's life and career I refer to: J. P. Lalardrie, "Hippolyte Morestin 1869–1918," *Brit J Plast Surg* 25 (1972): 39–41; P. Lecène and H. Mondor, "L'Oeuvre Chirurgicale de H. Morestin," *J Chir* 16 (1920): 1–8. The date of Morestin's death is variously given as 1918 or 1919.

10   See Long, "Les Blessés de la Face."

11   *Die Gegenwärtigen Behandlungswege der Kieferschussverletzungen*, vol. 1–10, ed. Christian Bruhn (Wiesbaden: J. F. Bergmann, 1915–17); and, for an English-language summation, see W. H. Dolamore, "The Treatment of Injuries of the Face and Jaws at Dusseldorf," *J Assoc Mil Dental Surg* 2 (1918): 137–46.

12   See H. Morestin, "Des Autoplasties en Jeu de Patience," *Bull de l'Acad de Méd* 77 (1917): 371. The technique had been described by colleagues Charles Nélaton and Louis Ombrédanne from Paris in the early 1900s. I refer the reader to the extensive text written by these two surgeons: Charles Nélaton and Louis Ombrédanne, *Les Autoplasties* (Paris: G.Steinheil, 1907). The two had also published a book on rhinoplasty (nose reconstruction) in 1904 and were quite well known in facial surgery circles. Ombrédanne, initiated into the intricacies of plastic surgery by his mentor, Nélaton, devoted much of his career to pediatric patients. See J. Glicenstein, "Louis Ombrédanne (1871–1956), Chirurgien Pédiatre et Plasticien," *Ann Chir Plastique Esthétique* 60 (2015): 87–93. Yet, Morestin used autoplasty to the fullest.

13   Hippolyte Morestin was quite prolific in the year 1915. I have used as examples of his work case reports presented by Morestin in volume 41 of *Bulletin et Mémoires de la Société de Chirurgie de Paris*, specifically the following (page numbers in parentheses): "Mutilation Complexe de la Face par Blessure de Guerre" (1622–27); "Grave Difformité de la Face Consécutive à une Blessure de Guerre" (1627–31); "Les Transplantations Cartilagineuses dans la Chirurgie Réparatrice" (1994–2046); "Difformités Consécutives à une Blessure de la Face

par Balle" (2241–43). *Bull Mem Soc Chir de Paris* 41 (1915). These articles are not included in the bibliography but are sufficiently referenced here.

14 D. L. Breton, "Handicap d'Apparence: Le Regard de l'Autre," *Ethnologie française* 21 (1991): 323–30.

15 "Le docteur Hippolyte Morestin," *Le Figaro*, March 15, 1917.

16 Lecène and Mondor, "L'Oeuvre Chirurgicale."

17 Muir, *Happy Hospital*, 145.

18 B. Haiken, "Plastic Surgery and American Beauty at 1921," *Bull Hist Med* 68 (1994): 429–53.

19 Breton, "Handicap d'Apparence."

20 McKenzie, *Reclaiming the Maimed*, 117.

21 A similar veterans' organization evolved in Weimar Germany after the war, called Deutscher Reichskriegerbund (German Reich Warriors' Association).

22 M. Gehrhardt, "La Greffe Générale: The Voice of French Facially Injured Soldiers," *Modern Contemp France* 26 (2018): 353–68.

23 Charles Valadier was no longer a French national and apparently did not want to join the American contingent at Neuilly-sur-Seine.

24 Varaztad Kazanjian (1879–1974) was a skilled surgeon in his own right. A naturalized US citizen, Kazanjian completed his oral surgery training at Harvard and sailed with the Harvard unit to France in 1915. He was retained by special permission with the British forces after the Harvard people had returned to the United States and developed a superb unit for maxillofacial trauma.

25 Both quotes from R. H. Ivy, "The Mysterious A. C. Valadier," *Plast Reconstr Surg* 47 (1971): 365–70, taken from H. D. Gillies and D. R. Millard, *The Principles and Art of Plastic Surgery* (Boston: Little, Brown and Company, 1957), 6. Robert Ivy himself was an American plastic surgeon of some notoriety. He, too, saw action in World War I and treated a number of Yanks with facial injuries. See also W. P. Cruse, "Auguste Charles Valadier: A Pioneer in Maxillofacial Surgery," *Mil Med* 152 (1987): 337–41. Despite his pomposity (or because of it), Charles Valadier was knighted in 1919.

26 Simon Shorvon and Alastair Compston, *Queen Square: A History of the National Hospital and Its Institute of Neurology* (Cambridge: Cambridge University Press, 2019), 166.

27 A. C. Valadier, "A Few Suggestions for the Treatment of Fractured Jaws," *Brit J Surg* 4 (1916): 64–73.

28 Lalardrie, "Hippolyte Morestin."

29 David Tolhurst, *Pioneers in Plastic Surgery* (Berlin: Springer, 2015), 37.

30 Quote taken from Suzanne Gehrhardt, "The Destiny and Representations of Facially Disfigured Soldiers during the First World War and the Interwar Period in France, Germany and Great Britain," (PhD thesis, University of Exeter, 2013), 104. This remark, according to Gehrhardt, was contained in a letter from Harold Gillies to Ralph Mllard, September 12, 1951.

31 W. F. Breakey and J. B. Mulliken, "Sir William Arbuthnot Lane and His Contributions to Plastic Surgery," *J Craniofac Surg* 26 (2015): 1504–07.

32   Lane actually expressed these feelings after the war, in 1918, during a visit to
      the United States. See F. Martin, "Visit of Three British Surgeons to America,"
      Boston Med Surg J 179 (1918): 135–38.

33   Reference for these figures: J. E. Edmonds, "Military Operations France and
      Belgium, 1916: Sir Douglas Haig's Command to the 1st July: Battle of the
      Somme," in *History of the Great War Based on Official Documents by Direction
      of the Historical Section of the Committee of Imperial Defence*, vol. 1, ed. Impe-
      rial War Museum and Battery Press (London: Macmillan, 1932), 483. Those
      numbers are much too precise. Likely, the full extent of the carnage will never
      be known. Many men were left dead and decomposing on the battlefields or
      simply disappeared in the bursts of exploding shells.

34   A detailed description of the Queen's Hospital, Sidcup, can be found in:
      L. W. Johnson, "Queen's Hospital for Facial and Jaw Injuries, Frognal, Sidcup,
      Kent, England," *US Naval Med Bull* 14 (1920): 17–65.

35   Harold Gillies, *Plastic Surgery of the Face* (Oxford: Oxford University Press, 1920), 5.

36   *Ibid.*, 7–12.

37   Gillies was not the only one to use such vascularized pedicles. The French
      surgeon Léon Dufourmentel popularized the pedicled flap from the temporal
      scalp to assist in reconstructing the chin, a flap that carries his name. Never-
      theless, Gillies is still credited for promoting the versatile pedicle flap for wide
      clinical use. See K. W. Marck, R. Palyvoda, A. Bamji, and J. J. van Wingerden,
      "The Tubed Pedicle Flap Centennial: Its Concept, Origin, Rise, and Fall," *Eur
      J Plast Surg* 40 (2017): 473–78.

38   Gillies, *Plastic Surgery of the Face*, 19–23.

39   *Ibid.*, 364.

40   *Ibid.*, 28.

41   Retouching of photographs to soften features and convey a better outcome
      than really occurred was claimed by at least one historian: Ana Carden-Coyne,
      Reconstructing the Body: Classicism, Modernism, and the First World War (Oxford:
      Oxford University Press, 2009), 96. There is nothing to suggest that in Gillies's
      textbook written for clinical use and not to necessarily promote his expertise.
      In fact, Sidcup archivist Andrew Bamji found some of the photographs in filing
      cabinets, long lost to the public. Hardly could they have been altered. See A.
      Bamji, "Facial Surgery: The Patient Experience," in *Facing Armageddon: The
      First World War Experience*, ed. Hugh Cecil and Peter Liddle (Barnsley, U.K.:
      Pen and Sword, 2003), 495.

42   Joseph M. Hone, *The Life of Henry Tonks* (London: W. Heinemann, 1939),
      114. In referencing Henry Tonks, I used additional sources: S. Biernoff, "Flesh
      Poems: Henry Tonks and the Art of Surgery," *Visual Culture in Britain* 11
      (2010): 25–47; J. Freeman, "Professor Tonks: War Artist," *Burlington Magazine*
      127 (1985): 284–93; J. P. Bennett, "Henry Tonks and His Contemporaries," *Br
      J Plast Surg* 39 (1986): 3–34.

43   This actually was a communication between Henry Tonks and the art critic D. S.
      MacColl, cited in Hone, *Henry Tonks*, 135.

44   Reginald Pound, *Gillies, Surgeon Extraordinary: A Biography* (London: M. Joseph, 1964), 27.

45   "The Queen's Hospital, Frognal, Sidcup," *Lancet* 2 (1917): 687–89.

46   Jason Crouthamel and Peter Leese, *Psychological Trauma and the Legacies of the First World War* (London: Palgrave Macmillan, 2017), 36.

47   Sister Catherine Black, *King's Nurse Beggar's Nurse* (London: Hurst & Blackett, 1939), 87. Benger's food was a mixture of wheat flour and an extract containing digestive ferments of pancreatic juice, usually served mixed with warmed milk. It was a staple of diet for the infirmed—easily digestible.

48   Elizabeth Walker Black, *Hospital Heroes* (New York: Charles Scribner's Sons, 1919), 56.

49   As quoted in Andrew Bamji, *Faces from the Front* (Solihull, U.K.: Helion and Company, 2017), 58.

50   "Soldier Craftsmen: Display of Works by Hospital Patients," [London] *Times*, December 9, 1917, 11.

51   Gillies, *Plastic Surgery of the Face*, vii.

52   Actually, Louis Ombrédanne served in the Verdun sector during the war and later at Tours and the Val-de-Grâce, practicing his innovative plastic surgery techniques there as well. See Glicenstein, "Louis Ombrédanne."

53   As quoted in F. Derquenne, "Deux Pionniers Français de la Chirurgie Esthétique: François Dubois et Raymond Passot," *Hist Sci Med* 49 (2015): 29–40. See also Raymond Passot's monumental *oeuvre*, *Sculpteur de Visages* (Paris: Denoël et Steele, 1933), from which this quote is taken.

54   See Noële Roubaud and R. N. Brehamet, *Le Colonel Picot et les Gueules Cassées* (Paris: Nouvelles Éditions Latines, 1960).

55   W. A. Lane, "Introduction," in Harold Gillies, *Plastic Surgery of the Face* (Oxford: Oxford University Press, 1920), vii.

56   Jay Winter, *Remembering War* (New Haven, Conn.: Yale University Press, 2000), 1.

57   Marjorie Gehrhardt, *The Men with Broken Faces* (Oxford: Peter Lang, 2015), 25.

CHAPTER NINE

1   I have used as my references for the life of Hugh Owen Thomas and bonesetters the following sources: Arthur Keith, *Menders of the Maimed* (London: Oxford University Press, 1919), 35–62; S. Wren and N. Ashwood, "The Life and Times of Hugh Owen Thomas," *Trauma* 12 (2010): 197–201; A. J. Carter, "Hugh Owen Thomas: The Cripple's Champion," *Brit Med J* 303 (1991): 1578–81; R. J. T. Joy, "The Natural Bonesetters with Special Reference to the Sweet Family of Rhode Island," *Bull Hist Med* 28 (1954): 416–41; S.-A. Phillips and L. C. Biant, "The Instruments of the Bonesetter," *J Bone Joint Surg [Br]* 93 (2011): 115–19.

2   See D. S. Macnab, "Hugh Owen Thomas (1834–1891)," *CMAJ* 45 (1941): 448–52.

3   *Ibid.*

4   "Crazy Sally" Mapp of Epsom (1706–37) was but one example. Characterized as an "enormous, fat, ugly, drunken woman," she nevertheless earned quite a

reputation for her work on bone and joint disorders. Her checkered career carried far and wide and even inspired a play: *The Husband's Relief; or the Female Bone-Setter and Worm Doctor*. See E. L. Strohl, "Crazy Sally of Epsom," *JAMA* 182 (1962): 268.

5   Richard Evan Thomas, son of Evan Thomas was informally referred to as Richard Evans or Richard ap Evan ("Richard, son of Evan"—a familiar Welsh custom).

6   For a colorful portrayal of Anglesey life in the 19th century, see "Periphery, Modernity and the Discovery of Wales in Travel Writing in German from 1790 to 1850," in *Hidden Texts, Hidden Nation*, ed. Kathryn N. Jones, Carol Tully, and Heather Williams (Liverpool: Liverpool University Press, 2020), 113–54, quote 126.

7   "Owen Roberts M.D., St. Asaph," *Brit Med J* 1 (1871): 409.

8   Membership in the Royal College of Surgeons was akin to the present-day certification by the American Board of Surgery, a warranty of competence in the surgical arts.

9   Hugh Owen Thomas, *Contributions to Surgery and Medicine*, vol. 3 (London: H. K. Lewis, 1887), 114–15.

10   See the 1883 report by Liverpool's "Special Commission," initially posted in the *Liverpool Daily Post* in January 1883 entitled "Squalid Liverpool." It later was reprinted in pamphlet form. Quote taken from 4.

11   As quoted in Keith, *Menders*, 37.

12   Thomas, *Contributions*, 3.

13   Hugh Owen Thomas, *Diseases of the Hip, Knee, and Ankle Joints* (London: H. K. Lewis, 1878), 98–99.

14   Thomas, *Diseases*, 185–86.

15   Quotes as expressed in Keith, *Menders*, 44, 47.

16   Quote taken from Frederick Watson, *The Life of Sir Robert Jones* (London: Hodder & Stoughton Ltd., 1934), 61. This was a major source for the life and works of "the nephew," Sir Robert Jones.

17   "Hugh Owen Thomas, M.D., M.R.C.S.," *Lancet* 1 (1891): 174–75.

18   His report appeared in the *Lancet* later in February. See R. Jones and O. Lodge, "The Discovery of a Bullet Lost in the Wrist by Means of the Roentgen Rays," *Lancet* 1 (1896): 476–77. Thurstan Holland was to become one of the prominent radiologists of Great Britain.

19   Watson, *The Life of Sir Robert Jones*, 134.

20   I have used as reference for these civilian results the article by W. L. Estes, "End Results of Fractures of the Shaft of the Femur" *Ann Surg* 56 (1912): 162-184.

21   R. Jones, "Mechanical Treatment of Compound and Suppurating Fractures Occurring at the Seat of War," *Brit Med J* 1 (1915): 101–02.

22   Claude Bernard, of course, was the architect of the *milieu intérieur*. Quote "machinery of life" from Samuel David Gross, *A System of Surgery: Pathological, Diagnostic, Therapeutic, and Operative* (Philadelphia: Henry C. Lea's Sons & Company, 1882), 114.

23   R. Liston, "On Fracture of the Neck of the Femur," in *Dissertations by Eminent Members of The Royal Medical Society*, ed. Douglas Maclagan (Edinburgh: David Douglas, 1892), 95–103. Liston presented his paper in 1820. In the days before

general anesthesia, the speed at which operations were done was critical. The London surgeon Liston was among the speediest, called by some "the fastest knife in the West End."

24 Quote and reference for these statistics from W. G. Macpherson, *Medical Services: Surgery of the War* (London: His Majesty's Stationery Office, 1922), 339, 354–55.

25 E. W. H. Groves, "The Life and Work of Moynihan," *Brit Med J* 1 (1940): 601–06.

26 H. Platt, "Moynihan: The Education and Training of the Surgeon," *Ann R Coll Surg Engl* 30 (1962): 220–28.

27 Watson, *The Life of Sir Robert Jones*, 150.

28 "Home Hospitals and the War," *Brit Med J* 1 (1915): 39–42.

29 Robert Jones published two articles on the care of femur fractures in late 1914 and early 1915. Both were concerned with the proper traction on the fracture and the need for rigorous wound care. See R. Jones, "Treatment of Fractures of the Thigh," *Brit Med J* 2 (1914): 1086–87; and Jones, "Mechanical Treatment of Compound and Suppurating Fractures."

30 Ann Clayton, *Chavasse: Double VC* (Barnsley, U.K.: Pen and Sword, 2006), 170.

31 *Ibid.*, 188.

32 Watson, *The Life of Sir Robert Jones*, 158.

33 See R. T. Austin, "Meurice Sinclair CMG: A Great Benefactor of the Wounded of the First World War," *Injury* 40 (2009) 567–70. Quote from Watson, *The Life of Sir Robert Jones*, 155.

34 D. M. Aitken, "The Treatment of Gunshot Fractures," *Brit Med J* 2 (1916): 213–15.

35 See E. M. Cowell, "A Method of Teaching the Front Line Application of Thomas's Splint by Numbers," *J R Army Med Corps* 33 (1919): 175–78.

36 Watson, *The Life of Sir Robert Jones*, 159.

37 See Alfred Keogh's "Introductory Note" in Sir Robert Jones, *Notes on Military Orthopaedics* (London: Cassell and Company, 1917), xiv.

38 Watson, *The Life of Sir Robert Jones*, 148.

39 H.M.W. Gray, *The Early Treatment of War Wounds* (London: Hodder & Stoughton, 1919), 49, 50. Gray had been consulting surgeon to the British Third Army during the war.

40 Statistics from Macpherson, *Medical Services*, 354–55; quote 339. About 10 percent of wounded needed an amputation outright. From these grievous injuries and the trauma of a thigh amputation, one third would die.

CHAPTER TEN

1 Thomas Hardy, *The Works of Thomas Hardy in Prose and Verse* (London, Macmillan and Company, 1920), 93.

2 George William Sherman, *The Pessimism of Thomas Hardy* (Madison, N.J.: Fairleigh Dickinson University Press, 1976), 41.

3 See also Ernest Brennecke, *The Life of Thomas Hardy* (New York: Greenberg Publisher, 1925), particularly 203–11.

4   T. R. Elliott, "Transient Paraplegia from Shell Explosion," *Brit Med J* 2 (1914): 1005–06.

5   C. S. Myers, "A Contribution to the Study of Shell Shock," *Lancet* 1 (1915): 316–20.

6   W. A. Turner, "Remarks on Cases of Nervous and Mental Shock Observed in the Base Hospitals in France," *Brit Med J* 1 (1915): 833–35.

7   For reference, see Janet Oppenheim, *"Shattered Nerves"* (New York: Oxford University Press, 1991), especially 79–109.

8   William Aldren Turner and Thomas Grainger Stewart, *A Textbook of Nervous Diseases* (Philadelphia: P. Blakiston's Son & CO., 1910), 523, 547.

9   T. R. Glynn, physician and pathologist in Liverpool, wrote on "The Traumatic Neuroses" in 1910 (*Lancet* 2 [1910]: 1332–36).

10   See J. Robinett, "The Narrative Shape of Traumatic Experience," *Lit and Med* 26 (2007): 290–311.

11   Lord Moran, *The Anatomy of Courage* (New York: Carroll & Graf, 1945), 20–21.

12   M. I. Finucane, "General Nervous Shock, Immediate and Remote, After Gunshot and Shell Injuries in the South African Campaign," *Lancet* 2 (1900); 807–09.

13   A. Wilson, "Notes on 150 Cases of Wounded French, Belgians, and Germans," *Brit Med J* 2 (1914): 806–07.

14   Quote taken from Simon Shorvon and Alastair Compston, *Queen Square: A History of the National Hospital and Its Institute of Neurology* (Cambridge: Cambridge University Press, 2019), 347.

15   J. S. Risien Russell, "The Treatment of Neurasthenia," *Lancet* 2 (1913): 1453–56.

16   For an early dissertation on neurasthenia see G. Beard, "Neurasthenia, or Nervous Exhaustion," *Boston Med Surg J* 3 (1869): 217–21. The term itself comes from the Greek νεύρο, meaning "nerve," and σθένος, meaning "strength."

17   H. Oppenheim, "Stand der Lehre von den Kriegs- und Unfall-Neurosen," *Berliner Klinische Wochenschrift* 54 (1917): 1169–72. For a discussion of Oppenheim's efforts to address traumatic neuroses see B. Holdorff and T. Dening, "The Fight for 'Traumatic Neurosis,' 1889–1916: Hermann Oppenheim and his Opponents in Berlin," *Hist Psych* 22 (2011): 465–76.

18   F. Rusca, "Experimentelle Untersuchungen über die trauma tische Druckwirkung der Explosionen," *Deutsche Zeitschrift für Chirurgie* 132 (1914/15): 315–73.

19   R. Gaupp, "Kriegsneurosen," *Zeitschrift f Neurologie und Psych* 34 (1916): 357–90.

20   R. Gaupp, "Hysterie und Kriegsdienst," *Münchener Med Wochenschrift* 62 (1915): 361–63.

21   *La Suicisse*, April 1917, in Stéphane Audoin-Rouzeau, *Men At War 1914–1918* (Oxford: Berg, 1992), 73.

22   *Grenanda*, April 23, 1917, in Audoin-Rouzeau, *Men at War*, 162.

23   For further biography, see D. R. Kumar, F. Aslinia, S. H. Yale, and J. J. Mazza, "Jean-Martin Charcot: The Father of Neurology," *Clin Med Res* 9 (2011): 46–49.

24   See M. S. Micale, "Jean-Martin Charcot and *les névroses* traumatiques: From Medicine to Culture in French Trauma Theory of the Late Nineteenth Century," in *Traumatic Pasts: History, Psychiatry, and Trauma in the Modern Age, 1870–1930*, ed. Mark S. Micale and Paul Lerner (Cambridge: Cambridge University Press, 2001), 123.

25   See also Mark S. Micale, *Hysterical Men* (Cambridge: Harvard University Press, 2008), quote by Charcot taken from 158.

26   G. Roussy and J. Lhermitte, *Psychoneuroses de Guerre* (Paris: Masson et Cie, 1917), 5–6.

27   Douglas T. Hamilton, *High-Explosive Shell Manufacture* (New York: The Industrial Press, 1916), 32–41.

28   See the excellent review by I. Cernak, "Understanding Blast-Induced Neurotrauma: How Far Have We Come?," *Concussion* 2 (2017): 1–19.

29   A. Bowlby, "Wounds in War," *Lancet* 2 (1915): 1385–98.

30   Millicent, Duchess of Sutherland, *Six Weeks at the War* (London: "The Times," 1914), 33–34.

31   Siegfried Sassoon, *Sherston's Progress* (London: Faber and Faber, 1936), 51.

32   For the effect of the World War on contemporary views of masculinity, see Joanna Bourke, *Dismembering the Male: Men's Bodies, Britain, and the Great War* (Chicago: University of Chicago Press, 1996).

33   For details of the career of Charles Myers, see F. C. Bartlett, "Charles Samuel Myers. 1873–1946," *Obit Notices R Soc* 5 (1948): 767–77.

34   See brief summary of her domestic troubles in "Duchess Married to Army Aviator," *New York Times*, January 24, 1920, 11. Despite the personal incentives for the duchess, service in nursing during World War I was highly desirable among British women with sufficient training to qualify. It was viewed as their patriotic duty and eagerly sought after. See the informative exposé by Janet S. K. Watson, "Wars in the Wards: The Social Construction of Medical Work in First World War Britain," *J Brit Studies* 41 (2002): 484–510.

35   Quotes in I. McDonald, "Gordon Holmes Lecture: Gordon Holmes and the Neurological Heritage," *Brain* 130 (2007): 288–98; and R. S. Fishman, "Gordon Holmes, the Cortical Retina, and the Wounds of War" *Documenta Ophthal* 93 (1997): 9–27.

36   See Ben Shephard, *A War of Nerves: Soldiers and Psychiatrists in the Twentieth Century* (Cambridge, Mass.: Harvard University Press, 2003), 47–49.

37   I used Charles Myers's frank and measured report of his experiences with shell shock in *Shell Shock in France 1914–1918* (Cambridge: Cambridge University Press, 1940), from whence the quotes were taken.

38   Henry Maudsley, *Body and Mind* (New York: D. Appleton and Company, 1871), 41–42.

39   S. Finger, P. J. Koehler, and C. Jagella, "The Monakow Concept of Diaschisis; Origins and Perspectives," *Arch Neurol* 61 (2004): 283–88.

40   See the three-part lectureship of Frederick Mott that appeared in *The Lancet*, February 12, 26, and March 11, 1916 (F. Mott, "The Effects of High Explosives Upon the Central Nervous System," *Lancet* 1 [1916]: 331–38, 441–49, 545–53).

41   *Report of the Committee of Enquiry into "Shell-Shock"* (London: His Majesty's Stationery Office, 1922), 93.

42   H. Wiltshire, "A Contribution to the Etiology of Shell Shock," *Lancet* 1 (1916): 1207–12.

43   As related by Frederick Mott, referring to his comments in "Preface" *Arch Neurology*, 3 (1907): iii-vii, contained in his publication "The Maudsley Hospital, Past and Present," *J Ment Sci* 67 (1921): 320.

44   The cases were originally slated for the neurological section of the London General Hospital but in January 1916, many of these patients were sent across the street to the new Maudsley Hospital.

45   For an extended discussion of the Maudsley Hospital, see Mott, "The Maudsley Hospital." Kraepelin was not impressed with Mott's plan and doubted it would materialize. He admired the man, though, and felt advancement in psychiatry in England would only occur through him. See E. Jones, S. Rahman, and R. Woolven, "The Maudsley Hospital: Design and Strategic Direction, 1923–1939," *Med Hist* 51 (2007): 357–78. The new Maudsley Hospital proper would not open to psychiatric cases until 1922.

46   See Frederick Mott, *War Neuroses and Shell Shock* (London: Hodder & Stoughton, 1919), 267–86.

47   See Mott, "Special Discussion on Shell Shock Without Visible Signs of Injury," *Proc R Soc Med* 9 (1916): i-xxiv.

48   See John Wormald and Samuel Wormald, *A Guide to the Mental Deficiency Act, 1913* (London: P.S. King & Son, 1913), quotes 8–9.

49   W. A. Turner, "Arrangements for the Care of Cases of Nervous and Mental Shock Coming from Overseas," *Lancet* 1 (1916): 1073–75.

50   See G. Elliot Smith and T. H. Pear, *Shell Shock and Its Lessons* (London: Longmans, Green & Co., 1917). See, too, R. Hemmings, "Rivers, Myers and the Culture of War Neuroses," in Robert Hemming, *Modern Nostalgia* (Edinburgh: Edinburgh University Press, 2008), 28–53.

51   Quotes from W. J. M. A. Maloney, "'The National' and Dr. F. E. Batten," *J Nerv Ment Dis* 49 (1919): 91–94.

52   Johanna, Louisa, and Edward Chandler, three orphans, raised £800 for a place to care for their paralyzed grandmother and others with the same affliction. They were aided by the Lord Mayor of London, David Wire, who was paralyzed as well. See B. Buford Rawlings, *A Hospital in the Making: A History of the National Hospital for the Paralysed and Epileptic* (London: Sir Isaac Pitman & Sons, 1913).

53   See G. K. York III and D. A. Steinberg, "Hughlings Jackson's Neurological Ideas," *Brain* 134 (2011): 3106–13; and C. Uff, D. Frith, C. Harrison, et al., "Sir Victor Horsley's 19th Century Operations at the National Hospital for Neurology and Neurosurgery, Queen Square," *J Neurosurg* 114 (2011): 534–42.

54   *Alienist* is an archaic term for psychiatrists, from the French *aliéné*, meaning "insane." Most worked in insane asylums. It distinguished them quite clearly from neurologists, or those directly concerned with diagnosis and treatment of neurological—not mental—diseases.

55   Edgar Adrian (later, Baron Adrian of Cambridge) would win the Nobel Prize for
      physiology in 1932 for his demonstration of the electrical activity in neurons.
56   E. D. Adrian and L. R. Yealland, "The Treatment of Some Common War Neu-
      roses," *Lancet* 1 (1917): 867–72.
57   L. Tatu, "Edgar Adrian (1889–1977) and Shell Shock Electrotherapy: A For-
      gotten History?," *Eur Neurol* 79 (2018): 106–07.
58   Elaine Showalter, *The Female Malady: Women, Madness and English Culture 1830–
      1980* (London: Virago, 1987), 181.
59   Lewis R. Yealland, *Hysterical Disorders of Warfare* (London: Macmillan and Co.,
      1918), 8–9; scene recreated in Pat Barker, *Regeneration* (New York: Random
      House, 1991), 227.
60   W. R. Russell, "Major Hysteria," *Brit Med J* 1 (1935): 872–76.
61   For a thorough discussion of electrotherapy see S. L. Gilman, "Electrotherapy
      and Mental Illness: Then and Now," *Hist Psychiatry* 19 (2008): 339–57.
      Even today, electroshock therapy is practiced for recalcitrant cases of severe
      depression.
62   See J. Bradley, M. Dupree, and A. Durie, "Taking the Water-Cure: The Hydro-
      pathic Movement in Scotland, 1840–1940," *Bus Econ Hist* 26 (1997): 427–37; and
      Jean Moorcroft Wilson, *Siegfried Sassoon: The Making of a War Poet* (New York:
      Routledge, 1999), 389.
63   Richard Slobodin, *W. H. R. Rivers* (New York: Columbia University Press, 1978),
      13.
64   W. Langdon-Brown, "To a Very Wise Man," *St. Bartholomew's Hosp J* 49 (1936):
      29–30.
65   Quoted in Langdon-Brown, "To a Very Wise Man.".
66   Sassoon, *Sherston's Progress*, 11, 50.
67   *Ibid.*, 50.
68   W.H.R. Rivers, *Instinct and the Unconsciousness* (Cambridge: Cambridge Univer-
      sity Press, 1920), 208 (italics mine).
69   Joseph Breuer and Sigmund Freud, *Studies on Hysteria*, trans. James Strachey
      (New York: Basic Books, 2000), 5–6.
70   Rivers, *Instinct and the Unconsciousness*, 208.
71   T.E.F. Webb, "'Dottyville'—Craiglockhart War Hospital and Shell-Shock
      Treatment in the First World War," *J R Soc Med* 99 (2006): 342–46.
72   See W.H.R. Rivers, "The Repression of War Experience," *Proc R Soc Med* 11
      (1918): 1–20.
73   P. Fox, "Confronting Postwar Shame in Weimar Germany: Trauma, Heroism
      and the War Art of Otto Dix," *Oxford Art J* 29 (2006): 249–67.
74   See S. C. Linden and E. Jones, "German Battle Casualties: The Treatment of
      Functional Somatic Disorders during World War I," *J Hist Med Allied Sci* 68
      (2013): 627–58.
75   Officially termed the War Office Committee of Enquiry into Causation and Pre-
      vention of "Shell-Shock."
76   *Report of the Committee of Enquiry into "Shell-Shock,"* 47, 94.

77 C. S. Myers, "A Final Contribution to the Study of Shell Shock," *Lancet* 1 (1919): 51–54.

78 T. Loughran, "Shell Shock, Trauma, and the First World War: The Making of a Diagnosis and Its Histories," *J Hist Med Allied Sci* 67 (2010): quote 112.

CHAPTER ELEVEN

1   See R. Barnett, "Influenza," *Lancet* 393 (2019): 396.

2   The 1918 influenza virus had many of the ancestral characteristics of the H1N1 human and swine virus. See J. K. Taubenberger, A. H. Reid, T. A. Janczewski, and T. G. Fanning, "Integrating Historical, Clinical and Molecular Genetic Data in order to Explain the Origin and Virulence of the 1918 Spanish Influenza Virus," *Phil Trans R Soc Lond* B (2001): 1829–39; see also J. K. Taubenberger and D. M. Morens, "1918 Influenza: The Mother of all Pandemics," *Emerg Inf Dis* 12 (2006): 15–22.

3   "Influenza," *Public Health Reports*, 33 (1918): 502.

4   Information taken from J. M. Barry, "The Site of Origin of the 1918 Influenza Pandemic and its Public Health Implications," *J Translat Med* 2 (2004): 1–4. The first report of Private Gitchell seems to have appeared in Adolph A. Hoehling's *The Great Epidemic: When the Spanish Influenza Struck* (New York: Little, Brown, 1961), 14–15. See also Catherine Arnold, *Pandemic 1918: Eyewitness Accounts from the Greatest Medical Holocaust in Modern History* (New York: St. Martin's Press, 2018), 36. Albert Gitchell recovered from his illness and died peacefully in 1968 at the age of seventy-eight.

5   E. L. Opie, A. W. Freeman, F. G. Blake, et al., "Pneumonia at Camp Funston: Report to the Surgeon-General," *JAMA* 72 (1919): 108–16.

6   Jessie Lee Brown Foveaux, *Any Given Day: The Life and Times of Jessie Lee Brown Foveaux* (New York: Warner Books, 1997), 145.

7   M. W. Hall, "Inflammatory Diseases of the Respiratory Tract," chapter 2, in *The Medical Department of the United States Army in the World War*, vol. 9, ed. M. W. Ireland (Washington, DC: US Government Printing Office, 1928), 84.

8   G. A. Soper, "The Pandemic in the Army Camps," *JAMA* 71 (1918): 1899–1909.

9   M. W. Ireland, "Report of the Surgeon General of the Army," in *War Department Annual Reports, 1919*, vol. 1 (Washington, DC: Government Printing Office, 1920), 2153–65.

10 M. W. Ireland, "A Fighter for the Cause of Health: The Military Record of Colonel Victor C. Vaughan," *J Lab Clin Med* 15 (1930): 878–84.

11 Ireland, "Report of the Surgeon General," 2159.

12 *Ibid.*, 2153.

13 *Ibid.*, 2149.

14 R. I. Cole, "The Etiology and Prevention of Influenza," *Rufus Ivory Cole Papers*, BC671 February 1946, Courtesy of The American Philosophical Society, Philadelphia, 3–4.

15 E. R. LeCount, "The Pathologic Anatomy of Influenzal Bronchopneumonia," *JAMA* 72 (1919): 650–52.

16   M. C. Winternitz, Isabel M. Wason, and Frank P. McNamara, *The Pathology of Influenza* (New Haven, Conn.: Yale University Press, 1920), 9, 55.

17   R. Pfeiffer, "Die Aetiologie der Influenza," *Zeitschr für Hyg und Infektionskr* 12 (1893): 357–86.

18   "German Bug Causes Influenza Physician Here Discovers," *Philadelphia Evening Bulletin*, September 20, 1918, 21.

19   See P. K. Olitsky and F. L. Gates, "Experimental Studies of the Nasopharyngeal Secretions from Influenza Patients," *J Exp Med* 33 (1921): 125–45. What Pfeiffer isolated was what we now call the bacterium *Haemophilus influenza*, a sometimes-normal inhabitant of the nose and throat but also a possible pathogen in cases of inflammation and disruption of normal respiratory defense mechanisms.

20   "Lessons of a Great Epidemic: The Pathology of Influenza," *Lancet* 1 (1919): 25–26.

21   Measures cited in Ireland, "Report of the Surgeon General," 2132–77.

22   Ireland, "Report of the Surgeon General," 2132–33. Toxicity is a form of sepsis, an infection that may completely overwhelm the body's defenses.

23   P. D. Olch, "Shields Warren : An Oral History," in *General History of Medicine, Oral Histories*, National Library of Medicine, Washington, DC, 11.

24   *Annual Report, Navy Department 1918/1919* (Washington, DC: Government Printing Office, 1920), 2425.

25   *Ibid.*, 2426.

26   *Ibid.*, 2431–55.

27   *Ibid.*, 2415.

28   A. G. Love and C. B. Davenport, "Immunity of City-Bred Recruits," *Arch Int Med* 24 (1919): 129–53.

29   *History of the U.S.S. Leviathan* (Brooklyn: Brooklyn Eagle Job Department, 1919), 92, 157–60.

30   Ireland, "Report of the Surgeon General," 3597–98.

31   W. J. MacNeal, "The Influenza Epidemic of 1918 in the American Expeditionary Forces in France and England." *Arch Int Med* 23 (1919): 657–88.

32   Anne Tjomsland, *Bellevue in France* (New York: Froben Press, 1941), 212.

33   See Meiron Harries and Susie Harries, *The Last Days of Innocence* (New York: Vintage Press, 1997), 391–92.

34   Ireland, "Report of the Surgeon General," 3415.

35   A. Trilla, G. Trilla, and C. Daer, "The 1918 'Spanish Flu' in Spain," *Clin Inf Dis* 47 (2008): 668–73.

36   The exact figure from the Army Medical Department was 23,937 and 42,350 respectively (A. G. Love, "Medical and Casualty Statistics," in *The Medical Department of the United States Army in the World War*, vol. 15, part 2, ed. M. W. Ireland [Washington, DC: Government Printing Office, 1925], 670–74).

37   M. W. Hall, "Communicable and Other Diseases," in *The Medical Department of the United States Army in the World War*, vol. 9, ed. M. W. Ireland (Washington: US Government Printing Office, 1928), 61–169, figure on 67.

38   F. Heckel, "La Grippe Épidémique Actuelle," *L'Illustration*, November 2, 1918, 425.

39   See P. Darmon, "La Grippe Espagnole Submerge la France," *L'Histoire* 281 (2003): 79–85.

40   Figures from K. D. Patterson and G. F. Pyle, "The Geography and Mortality of the 1918 Influenza Pandemic," *Bull Hist Med* 65 (1991): 4–21.

41   And British. Over 160 of their medical officers died in 1918—all of them accounted for by the influenza pandemic. Almost 105,000 civilians would succumb. See "The Military Medical Services in 1918," *Brit Med J* 1 (1919): 131–33; and M. Bresalier, "Fighting Flu: Military Pathology, Vaccines, and the Conflicted Identity of the 1918-19 Pandemic in Britain," *J Hist Med Allied Sci* 68 (2013): 87–128.

42   See O. Lahaie, "L'Épidémie de Grippe Dite 'Espagnole'et sa Perception par l'Armée Française (1918–1919)," *Revue Historique des Armées* 262 (2011): 1–10.

43   F. Heckel, "La Grippe: Son Traitement Préventif, Prophylactique et Abortif," *L'Illustration*, no. 3946, October 19, 1918, 373.

44   Joan Freixas, *Traitement de la Grippe* (Paris: J.-D. Baillière et Fils, 1919).

45   C. Flügge, "Ueber Luftinfection," *Zeitschrif f Hygiene Inf* 25 (1897): 179–224.

46   J. Mikulicz, "Das Operiren in Sterilisirten Zwirnhandschuhen und mit Mundbinde," *Zentralbl f Chir* 24 (1897): 713–17.

47   See B. C. Doust and A. B. Lyon, "Face Masks in Infections of the Respiratory Tract," *JAMA* 71 (1918): 1216–19.

48   Alfred W. Crosby, *America's Forgotten Pandemic: The Influenza of 1918* (Cambridge: Cambridge University Press, 2003), 26. Another name used was *Schnupfenfieber*, which, literally translated, means "runny nose fever." *Katarrh*, or "catarrh," refers to the syndrome of copious upper respiratory tract secretions either nasally or pulmonary or both that usually accompanies upper respiratory tract infections.

49   General [Erich] Ludendorff, *My War Memories, 1914–1918*, vol. 2 (London: Hutchinson & Co., 1921), 617, 638.

50   The General Service Schools, *The German Offensive of July 15, 1918* (Fort Leavenworth, Kan.: The General Service Schools Press, 1923), 288.

51   Rudolf Binding, *A Fatalist at War*, trans. Ian Morrow (Boston: Houghton Mifflin Company, 1929), 241.

52   "Germans with Fever Drop in Their Tracks," *New York Times*, July 9, 1918, 7.

53   "Kaiser Ill of Influenza," *New York Times*, July 11, 1918, 2.

54   "General Ireland Returns," *New York Times*, October 29, 1918, 4.

55   *War Department Annual Report*, vol. 1, part 3 (Washington, DC: Government Printing Office, 1920), 3237.

56   A. N. Stark, "Medical Activities of the American Expeditionary Forces in the Zone of the Armies," *Mil Surg* 47 (1920): 154–76.

57   Richard Derby, *"Wade in, Sanitary!": The Story of a Division Surgeon in France* (New York: G.P. Putnam's Sons, 1919), 172–73.

58   Francis P. Duffy, *Father Duffy's Story* (New York: George H. Doran Company, 1919), 290.

59   Quoted in Nicholas Best, *The Greatest Day in History* (New York: PublicAffairs, 2008), 271.
60   See J. J. Keegan, "The Prevailing Pandemic of Influenza," *JAMA* 71 (1918): 1051–55. See also N. J. Blackwood, "History of the U.S. Naval Hospital, Chelsea, Mass., 1915–1918," *US Naval Med Bull* 14 (1920): 311–38.
61   W. T. Vaughan, "Influenza A Epidemiologic Study," *Am J Hygiene* (1921): 127–73.
62   "Weekly Reports for March 14, 1919" *Public Health Rep* 34 (1919): 491–541, figures 505.
63   Soper, "The Pandemic in the Army Camps."
64   "Weekly Reports" 34 (1919): 505.
65   *Ibid*, 505.
66   F. Aimone, "The 1918 Influenza Epidemic in New York City: A Review of the Public Health Response," *Public Health Rep* 125 (2010): 71–79.
67   W. S. Pugh, "Education and Sanitation Aboard Ship," *US Naval Med Bull* 13 (1919): 254–66.
68   From Nancy K. Bristow, *American Pandemic: The Lost Worlds of the 1918 Influenza Epidemic* (Oxford: Oxford University Press, 2012), 93.
69   K. H. Grantz, M. S. Rane, H. Salje, et al., "Disparities in Influenza Mortality and Transmission Related to Sociodemographic Factors Within Chicago in the Pandemic of 1918," *Proc Natl Acad Sci USA* 113 (2016): 13839–44.
70   "Weekly Reports" 34 (1919): 505.
71   C. M. Stetler, "The 1918 Spanish Influenza: Three Months of Horror in Philadelphia," *Pennsylvania History* 84 (2017): 462–87.
72   Bristow, *American Pandemic*, 156.
73   Taubenberger, "1918 Influenza."
74   Rudyard Kipling, *Twenty Poems* (Toronto: The Macmillan Company, 1918), 15–16.

CHAPTER TWELVE

1   Lettie Gavin, *American Women in World War 1: They Also Served* (Niwot: University Press of Colorado, 1997), 169. Mary Merritt Crawford (1884–1972) was a surgeon by training and the only woman physician to serve at the *Ambulance Américaine* in Neuilly-sur-Seine, where she worked for one year during the war as an anesthesiologist.
2   J. Mueller, "Changing Attitudes Towards War: The Impact of the First World War," *Brit J Political Sci* 21 (1991): 1–28.
3   Jared Diamond, *Guns, Germs, and Steel: The Fates of Human Societies* (New York: W. W. Norton & Company, 1997), 215.
4   Louis Mairet, *Carnet d'un Combattant* (Paris: Éditions Georges Crés, 1919), 271.
5   M. Howard, "World War One: The Crisis in European History—The Role of the Military Historian," *J Mil Hist* 57 (1993): 128–29. See a detailed discussion of the significance of the Great War also in A. Sked, "Epochenwende Erster Weltkrieg: The Historical Significance of the First World War," in *Die Habsburgermonarchie*

1848–1918, ed. Helmut Rumpler and Ulrike Harmat (Wein: Austrian Academy of Sciences Press, 1987), 21–47.

6   Jack J. Roth, *World War I: A Turning Point in Modern History* (New York: Alfred A. Knopf, 1967), 109.

7   M. Harrison, "Medicine and the Management of Modern Warfare: An Introduction," in *Medicine and Modern Warfare*, ed. Roger Cooter, Mark Harrison, and Steve Sturdy (Amsterdam: Rodopi, 1999), 1–27.

8   L. S. Pilcher, "The Influence of War Surgery upon Civil Practice," *Ann Surg* 69 (1919): 565–74.

9   A. Bowlby, "On the Application of War Methods to Civil Practice," *Proc R Soc Med* 13 (1920): 35–48.

10   Diamond, *Guns, Germs, and Steel*, 424.

11   The 19th-century experimentalist Claude Bernard insisted that internal harmony was maintained by efforts of the human *milieu intérieur* to counterbalance outside stresses, which he termed the *milieu extérieur*.

12   Peter C. English, *Shock, Physiological Surgery, and George Washington Crile* (Westport, Conn.: Greenwood Press, 1980).

13   See Kenneth M. Ludmerer, *Time to Heal* (New York: Oxford University Press, 1999), 30–39.

14   Harvey Cushing, *From a Surgeon's Journal* (Boston: Little, Brown, and Company, 1936), 501.

15   D. E. Rowe and R. Schulmann, "The First World War and Its Impact, 1914–1921," in *Einstein on Politics*, ed. David E. Rowe and Robert Schulmann (Princeton, N.J.: Princeton University Press, 2007), 61–92.

16   J. A. Blake, "The Influence of the War Upon the Development of Surgery," *Ann Surg* 69 (1919): 453–65.

17   W. D. Haggard, "The Medical Profession and the Great War," *Trans Southern Surg Assoc* 30 (1918): 7.

INDEX